MW01436034

In Praise of *Spirit Made Smaller*

Set against the dramatic backdrop of Alaska, Phillip Douglas's sensitive portrayal of a father desperately seeking the cause for his young son's illness and eventual death and his attempt to understand the reasons his wife, Maren, abandoned him and their child, stands in stark contrast to the landscape. From fraudulent science, emotional aloofness and narcissism, climate change, and polygamy, Douglas's range of topics is as broad and varied as the land his characters inhabit. He takes the reader to a fly-in camp in the Seven Sisters, to a Potlach in an Athabascan village on the Chitina River, and back to the Alaska Pacific University campus in Anchorage. All the while, the reader seeks with Gharrett Graywood the clues to his son's mysterious illness, is privy to the outrageous proclamations of the brilliantly eccentric Cashel Goodlette, and revels in the philosophy and wisdom of Monroe Bearhead, both men connected with the university's faculty.

Douglas relies on his own medical background and practice to explore the possible causes of Bobby's illness and death, treating the reader to both standard and cutting-edge concepts in medicine, presented clearly, which require no previous medical background to be easily understood.

Graywood's fear as he watches his son deteriorate, his ever-present grief at the loss of his son, and his growing bewilderment and anger at Maren's seeming indifference, even as her child lies in his coffin, tie this unlikely cast of characters with their talents and eccentricities into a well-honed work, one worth reading.

Gretchen Diemer, Poet
Between Fire and Water, Ice and Sky, NorthShore Press

To Molly,
The best of all the world!
Doug

Spirit Made Smaller

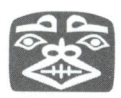

PHILLIP
DOUGLAS

Phillip Douglas

BOOK PUBLISHERS NETWORK
Changing the World One Book at a Time

Book Publishers Network
P.O. Box 2256
Bothell • WA • 98041
Ph • 425-483-3040
www.bookpublishersnetwork.com

10 9 8 7 6 5 4 3 2 1
Printed in the United States of America

LCCN 2014930791
ISBN 978-1-940598-23-9

Editor: Julie Scandora
Cover Designer: Laura Zugzda
Typographer: Marsha Slomowitz

To
Abel and Melissa
and how we spoke up for each other
in our respective worlds.

CHAPTER ONE

Eleven Candles

Bobby had lost consciousness at the birthday party, and paramedics rushed him to Providence.

What if it's a seizure? The way Rachel choked out what happened over the phone … it might be. Blasted damn traffic lights!

"Learn to drive, you fools," cursed Doctor Graywood, from Elmendorf Air Force Base to Glenn Highway. He broke speed limits big. If pulled over, he'd pressure the patrolman for an escort and pay the tickets later.

Passing out or having a seizure denoted only symptoms. Biting his lip, Graywood flashed through possible causes for an eleven-year-old: infection, expanding tumor, ruptured blood vessel, new onset diabetes, idiopathic … or something wrong with the heart.

Screw it.

He ran two more red lights. No sirens. Not yet.

Children's Hospital shined as a jewel in the silver-taupe tiara of Providence Regional Medical Center, adjacent to the University of Alaska Anchorage. It shared a front loop of road with the Medical Arts Pharmacy. A faded ring of shrubs tucked in the circle's apex surrounded a statue of Jesus Christ, arms halfway raised, starting to signal a touchdown in the garden's end zone.

Summer construction had closed the facility's main entrance. Loathing the obstruction, Graywood parked in the staff lot and blew past Admitting Registration and the descending escalator to the cafeteria. The pediatrics ward occupied the third floor.

"Hi, Doctor Graywood," said a pert pharmacy tech, stepping with him into the elevator. She clutched a basket of intravenous chemotherapy solutions.

"Hello, Julia," Graywood acknowledged. Mortified by what he'd find above, he peered at the seven IV bags.

"You gave a fabulous speech at your retirement party."

"Thanks," Graywood uttered. Odd she'd mentioned the event five weeks ago. He'd quit the Public Health Service to work for the Department of Justice.

"We don't see you here too often. You miss us?"

"Sure," he said, suppressing the knots kinking inside from prostate to windpipe. He'd come only to discover what had happened to his son.

A synthetic grey rock formation with a stuffed cloth walrus plus a half-dozen wooden seagulls greeted those who entered floor three. Graywood checked the nurse's station for his child's room. He'd been taken to radiology.

"We were expecting you," said Helen, the charge nurse. "Here's what we've done for Bobby so far."

Cocking her head, she keyed the medical record's blood and ECG results. "He's getting a CT scan, but they're running a bit behind. Doctor Timm wants to observe overnight and prep for an EEG tomorrow morning."

"Thanks, Helen," Graywood said, taking over the monitor. He scrolled the screen into catalogs of data waiting assembly to where one life might crash and burn. Others marred.

ECG—normal sinus rhythm. Oxygen Sat—99%. CBC—normal. Liver/Kidney Panel—pending.

What's wrong with him?

Helen interrupted, "If all goes well, he'll be discharged tomorrow afternoon."

"Is Doctor Timm here?"

“Called to ER. But there’s a woman in the waiting room who came with Bobby.”

Graywood joined her.

“Gary, I’m so sorry what’s happened,” she said, voice tight with tears. Petite Rachel and staunch Graywood held each other. Both vulnerable.

The waiting room depicted a Gold Rush theme of an old mining claim. A play cabin commanded one corner for preschool children to duck in and out. A mountain mural of a sluicing operation with a sourdough prospector on horseback leading two pack mules colored the adjacent walls. One row of seats appeared as painted mine tailings. A massive fake rock ruled the room’s center with one copper and three yellow-colored nuggets half-exposed for young, would-be prospectors to excavate. A plastic ore cart for pulling kids tilted on its side from a broken wheel.

“Rachel, what happened? They told me Bobby went for a CT scan.”

“He just passed out watching TV before the party,” she answered. “I couldn’t get him to move. It seemed like ages, Gary. I made sure he was breathing and called 911.”

“Does Doctor Timm know what happened?”

“I’m pretty sure,” she quavered and forced a cough to cover it.

Anxiety waves gripped Graywood down to his marrow. Doctor Timm had ordered a medical workup for non-traumatic, sudden loss of consciousness that centered on the heart, metabolism, and brain. Jaw muscles pulsed over his grinding teeth. “Thanks, Raych, for taking care of my boy.” He swallowed twice to wet his throat. “I’ll wait it out now. You can go home.”

She seized his hand. “I’m going for Cub and coming straight back.”

His thankful eyes affirmed her caring intent. Cub, her son, was Bobby’s best friend.

Bobby’s mother, Maren, worked in Baltimore or New York whenever determined by her strict deadlines. Graywood resolved to gather everything about their son’s medical workup before emailing her. That’s how she’d want it—concise, complete, and distant—if she wanted it at all.

He joined Bobby in radiology. Three patients were triaged ahead. For some reason, the second machine remained offline.

Bobby had fallen asleep on the gurney. *Let him rest.* Graywood stared at his beautiful boy under the lights coloring his blond hair like the sun had done on the beaches at Kauai four years ago.

He retreated into memories of their island adventure ... as far away as a father and son could get from here.

The vacation unfolded within 2007's spring break for Bobby's first-grade class. Graywood wanted to take him to a warm spot. More so, he craved a time out from Bobby's school. At the last parent-teacher conference, Graywood was informed his child demonstrated signs of attention deficit hyperactivity disorder.

Bobby had fallen behind in reading and blasted pell-mell through school like a runaway locomotive whenever permitted to leave his seat. Graywood tolerated the kinetic surges at home—rolling over furniture and whatever else got in the way—but Bobby could "do still" when ordered or be captivated with the right video game. Perhaps ADHD was overly applied to any rambunctious child. Graywood needed convincing.

The Garden Isle doubled as Kauai's other name. The oldest in the inhabited Hawaiian chain, it was born five million years ago from lava propelled through a rift in the Pacific tectonic plate. On a map, the island seemed a nibbled cookie—a rough, 553-square-mile circle enveloping several micro-climates and features including beaches, mountains, plains, desert, and rain forest. Combined, they simplified into two descriptions for tourists—wet on the windward east and north, dry on the leeward west and south. Kauai's extinct volcano, Mount Waialeale at 5,148 feet, dominated the center. High enough to condense water-laden trade winds into thick clouds, the summit collected annual moisture that averaged 451 inches. Like water exiting a giant sprinkling can, the resplendent rain ribboned off the inactive cauldron into scores of waterfalls and nourished the island's abundant flowering flora.

The Alaskan Airlines flight from Anchorage, with a Honolulu transfer, deplaned Graywood and his son at Li'hue. Both gasped from the squeezing impact of the island's humid heat.

Like his dad, Bobby rolled a carry-on down the ramp toward baggage claim. Entering the main concourse, he challenged a fellow travel mate, a boy of eight years, to a suitcase-push race along the corridor. Graywood nixed the contest and photographed the pretend drag racers instead.

Graywood had a ton of Bobby pictures. Stored on computer files, backed up to discs, and processed into six hardcover scrapbooks, they documented each year of the child's life. He'd take three hundred on Kauai and select the best for album number seven.

He'd mailed four miscellaneous, spliced sheets to Maren when Bobby was two years old but never had heard if she'd received them. One day, he hoped to show them all to her.

Graywood and Bobby drove their rental car along Highway 56 to their north-shore destination of Hanalei. Graywood had picked this location after an Internet search revealed its gentle, mile-plus beach enclosed by a reef-protected bay. No jagged rocks or shore coral to threaten injury to swimmers. Co-workers who'd visited Kauai raved about how Hanalei played out fewer knots of tourists, compared to the island's southern wedge shouldered on the Li'hue and Poipu shores.

More important, the bay was the home for the mystical "Puff, the Magic Dragon." The Peter, Paul, and Mary folksong had frolicked in Graywood's mind since he'd been Bobby's age yearning to tour Puff's domain. What better way than with Bobby to behold the spellbinding terrain through his boy's priceless eyes.

"Bobby, what year were you born?" Graywood glanced at the rearview mirror seeing the child's car-seat-strapped reflection.

"Ahhh, you know that, Dad."

"Yeah, I guess so … sometime 2000, right?"

"My birthday's September 16, 2000," corrected Bobby.

"Did you know that 2000 on the Chinese calendar is the year of the dragon?"

"Ohhh … really?" Bobby leaned forward as far as possible.

"Yep."

"Wow! I'm a dragon," he roared and blew pretend fire.

"That you definitely are," whispered Graywood. Louder, he added, "Does your teacher think you're a dragon?"

"I hope so."

Sensing the line of talk wouldn't lead to the behavior point he wished to make, Graywood swallowed and accepted Bobby's newfound character insight. "We're going to a place where we might find a scary, awesome-looking dragon."

Bobby jolted back and pulled up hands to cover chest and neck. Back-seat stillness held despite the traffic through Wailua and Kapa'a. "Dad," a tepid voice questioned, "is it a big dragon?"

"I really think so, the biggest in the whole world."

"Oh … uh … what does it eat?"

"Don't know," Graywood teased, tempted to say dragons like munching on irritating first-grade teachers and maybe little girls. But he punted, saying, "There're loads of chickens pecking away along this road. Maybe the dragon eats them."

"Just chickens?"

"Yeah, I bet only chickens. He doesn't eat little boys or girls. At least not boys."

Reassured, Bobby's bravado returned. "I hope the dragon roars real loud."

"So how do you think it roars?"

"Rarrrhhhhh!" he boy-blasted, hands cupped like a megaphone to his mouth.

"That's a strong one. I'm pretty sure the dragon wants to roar and roar with a younger dragon just like you."

"Dad, how much longer?"

From experience Graywood gave high estimates. "Probably an hour." Audible deflation swirled the back seat. Graywood instructed, "Dragons have been around for a long, long time, Bobby, and are very patient creatures. Do you feel like a dragon?"

"Yeahhh!"

"Can you do patient like a dragon and wait an hour and watch all the scenery go by?"

"I can do it, Dad."

"Then I bet Puff will be proud of you."

Red African tulip trees, ivory plumeria buds, descending trains of purple bougainvillea, and bunched hibiscus in crimson and lemon bordered the two-lane road.

Dragon boy grew hungry halfway to Hanalei. They stopped for taro fries and barbecued hamburgers ground from buffalo at the Ono-Char burger stand in Anahola. They ate at an outside table among the roaming feral chickens and two stray cats begging for pieces. Bobby threw crumbs to the piebald tom and cobby queen, but adroit fowl got them first.

An island without predators, concluded Graywood, and chickens owned it. Kauai had become heaven on earth for this avian race, and he mused on a pitiful flock somewhere at a Tyson's food plant praying for reincarnation here prior to their processing into parts.

Belly pangs vanquished, they motored past the Kilauea lighthouse turnoff and a group of Norfolk pines—straight enough for ship masts—marking the entrance to Princeville. Heeding the bluff's fishtail route down the gorge to a one-lane bridge spanning the Hanalei River, they waited their turn to cross. Taro fields covered the opposite lowland. Graywood had never seen so many shades of green, all tropical fresh from afternoon showers.

They arrived. Hanalei faced north at the midpoint in its sheltered bay. Three hunches of interlinked mountains sprouted rain-chiseled ridges to wall off the area's southern and western flanks. Eons of weather had sculpted cliffs, folds, and verdant valleys formed from the massive lava formations. The Bali Hai spire stood sentinel-like off the Na Pali coast wearing a flattened cloud like a beret. Gentle azure swept the lagoon to cap the palms. Farther out, an alabaster ketch sailed into an arched rainbow.

They'd found Eden.

Graywood had booked a studio apartment with full kitchen and lanai at the Hanalei Inn—a long block from the beach. The Ching Young Village stood a minute's walk away with shops, real estate offices, and grocery store. Graywood intended to cook most meals but deferred buying food until Bobby expended pent-up energy on the beach. Changing to swimming trunks, father and son raced to the waves.

Negotiating the concave shore, they aimed for the metal-roofed pier that sheltered an outer mooring. From the quay, two weathered fishermen cast lines opposite a convoy of ocean kayakers.

Bobby dashed seaward and plunged the crests with abandon. He swam with skill beyond what he'd learned at the Anchorage indoor public pool. Graywood picked up and discarded driftwood walking sticks.

Sunbathers dotted the sand reading paperbacks or slept on beach mats and blankets. Beneath a turquoise umbrella, a mother breastfed her infant. Surfers caught six-foot waves a hundred yards out, and younger daredevils boogie-boarded smaller swells. Graywood realized he'd have to buy one for his boy.

At the wharf, Bobby waded the swallow water and stroked a magenta-colored kayak, roped to a concrete pillar. Graywood leaped on the dock and approached the fishermen for the fabled location of the dragon, Puff. One opened a toothy smile to affirm fielding this query many years.

"Look 'cross the bay b'yond my line," he nodded west. "See tha' hill by the curl with tha' brown spot?"

"The one like a triangle top?" asked Graywood.

"Yah, man, that's Puff's head an' his horns some say. He's in long sleep now. Tha' brown spot you see's his good eye closed." The angler reeled the hook and added, "See tha' hump an' ridge joinin' tha' head?"

"Yeah," said Graywood, scanning the expanse.

"Tha' hump's the shoulders an' both arms folded in, an' tha' ridge's the neck."

The second fisherman joined them after locking a pole into an alloy rod holder, bolted to the pier's railing.

The toothy one went on, "The middle hump's the back with wings folded, an' tha' third's his backside with the legs under. His tail go way 'hind that one, way down the river. Man, from here you can't see him all."

"He encircles over half the bay," said Graywood, head rotating the described arc.

"Yah, he's grand one. He *moo nui,*" said the toothy man.

"*Moo nunui,*" emphasized the other angler, face nodding.

Graywood assumed moo nui and moo nunui to be Hawaiian terms for size and determined to buy a translation dictionary. It might be fun to rattle some to the staff back in Anchorage too.

"Thanks for the info. I'll pass it on to my boy."

Both men grinned and switched to busy their lines.

Graywood spotted Bobby on the beach playing tag with an older boy and smaller girl almost his size. He made friends easily. But it'd disappoint to tell how the mighty Puff was a semi-circle of hogbacks and bulges on the sunset side of Hanalei Bay. Instead, Graywood waved him over and conjured a story to wonder-pop the boy's eyes.

"Say there, Bobby, I just got all the news about our dragon, Puff."

"When we gonna see him?"

"I don't think we can for a while."

"Why?"

"Puff's a huge sleeping dragon who blows in the mist, and he lives beyond the great mountain in a secret cave on the wild side of the island."

"Ohhh ... Why's he's sleeping?" asked Bobby, lips pouting. He kicked an eroded sand castle.

"To build up all his magical powers."

"How big's Puff?"

"It's time to go back and fix some supper so you'll get bigger when mighty Puff wants to meet you."

"When, Dad?"

"Whenever he decides to wake up."

They sifted back to the inn, and Graywood spun out more threads of Puff's tale.

That evening on the lanai under the half-filled moon, Graywood thought of Maren.

Bobby's mother worked in the fashion industry. With the physical presence of a cover-girl, she could parade the runway, but her temperament was better suited for shaping the other models into the evolving ethers of avant-garde trends.

Maren field-marshaled three eastern, overlapped regions of women's fashion houses headquartered in New York City whose trademarks Graywood never recalled. Always on the sprint to Boston, Philadelphia, Baltimore, Washington, DC, and as far south as Savannah, Georgia, Maren remained elusive.

Their divorce was finalized one month prior to Bobby's first birthday. Thereafter, she'd remained petrifyingly aloof until two years ago when she'd turned lukewarm and accessible toward Graywood, but only on the Internet. She refused to disclose her cellphone number.

Graywood uncovered it. He never called.

She'd spoken to him only one time after the divorce—the day the Manhattan twin towers had collapsed in 2001. She'd kept silent despite Graywood's attempts to reach her through her parents. In four years, he'd heard nothing from her or her family, except the time Maren's father had sent a note attached to a copy of her mother's obituary in 2003: Bobby's grandmother had died from pancreatic cancer and never held her grandson.

But eighteen months ago, Maren mailed a beautiful, handwritten thank-you card for receipt of the two crates of shoes she'd left in Alaska—Graywood finally had shipped them via her father's address. Cautiously, he restarted weekly communication employing concise Monday emails to summarize Anchorage events and update their son's progress in all things. Her terse replies, every month or so, lacked any references to Bobby.

Then last Christmas, remarkably, she'd sent a holiday card wishing them both a Happy New Year 2007. Had she changed? Although wary and perplexed, Graywood grasped carpe diem and pursued a family reunion. He assembled a photo compact disc of Bobby growing up and the improvements made to their house. Praying she'd accept, Graywood priced three airline tickets for the week on Kauai and mailed an elaborate invitation and flight itinerary with the picture CD.

He envisioned a warm, enjoyable experience getting reacquainted and imagined future reunions lasting longer. Bobby would know his mother—and she might love him—not to the degree his father did, yet enough to show some kindness.

She declined. Her brusque response dictated no future pictures. Always the blithe blossom on briar, Maren destroyed Graywood's fantasy. Her opened palm at Christmas, holding so much promise, had gnarled into a splay of bleached bones by spring. Heartbroken for his son, Graywood revealed none of the busted hand he'd overplayed.

The Kauai journey had transformed from an anticipated harmonious reunion into necessary odyssey to escape from the mindset of Maren. Deep within, Graywood had to finish his endless good-bye to what she'd brewed six years ago.

A wild rooster announced Kauai's dawn.

Graywood rented a tan-colored boogie board for the week. If bought, he reasoned, what good would it do in Anchorage?

With the board's Velcro cuff wrist-tethered, Bobby attacked the waves and mastered prone rides. As the sun pranced overhead, the incoming surf ripened to four feet waves. But five-foot swells, if not caught right, flipped him on the swash marks.

"Dad, that one dirted up my nose," Bobby sputtered, pinch-faced, spitting sand and saltwater.

"You okay?" queried Graywood, suppressing a grin for the boy's bravery washed amuck.

"They're really good waves, but it's so hard," said Bobby, spewing beads of sea from his nostrils. "The strap gets in the way, and your head hits the board when you wipe out. And it gets in front of you, and you got to go under and get it."

"That's a whole lot to handle," replied Graywood, holding back chuckles.

"I don't wanna use the strap. I wanna stand."

"Well … it's lunchtime," said Graywood. "Let's take a timeout from boarding." He needed the pause to construct the reply on how the tether would be always wrapped around Bobby's wrist while boarding … or an ankle.

"Can I do some more?"

"Yeah, but not today. We're going to Kapa'a to get gear for snorkeling tomorrow."

"Yippee! Let's go now."

"After lunch." Graywood wanted to buy a Hawaiian dictionary too. He remembered a large shopping complex near there when they'd driven out the first day. It should support a decent book store.

The Whaler's General store at the Coconut Grove Center displayed everything a tourist needed. Graywood paid cash for the hand-sized dictionary, but when they stopped at the ABC Store on Kuku Street, the plan to buy snorkeling equipment took a detour. ABC had packaged masks in three sizes. However, the gracious saleswoman mentioned Snorkel Bob's down the road rented by the day or week. And fitted gear might be best for a young boy. Like the boogie board, it didn't make sense to buy what Bobby would outgrow or never use in Alaskan waters. Graywood pulled out the dictionary and thanked her.

"*Mahalo nui* for the tip."

"*Kipa mai*," she replied, face lighting up.

They backtracked to Snorkle Bob's, and Graywood noticed the Island Hemp and Cotton Company kitty-corner from the ABC Store advertising a T-shirt close-out sale. It intrigued him that they sold clothes fashioned from hemp, and he wondered if one might ever smoke the shirt off his back. The pondering got nipped off by Bobby's pleas to hurry to Snorkle Bob's.

Graywood's son was a doer, not a be-er. The "be still" command didn't make a dent on Bobby's lively behavior, but a no-nonsense "do still" worked for a few minutes. Yet on his own at Snorkle Bob's, he attentively sat and followed every instruction.

Two months earlier at the school conference, Bobby's first-grade teacher, Mrs. Weere, had inferred he acted ADHD-like. Like tainted soda fizzing from a can, Graywood's head replayed her acidic, confident summation. "Bobby most likely had a mild form in kindergarten, Doctor Graywood, but now it appears to BE increased to a moderate degree."

That damn BE *word again*, Graywood had thought at the time. Now he watched Bobby meticulously place the goggles over his face. "Nothing like ADHD had existed a hundred years ago. And how much abided in China or Japan today?"

Graywood suspected there weren't many Asian children medicated for it. He'd research the prevalence in other cultures once they'd returned home.

On the initial try, Bobby positioned mask and air tube for a tight seal. To verify, the fitter instructed taking them off and starting over.

Astringent, Graywood still couldn't get past Mrs. Weere's veiled warning: "A child who loves to read will do well in life. Unfortunately, Bobby doesn't wish to read."

Graywood tried to rationalize it down. *I don't remember BE-ing hooked on reading when I was six and a half. Is better reading ability a cultural goalpost change from the last century to this one? If you read below average as a kid today, are you labeled with a disease, where a hundred years ago you weren't?*

Bobby's second attempt donning the equipment received copious praise from the assistant. Nothing physical daunted his boy … he just sparkled. Now it was his dad's turn.

"Was it hard to do?"

"Nah, Dad. You can do it."

In the morning, they drove to a snorkeling spot near Haena State Park the locals called Tunnels Beach. Graywood lugged the boogie board as the backup sport *du jour* should the swells crest too high, but the transparent water lapped low. Where not covered by creeping strands of naupaka, the beach roasted their feet. Graywood taught Bobby an old trick he'd learned on the Oregon coast as a boy to twist each foot, balls first, down into the sand to get to cooler layers. He unpacked both snorkel sets and spread anti-fog gel on the insides of the masks. Bobby needed no help donning the gear, only a reminder to stroke with soft fin motions to avoid spooking the reef fish.

Floating prone and exchanging air through the tubes, they eased aside a pinktail triggerfish into a school of striped, black-and-white convict tangs. Graywood forgot to bring fish food, so the group showed no interest, instead of darting about for an easy meal.

The looming shadow of a larger creature joined them. Graywood surfaced and watched Bobby tread submerged behind it. He followed the green sea turtle twenty yards before popping up screaming it was a baby dragon. Graywood replied it was a distant cousin to the great Puff and to keep careful not to stress or touch it because Puff fiercely protected all his little cousins.

As morning advanced, other snorkelers joined to make a human flotsam. Either from anxiety or boredom to do something else, Bobby ceased swimming and paced the beach. Where sand abutted a lava tide pool and encased a deep scoop of sea decorated with weed ribbons, he discovered three turtles sunning. Electrified, he bounded back.

"Dad, I've found the cousins' hideout!"

"What?"

"Puff's cousins. Three of them. I've found the cousins!" he stammered, half-garbled.

"Then be very hushed about it, Bobby. Do some respect and stay away. Can you DO that? Hideouts are supposed to be secret places and not yelled about."

"But, Dad, it's exciting! I promise not to hurt 'em."

"Keep away. Don't disturb them." Graywood returned to studying the dictionary yet sideways observed Bobby sneak away. Every six steps or so, he'd pause to scan over each shoulder to verify no one detected the route.

Graywood sighed and located the Hawaiian word for turtle. He didn't want Bobby telling everyone he'd found the cousins. It reminded him of Maren whenever she complained of feeling premenstrual; calling her pending period "a visit from the cousins" had been vogue for her clique when they'd entered adolescence. She hated her cousins coming, turned more tolerant after they'd arrived, and grew elated once they'd left.

Bobby raced back. "They're still there!"

"The official dragon word for the cousins is *honu*," instructed Graywood. "Puff wants you to call them honu."

"*Honooo*," Bobby repeated, bright-eyed, and dashed off.

Horselaughing, Graywood mused on Maren moaning about turtles, her honu, whenever they came to visit.

Bobby bolted to a family by the shore where the brother and sister had built sand castles. He started his own. The smaller of the two, the girl, lent Bobby a Frisbee to mound material to catch up. Neglecting her brother, she helped the zesty new friend. They worked as a team. She brought Frisbee-filled loads, and Bobby molded the rising knoll. They reminded Graywood of his romping with others on Oregon beaches by Coos Bay.

Watching them, another Maren image bloomed of what might have been: Graywood had hoped for two children after proposing. She'd left six years ago. How could a wife and mother commit such a deed? The bewilderment had burned as sizzling asphalt that purged the throat down into hell-hotted farts. His dream world would have been complete had Bobby a younger sister; tangible were both she and Maren here now.

The girl and Bobby quit the sand pile and crept like slinking robbers to the tidal pool. He must have told her the secret about the turtles. Honu, Graywood hoped he'd remembered, not the cousins.

Graywood ambled to the abandoned brother and asked for his parents. He pointed to a couple stretched on reed mats beneath a ginger-blossom-red canopy.

"My name's Gary Graywood," he introduced. "Looks as if my son joined your girl and boy in a major construction project."

The three adults exchanged their children's names, Annie and Justin plus Bobby, and other details. From Seattle, they relished the escape from its dreariness. Mentioning he'd attended medical school there, Graywood confirmed the city's dismal springtimes. The wife asked where Bobby's mother might be. Graywood simply replied shopping.

Meanwhile, Justin had searched for and linked up with Annie and Bobby. For the rest of the day, each adopted a sleeping honu to watch over. An honorary honu guard schedule was negotiated with detailed rules and penalties. It lasted no more than ten minutes when implemented—derailed by hunger, Frisbee tosses, shooting whale spouts from humpbacks before sea-flapping their majestic flukes, or castle reconstructions made necessary by the relentless incoming tide.

Observing the cacophony of actions and sounds, Graywood resolved every Maren memory had to be erased. No more storage of her on folders or websites in his brain—access denied. Outdated files had to be deleted. Six years of limbo had been too much. She'd become a mirage lacking any chance of flesh. She'd never come back. From now on, he'd embrace only the trite summary she'd pronounced upon departure from Anchorage's airport: "Gary, you and Robert would be better off with a woman who's truly into you both, rather than me staying here going through the motions."

The afternoon at Tunnels Beach repeated the morning.

Secured in the car seat, Bobby slept exhausted on the return to Hanalei. In a cord of vehicles waiting turns to cross the one-lane bridge over a languid Wainiha River tributary, Graywood closed both eyes and drained from his heart the final ounce of Maren. Love was supposed to endure disappointment. He'd suffered enough. Mercifully, he'd accept being better off as a single parent.

A nocturnal downpour splattered the mountains and thickened the waterfalls.

Bright morning hues in Eden—from red-torch ginger to orange bird-of-paradise to purple-plus bougainvillea—bedecked the softened air. Graywood breathed in color for the first time.

For the remaining days, Graywood paired morning Hanalei beach activities with afternoons of exploration. After each boogie-boarding session, Bobby pestered to jump off the pier's end. Graywood diverted him toward safer thrills knowing clever distractions snipped off diving impulses. Once Bobby's energy faded with the afternoon sun, he forgot the conquest.

The March surf slammed too rough to dare a Zodiac motorboat to Na Pali sea caves and dart among the spinner dolphins. Instead, father and son hiked to Queen Emma's Baths, a series of eroded tidal pools patrolled by elusive crabs below Princeville's bluff. Climbing the gigantic basalt blocks reminded Graywood of the time prior to Maren when he and his business partner, Piper Gunlock, had tethered up to rappel off Spencer Glacier in the Chugach Mountains east of Anchorage.

Once more he embraced Piper's sage instructions: "If you lead, when you see a rock, step on it 'cause it's been there a helluva long time lying on good ice." A glacial stone implied solid support, compared to a snow-covered crevasse giving way to drop a soul a hundred yards or more.

Graywood didn't need Piper's guidance or ice pick and taut ropes for Kauai's pumice, yet he compared the brown-black, volcanic slabs to the sooty ice floes and gingerly led Bobby over the driest surfaces to minimize slips and scraped skin.

The afternoon prior to their departure for Anchorage, they explored the Kilauea Point Lighthouse and National Wildlife Refuge. Turning onto Kilauea Road into the town by the same name, they spotted a farmer's market in an open field beyond the post office. Tourists and locals mingled among the back-ends of pickups and vans, half-sheltered by blue, maroon, and tent-green sunshades over red earth and tamped-down grass. Vendors sold pineapples, limes, flavored goat cheeses, mixed flowers, organic lettuce, basil, Thai eggplant, Chinese parsley, avo, and purple sweet potatoes.

A machete-wielding man attended a truck brimming with coconuts and chopped-off ends so buyers might suck the tepid, sweet liquid through a straw. Graywood ordered one for his boy. When handed the coconut, Bobby almost dropped it from excitement. The merchant gave the shaka sign to hang loose. Bobby repositioned the coconut tight under one arm and ably shook the gesture back.

Kilauea Point Lighthouse and National Wildlife Refuge occupied the island's northern tip. Built on the bluff in 1913, the lighthouse had operated the largest clamshell lens in existence. An automated beacon replaced it sixty years later. Offshore squatted a chalky splotched island—the bird sanctuary splattered in weather-bleached avian excrement.

Graywood and Bobby took the self-guided tour. With binoculars signed out from the park ranger, they identified the birds winging overhead or roosting windward on the neighboring scarp. A tolerant pair of nene, the Hawaiian state goose, waddled the path ahead and ignored Bobby's closer approaches. Water spout sightings beyond the sanctuary island distracted him from the geese. Magnificent head and pectoral ocean-surface slaps confirmed two rival whales engaged in a cetacean courtship of a third.

Two wedge-tailed shearwaters looped the blue sky. Graywood followed the loud groaning pair to their nest, but the graceful soaring of a Laysan albatross hijacked his eyes. The white-feathered adult with charcoal-brown tail displayed a majestic, seven-foot wingspan. Yawing and arcing like a prop pilot over vast cornfields, the bird choreographed with the updrafts and veered toward a grassy runway near the cliff.

Graywood broke off to confirm Bobby still enmeshed by the whales. When he returned to the albatross landing site, he found two. Wooing to lay claim to the other, they bobbed heads and sky-pointed beaks. The two-part ritual repeated. Graywood imagined hearing their copious exchanges of bill clackings, whistles, and oo's.

It hit him hard—the explosive psychic release and its reminder it was time he saw other women. Out of self-deception, he'd cemented away his feelings for other women in hope Maren might someday return. He'd conjured the excuse of raising Bobby on his own to exclude dating, its risks, and hurts.

Peeling down to a deeper honesty, he'd perpetuated the outright fantasy of Maren returning as the convenient, social checkmate. But on the drive back from Tunnels Beach, he'd finished her off. Maren was over …

"Dad, whatcha watching so long?"

The moment broken, Graywood's jaw lowered, yet he glanced sideways at the mating birds.

"Dad, you look kinda funny."

"I guess I do." Graywood returned the binoculars to his eyes. The albatross duo circled in a bonding dance.

"How long we gotta stay here?"

Graywood ignored his child. Clenched in revelation, he hoisted himself out of the mental box he'd created. Six years of confinement ended. Blood surging, wings unclipped, he soared.

And he beheld his son's bright face. "I think it's time we moved on, Bobby."

"Good. I'm hungry."

Graywood breathed the fullness in release and uttered, "Me too."

They handed in the binoculars and strolled to the parking lot.

"Dad, you take so long to do things."

"You're right, Bobby."

He had lost what he had come to lose.

The computed tomography scan whirled to completion, and Graywood wheeled Bobby to his room. For the moment, all that was known was an eleven-year-old boy had suffered a prolonged period of unconsciousness called syncope. Graywood remained with him overnight at Children's Hospital.

Rachel and Cub returned. They reported before the party Bobby appeared tired and confused but showed no weaknesses in the arms and legs once he'd regained consciousness. Yet Doctor Timm's examination of Bobby revealed a component of neurocardiogenic syncope—the positive tilt-table sign—suggesting dysfunction within the autonomic nervous system where certain nerves functioned not fast enough to respond to common environmental stresses, such as standing quickly after lying down. Thankfully, no brain tumors were visualized on the CT.

Bobby's normal blood tests excluded diabetes, hypoglycemia, and other metabolic diseases and shifted Doctor Timm to prospect on Bobby's heart for cardiac causes of his passing out. She ordered an echocardiogram to assess for heart valve and muscle malfunctions that might manifest initially as syncope.

The result came back normal, same as Bobby's electrocardiogram. Combined, they ruled out congenital and genetic cardiac diseases.

Switching diagnostic focus to Bobby's brain, the low intensity impulses recorded on the EEG lacked a definitive abnormal pattern and were interpreted equivocal. The absence of a seizure premonition insinuated an intermittent, cardiac rhythm disturbance or a rare, hereditary, neurodegenerative disorder as a possible cause for Bobby's syncopy.

Doctor Timm emphasized to Graywood 40 percent of syncopal episodes remained unexplained after lengthy and careful examinations. Such might be the case with Bobby. She deferred labeling his condition anything other than an undefined loss of consciousness, probably neurologic in nature. He was discharged the following afternoon.

Relieved to get Bobby back, Graywood drove his son home and willed the belief that everything would be grand ... like the time little four-year-old Bobby brought home his pet cat.

Graywood braked the Subaru in front of Rachel's house to collect his boy after work.

Gleeful Bobby chugged out the front door holding a shoe box. "Dad, look what Cub gave me."

Footwear from Cub didn't make sense. Graywood craned to peer inside and detected a tortoise-shell kitten.

"Can we keep him? Can we, Dad?"

Graywood hesitated.

"Dad, he's just like Rum Tum you tell me at night. It's him, Dad. He's Rum Tum."

A tiny feline paw snagged the cardboard edge. Two innocent eyes entranced a new keeper.

"I don't know. It's pretty small." Graywood rubbed the soft fur between the ears. "It'll need a whole lot of love and care from you, Bobby. Really, a whole lot."

"I love him, Dad! I promise I take care of him. I really will."

"You know it'll need your care every day."

"I take really good care of him, just like we do each other."

Astonished by that comeback, Graywood placed an index finger under the kitten's chin. *Your child's growing up when he starts believing he's taking care of you.* "So you think this tiny one wants to come home and live with us?"

"Oooh, I do. I really, really do!"

"What makes you think it'll want to be called Rum Tum?"

"'Cause I dream Rum Tum looks like him, just bigger."

"Bigger?"

"Way bigger."

"Maybe," teased Graywood, "too big to sit in the kayak with Rum Tum's buddy, little Aleutian girl?"

"No, Dad, not that big."

"You'll promise to help him get bigger."

"I promise."

"Every day?"

"Every day."

Graywood stroked the kitten's back and lifted it from the box. It rasped a scratchy, high-pitched plea.

"Leave him with me and say good-bye to Cub and Mrs. Rachel."

Accelerating to warp drive, Bobby rocketed toward the house screaming gobs he got to keep Rum Tum.

"And thank them for watching you and for Rum Tum," yelled Graywood.

The kitten meowed. Cradling it, Graywood admired the yellow-brown eyes. "So you're the teeny blessing sent to help me raise Bobby, eh?"

He double-checked for ear mites and palpated the neck and abdomen for nodes and masses. He pulled up the tail and confirmed a healthy female. "Well, little one, we'll have to see how your Bobby handles this when we take you in for shots. I'm counting on you to be a good role model on that 'cause he hates them screaming-bad. That'll be the first thing you'll teach him."

Bobby barreled to the car. "I'm ready to go home with Rum Tum."

Graywood placed the kitten in the shoebox and handed them to Bobby. "Be careful holding her."

The "her" went right past the boy. He held the precious cargo like treasure and scrambled into the safety seat. With a tooth-wide smile, Graywood buckled them in. Rachel giggled at the front door when Graywood waved all okay. The rearview mirror revealed a quiet boy cherishing a new companion.

"Ahh ... say there, Bobby?"

"Yeah, Dad?"

"We've got a big problem."

"What?" Afraid, Bobby clutched the shoebox.

"There's something wrong with the kitty-cat."

Silence. Rounding the corner Graywood suspected Bobby's dread having to take the animal back.

"Your kitty probably won't want to be called Rum Tum."

"Oh no, Dad," Bobby returned, with relief. "He's my Rum Tum."

"Are you sure?"

"He's the most Rum Tummmmy-ist there is!"

"So how do you know?"

No answer. Bobby focused exclusive attention on the furry one.

Graywood drove the rest of the way appreciating the rare backseat silence. When they entered O'Malley Drive, he asked, "So ... isn't Rum Tum a boy cat?"

"Yeah, we're gonna be best buddies."

"Well, I think it's important to know I've looked at your kitty-cat, and she's a girl."

Dead air. They passed the Alaskan zoo, the golf course, and their church. Repeated mirror glances revealed Bobby's intense stares into the box. Graywood exited onto Upper O'Malley Road and feared the boy might wish to return the animal to Cub because of the wrong sex.

Not a sound.

They entered Snowline Drive.

"How's the kitty-cat done so far?" asked Graywood, the question meant about Bobby, not the kitten. He employed the strategy where parents often inquired about a child's toy or pet—such as Rum Tum, or the kitten in this case—but actually referred to their offspring's condition.

"Dad, help me pick her name."

Relieved by the request and this one, no less, Graywood guided them from the Subaru, unlocked the garage side door, and entered the kitchen. Bobby followed holding the carton like a rare jewel.

"Well, Rum Tum likes rum in his tummy," Graywood said, flipping on a light. "What do you think she'd wish in her tummy?"

"What's like rum?"

"Oh, there's vodka, Martini, bitters, port." Graywood warmed the left-over chicken pasta and boiled a package of frozen peas.

"Are there other things?" Bobby asked, disappointed with the choices.

"Well, what about whiskey, gin, Chianti, brandy … uhmm, not Chianti; that's a wine." Graywood sensed Bobby's search for a name that flowed as easily as Rum Tum. Chianti Cat seemed okay but was a tongue-twister for a four-year-old. Graywood assessed the feline's whiskers and offered, "How about Whiskey Whiskers and shorten it down to Whis-Whis?"

"Dad, that's not a girl's name."

"Yeah … it doesn't sound too good."

Graywood passed by choices to do with Martini and returned to Chianti, rolling it over in word combinations. Three syllables in Chianti; Rum Tum, only two. What dribbled off the tongue with cat besides Chianti? Then he realized they had no cat food.

"Bobby, we forgot to get some kitten chow on the way home."

"Dad, her box's all wet."

Graywood grabbed today's unread newspaper, plopped the kitten on it, and noted to buy a litter box too. "Bobby, go upstairs and bring one of the empty shoeboxes out of the guest bedroom's closet."

The car version of the getting-ready-to-go-somewhere routine from home switched into rapid mode, this time with three travelers instead of two because Bobby refused to part with the kitten. Graywood lined the shoebox, punched six holes into the lid, and instructed Bobby to hold the container upright with the tiny one hidden inside while they shopped for kitty's food, comb, a toy, cat litter and box, and a collar to wear in a couple of months.

They pulled off the shopping caper without discovery, although the single cat toy multiplied to six: one for each day of the week with all to be played with on Sunday. Indeed, Bobby had negotiated well for her.

For nine days, they tested dozens of titles on the tortoise-shell, but candidates such as Bourbon Ball and Torty Tail missed taking hold. Even the Rum Tum bedtime stories attempted to find a name. At the end of one goodnight narrative, Rum Tum roared that he loved rum in his tummy as much as the kitty might love rum or brandy in her belly.

Bobby jounced upright off the pillow and declared, "Dad, that's it."

"What?" returned Graywood, breaking out of Rum Tum's alto voice.

"Brandy Belly, that's her name."

"Well I don't know if Rum Tum agrees to the belly part," Graywood said. His mind replayed the two words. A sobriquet flashed, and he proposed, "Brandy Belly is too much like Rum Tum's tummy. How about shortening it to Brandy Belle?"

With a wide-mouth grin, Bobby agreed and hugged his dad.

Bobby and Brandy Belle reunited after the overnight at Providence.

Graywood prepared mac and cheese and peas for dinner yet hedged emailing Maren regarding their child's unexplained syncope. For dessert, father and son wolfed down saved birthday cake once Bobby had blown out the eleven candles in a single puff. Per routine, they executed kitchen cleanup and cat maintenance duties before Graywood coached the boy through leftover homework, capped off by reading aloud from the *Spider-man* comic Brandy Belle had bought for Bobby's welcome-home present. Prior to bedtime, they competed in video bowling games on the great room's big screen.

Graywood assessed for subtle changes in Bobby's brain function throughout the evening activities and detected nothing abnormal. Everything appeared well. Confident, he withheld contacting Maren.

Later that evening, once Bobby was in bed, Graywood reviewed everything Bobby had done since he'd started school. O'Malley Elementary turned out to be not what he'd expected …

Graywood couldn't believe it! The first-grade teacher, Mrs. Weere, had just implied his son had attention deficit hyperactivity disorder. Distraught, he determined to medically refute or validate her assessment of Bobby's behavior.

Attention was defined as directed awareness. For Graywood, ADHD, if it truly existed, was a deficit in directed awareness. Negating the deficit, as he understood Mrs. Weere, was necessary to succeed in today's school environment.

But Bobby's a doer—amazing blond hair and wide blue eyes, charging by with every strand a-flying—not a "be-er." "Be still" doesn't work too well, but "do still" does, at least for a little while. "Out, go outside, run in the yard," I've yell more than three times a day, but I love when he rushes like a colliding train for hugs.

Cub's father, Piper Gunlock, had kidded Graywood about the number of BTUs in energy Bobby expended whenever the two boys played together. Piper called them "Bobby thermal units."

"Bobby's a brave little soul," reasoned Graywood, out loud. "Yes, he's impulsively brave at times. That happens. But in kindergarten he wasn't the worst of the *kindergargoyles*—those pint-sized cherubs yearning to escape from enforced tedium inside classrooms just wishing to unleash pent-up bouts of jumping, running, bashing, and bursting in the brilliant world of boyhood for a few moments. Yes, if they gave a grade for adhering to tenets of quiet time, Bobby would've failed."

But what's that got to do with reading ability? Mrs. Weere's worried he's a poor reader in class. For Christ's sake, I don't remember doing a whole lot of reading aloud in damn first grade when I grew up!

Oh, good God, calm down. She means well. You can work on it with him at home. Get him to tell what he's learned in school and read something out loud to you and Brandy Belle after dinner each night.

With the basic plan of attack, Graywood layered on the medical perspective. Bobby had two ears. If different streams of information got delivered into each one, to which would he attend? Which would he choose, and which should be relegated to background noise?

Could he even do that? Adults managed it all the time at receptions and cocktail parties. But did Bobby need more help filtering out what to ignore and what to concentrate on to assist proper attention direction, especially at school?

ADHD was a diagnosis of exclusion. All other potential causes for poor school performance had to be sought and ruled out before so labeling a child. If a potential impairment was discovered, it had to be treated, and the student's performance reassessed.

Specialists evaluated Bobby's eyes and ears. They confirmed normal sensory system functions.

Perhaps Bobby had been exposed to a substance that interfered with appropriate classroom behaviors. Could his hyperactivity be secondary to hyperthyroidism, or might the attention deficit have resulted from elevated blood-lead levels? Or were they red herrings? Graywood wanted everything checked.

He bribed Bobby to surrender four tubes of blood to measure thyroid hormones, lead levels, serum chemistries, and PBDE. Graywood had to spell out polybrominated biphenyl ether on the laboratory slip to insure the sample was sent to the correct reference laboratory.

A fire retardant, PBDE was manufactured for furniture cushions, electronics, mattresses, and carpet padding. Its dust, if consumed or inhaled, mimicked the effects of thyroid hormones. Long-term exposure had been theorized to cause an overactive thyroid gland: the Environmental Protection Agency had noted a curious epidemic of hyperthyroid disease among exclusively indoor pet cats and found they harbored higher tissue levels of PBDE. EPA had concluded more studies were needed to determine the full connection between PBDE exposure and cat hyperthyroidism, yet they also speculated humans, particularly infants and toddlers, might face the same health dangers from this flame retardant's particles. If Bobby's PBDE or thyroid tests had returned abnormal, Graywood resolved to test Brandy Belle for PBDE as well.

High blood-lead levels in children adversely affected maturing brains and reduced IQ scores. To limit exposures, lead had been banned since the 1970s from paints and motor fuels.

The Graywood house on Snowline Drive was constructed in 1991—building codes in effect should have prevented utilization of leaded paints and other materials. Perhaps the prior owner or a subcontractor might have illegally applied them before Graywood and Maren had purchased the home in 1999. If so, Bobby's indoor rambunctiousness may have caused sufficient exposure to flaked lead that later compromised classroom learning.

When the laboratory results came back, all gave normal values for Bobby's peer group. Bittersweet, Graywood worried over the ADHD label tattooed to his boy. He mined Internet sites and consulted with Bobby's pediatrician, Doctor Natalia Timm, for assistance.

She theorized Graywood's son might possess a subnormal ability to sift in and filter out environmental and social inputs, or more to the point, to elect and select his attention to whatever needed to be done to succeed in school. Compared to the majority of his first-grade classmates, the maturation in the executive part of his six-year-old brain—the prefrontal cortex responsible for impulse control and abilities to learn from mistakes, exercise judgment, and perform higher-order societal functions—had not yet met the modern expectations for his stage of development.

Bobby was too sensitive. The deluge of environmental inputs easily overcame him. For skills society now judged critical—such as quiet reading at a work station—his concentration prowess appeared lacking. Bobby's sub-par focus on higher-order tasks, setting realistic goals, and carrying through step by step to completion were handicaps. Twenty-first century culture expected much from its children.

And Doctor Timm provided insight into ADHD mechanics. As a pragmatic empiricist, she offered an analogy based upon what had befallen NASA's Deep Space 1. In the 1990s, NASA pushed the cutting edge of space exploration and designed an unmanned space vehicle that employed an auto-guidance system linked to ion propulsion engines for a rendezvous at an asteroid beyond Jupiter.

Once launched, the mission did not unfold as planned. The probe drifted in space. It could not triangulate its position, making it unable to execute the programmed course to the asteroid.

NASA discerned too much diffuse starlight hampered the triangulation put into the auto-navigation system—too many bright points coming from every direction existed in the navigational camera. Once NASA radioed the probe fresh operating instructions to rank and disregard the light-flare noise, Deep Space 1 fired up and proceeded on the projected course.

Doctor Timm compared Bobby's social navigational system to Deep Space 1's. Too much raw information confused and frustrated him. Adding a long-acting form of Ritalin or a pristine drug, such as Adderall or Strattera, to aid brain function appeared equivalent to NASA transmitting updated operating instructions into the spacecraft. Ritalin would sharpen the nervous system's abilities by speeding up the brain's inhibitory part to sort and disregard superfluous inputs. It would allow Bobby to concentrate on the task at hand.

Graywood wobbled side to side sitting across from her … but finally agreed. Even the smartest piece of equipment devised by man could not handle the excess inputs from outer space without help in order to follow its planned course. So be it with Bobby.

"Which med is best for him?" queried Graywood.

"A generic, extended-release form of Ritalin," recommended Doctor Timm.

"Not a newer brand name?"

"We could do that, but compared over time to Ritalin, they don't show a meaningful difference in tuning out the majority of distractions and improving a child's concentration. And since Ritalin's been on the market decades longer, it has much more clinical data. It's the one I prescribe the most and feel comfortable to start."

"Makes sense," said Graywood, voice hanging back.

Doctor Timm swiveled her leather chair and entered an electronic prescription in the desk computer.

"Bobby's got garden-variety ADHD," she spoke, percussing keys, "not too severe, but enough so Ritalin should help."

"Remind me of side effects?" asked Graywood.

"To minimize those, we'll see how he does on the standard starting dose and watch for changes in appetite and sleep. We'll monitor growth curves, too. Those are the notable ones."

She printed a side-effect profile and handed it to Graywood. "As you can see, there's a bevy of rarer ones too. We'll switch to a newer brand if any occur or the ones I've mentioned happen and become intolerable for Bobby." She clicked to review Bobby's growth chart.

"Do the newer drugs have fewer side effects than Ritalin?" asked Graywood.

"That's what the drug reps say," she replied, "and so far, some are a tad better on having fewer unwanted ones." Her head lifted from the monitor to catch Graywood's eye, and she added, "However, they don't have as many cumulative years of clinical practice usage like Ritalin, so we don't yet know all their unknowns. We probably know everything there is about Ritalin since it's been around so long."

Dr. Timm intentionally left out that medications, such as Strattera, were still under pharmaceutical patents and more expensive.

Graywood accepted the logic for beginning an agent prescribed for decades. It seemed less inclined to harbor unknown complications compared to one just brought on the market. That was the constant rub against the medical-pharmaceutical-industrial complex.

While waiting to fill Bobby's prescription, Graywood pondered the dilemma. An advanced therapy got FDA approval after its maiden clinical trials on a thousand or so young and middle-aged people. They suffered only the ailment being evaluated and took no other pills. But once the government authorized the treatment for the general market, the fresh medication was available to everyone with the same condition regardless of age or illness status, including senior-aged patients who often each imbibed six or more concurrent drugs for other health problems. At that point, the truer clinical trial commenced—conducted in the thousands of doctors' offices across the country on tens of thousands of less healthy patients. Out of that broader scope derived the honest range and severity of adverse side effects, which confirmed or damned the initial FDA clearance for public use. Repeated history bore out the disparities—unknown inherent dangers in prescriptions such as Ephedrin, Vioxx, Accutane, and Phen Fen had their commercial uses restricted or withdrawn years after they'd obtained FDA approval.

Viewing Anchorage's distant streetlight aura from the deck at home, Graywood mulled over how complicated this century had become. Bobby needed help from Ritalin to concentrate. A hundred years ago, kids like him didn't ingest a brain drug for school simply because society operated on fewer inputs stampeding in from all sides.

Yet the overwhelming harshness of multiple information levels harnessed into today's culture mandated a better mind filter—many children couldn't get by on the low capacity screeners wired into their heads at birth that had been socially adequate for their ancestors. Today, having a minor-league input-sifter meant getting branded with ADHD and taking one or more of its medications. If Mark Twain's Huckleberry Finn had lived now, he'd have been so marked as well … like Bobby.

Graywood acknowledged ADHD's spectrum of wide-ranging intensity and believed, at most, his son's symptoms were moderate. Bobby acted more distractible than normal yet fell behind in class not enough to repeat first grade.

Thankfully, Bobby displayed nothing as tragic as a variant of autism, the dreaded umbrella of human social disorders that began in early childhood and persisted lifelong. This illness group commanded a good portion of Alaska's special education effort and had no single treatment. In contrast, most ADHD could be managed by a drug schedule linked to school attendance whenever attention and concentration were most needed.

And Graywood chewed over ADHD's contribution to No Child Left Behind and the lofty goal of universal academic proficiency. He suspected the federal mandate had created unintended consequences in ADHD's labels liberally applied on marginally performing children. From discussions with principals and teachers, Graywood concluded this law, and the threat to withhold funds to districts with poor academic performances, had forced the public school systems to concentrate on those students lurching between success and failure on statewide tests. Teachers struggled to meet annual proficiency goals and had the greatest incentive to bring failing students up to minimum passing scores. If a drug such as Ritalin possibly helped, it almost certainly got recommended.

Graywood acquiesced to Bobby taking a pill to avoid placement in the lower expectation classes. His son did poorly with concentration and reading, and Mrs. Weere proclaimed he needed tutoring or a drug or both to pass future reading and arithmetic assessments. Still Graywood doubted the veracity in this evolving piece of pedagogy. Was there a true epidemic of ADHD in the United States? Or had it become a social inclination to reclassify common and ordinary behavioral problems under this abnormal title?

It troubled Graywood: a derived social scheme blunt-sorted large numbers of young boys and girls into taking powerful prescriptions. Yet the weight of evidence that medication might help more than harm Bobby had persuaded Graywood to submerge doubt. One statistic motivated utmost: 30 percent of kids with ADHD did not finish high school.

With Ritalin, Bobby responded less to every whim, and his brain shifted up a notch to the long-term planner mode required for every primary school student in America. He thrived without any known side effects.

CHAPTER TWO

Bobby's Pilots, Storytellers, and Matrons

Viewed from the North Pole, Alaska dominates the northern hemisphere, and Anchorage is almost equidistant between two major financial capitals: from its international airport are New York City, 3,385 miles, and Tokyo, 3,434 miles.

Anchorage is Alaska's economic and population core. Its eclectic skyline reveals a juvenile boomtown in perpetual transition as the northern Pacific's regional hub and gateway to the Arctic Ocean.

Once an outback junction between the gold fields in the south and the Matanuska and Susitna valleys to the north, Anchorage was designated by the US government in 1915 as headquarters for the railroad connecting the territory's interior mineral claims and coal fields to the port of Seward on the Gulf of Alaska. The small town hiccupped an unexpected expansion when the Japanese invaded the Aleutian Islands in World War II, and it spurted with reconstruction subsequent the devastating 1964 Good Friday earthquake.

Oil discovered in Prudhoe Bay on Alaska's North Slope had rocked the state's major borough far greater than any gigantic earth tremor. Oil brought world-class wealth, and Alaska became a gargantuan sluice where everyone searched for real and imaginary stars of gold. Happily accepting the growth greased by the region's fossil fuel extraction, Anchorage led Alaska's heady development and pimped itself as the Capital of the North Pacific and Beyond.

But the proud urban complex grieved for its lost nature-bound traditions and vanishing tranquility. Grey citified blocks, woven in random dull stones, looked out of place with the grand sweeps of steadfast mountains ringing the horizon.

One still found the rougher, hell-raising sides of town where Native Americans barely were tolerated. Prejudice might end in another decade or two of pell-mell growth ... replaced by other unbridled anxieties.

Like Los Angeles or New York City, "Los" Anchorage had become a community where people remained lonesome together, where each Alaskan skinned out his or her befitting portions of nineteenth and twentieth century folkways to shoulder into the twenty-first.

Gharrett Graywood had an unremarkable birth in Coos Bay, Oregon, but didn't stay there long. Grasping for good-paying construction work, his father moved the family to Anchorage after the 1964 earthquake.

Badly burned when four years old from a kitchen fire, Graywood needed skin grafts on his right leg and a year to heal. His mother hired on as a teacher's aide once he'd entered primary school. He loved learning from picture books, and his parents bought him a Polaroid camera for his tenth birthday and urged capturing the world with it.

Thereafter, Graywood's father contracted a virus that inflamed and weakened the heart muscle into a fading pump. Despite extended treatments in Anchorage and Seattle, the inefficient cardiac pulsations failed to clear blood backed up in the lungs. He drowned in his own fluids. Graywood's mother never remarried.

With no teaching jobs in Oregon or Washington, mother and son returned to Anchorage. State coffers, flushed with Prudhoe Bay drilling royalties, had expanded the resources for Alaskan public school systems. The small life insurance annuity on Graywood's father supplemented family income, and an annual payment each legal resident received from North Slope oil taxes—the vaunted Permanent Fund—also helped.

Once Graywood had finished a biology degree at the University of Alaska and gained admission into medical school, he orbited three overlapping spheres: a boatload of student loans, a future as a physician, and an ailing parent riddled by lung cancer.

His mother had inhaled three cigarette packs a day due to teaching pressures, her husband's unexpected death, and Alaska. Graywood shuddered whenever hearing her spiked-like spasms and wished to God he could cough for her. She died the month after his college graduation ceremony.

Lacking funds for medical school, Graywood garnered a federal Health Professional Scholarship and maneuvered to pay back its service obligation through the Public Health Service rather than the military. After a family practice residency, he served two years on loan to the National Indian Health Service at a stand-alone clinic in southwest Alaska, operated by the Bethel Indian Corporation. There he sustained patients with diverse illnesses and provided supervision for the remote village health aides, midwives, alcohol and drug counselors, and aeromedical evacuation teams.

When he obtained a Masters of Public Health degree in 1996, Graywood assumed regional supervision of the public health clinics throughout southwestern Alaska. A promotion eighteen months later conferred the deputy directorship of all the Alaskan clinics plus a transfer from Bethel to Anchorage.

The new position required extensive liaison to isolated facilities across the Forty-ninth State. To negate delays and lessen daunting travel times, he sought a fixed-wing pilot's license, planning to purchase a single-engine airplane.

Tolerant, kind, and openhearted, he believed it superior to manage personnel and resources face to face and not rely solely on starched radio and landline communications. He enjoyed meeting the gallant, frontline subordinates serving on Alaska's periphery. Likewise, they appreciated visits from the boss who'd fashion the extra time to fly to the far-flung bailiwicks—a courtesy rarely done by prior leaders. Graywood expected the best from everyone—and usually got it.

For a flight instructor, Graywood hired Piper Gunlock. As a bush pilot, Piper managed adversity with outward aplomb, and Graywood envied his stubborn strength.

Piper made a livelihood transporting tourists, sportsmen, and freight to remote areas in a de Havilland DHC-2 Beaver. On the lookout for extended work, he submitted competitive bids for multiple-day commercial and governmental contracts to move clients, cargoes, or work teams across the hinterlands.

Once he'd flown a National Geographic team around Denali to complete an expedition. On another deal, he'd supported a Hollywood film crew shooting a three-month-long documentary about migrating birds of the tundra. He befriended one of the science advisors who, in turn, had recommended him to Doctor Cashel Goodlette at the US Geological Survey Office in Anchorage.

One of Doctor Goodlette's federal grant proposals had received last-minute approval to study climate change. Hard-pressed, he needed a crafty, reliable aviator to reposition data-collecting equipment in and out of twenty-three adverse locations hugging the North Slope prior to the fiscal year end. Piper made it happen, and Goodlette thereafter employed him as the primary back-country conveyance.

A charter member of the Chugach Air Volunteer Search & Rescue, Piper also listed availability on three rosters posted at the Merrill Field control tower for emergency transfers, evacuations, and urgent medical supply deliveries. Other registries had him as backup for routine hauls on fixed-wing, single- and twin-engine aircraft.

Word of mouth recommendations negated Piper's need to advertise as a flight instructor. Students sought him. He squeezed in the pilot training sessions with his unpredictable transport schedule.

Piper emphasized how to take risks in the air: his motto was, "Always prepare for calculated risks, and those will be handled well. It's risk you don't calculate for that'll kill you."

Two common hazards Piper hammered home involved the seasonal weather changes for thaw in the spring, and freeze-up in the fall. Unpredictable transitions between winter's perpetual dark and summer's long days compounded any flight plan—a pilot taking off on frozen ground might land on soft, soggy earth. The main challenge centered on selecting the correct landing gear for both ends whenever conditions dramatically altered. In winter, thick ice remained the pilot's friend, and attached skis allowed graceful approaches onto frozen lakes, but ice became the enemy once thinned too much into spring.

Simply put, the most important act in flying was the approach. At each touching down on whatever posed as the runway, Piper expressed, "It's God's will we got here again."

"Gary, I do this only for a few of my beginning students," said Piper. "I'm gonna show you how to fly from point A to point B with my method of blendin' to air currents, which Mother Nature gives us. I can tell you're up to it. So you ready for my first question?"

"Sure."

Out of the blue, Piper asked, "Do you think I'm mad?"

"No," replied Graywood, stunned. "Why should I?"

"Good. Always remember never sit next to a pilot you think's a madman."

"That makes sense."

"Damn straight it does," agreed Piper. "First you'll learn basics on a Cessna 152 at Merrill Field, and then we'll handle instrument flying with the 185."

"When will I fly a floatplane?"

"Well," paused Piper, eyes dancing with excitement, "you gotta first solo on wheels. Damn floats are a tricky pair of bastards and a whole skill level up. For that, we've gotta fly out of Lake Hood, but it'll cost you more."

"To fly anywhere, that's my goal."

Piper raised a hand to stroke his long neck weighing the opportunity Graywood presented. He needed to assess this doc's commitment to serious aviation.

"So, Gary, the key to keepin' yourself flyin' and alive in Alaska is knowin' your limits. You know the limits on your plane and match 'em to the limits weather gives each goddamn day and every goddamn hour. And always remember those goddamn limits can shift a helluva lot in ten minutes, 'specially round thaw and freeze-up. To survive, you gotta let yourself go and get kinda like the air 'cause air density gives wing lift, and weather and altitude make density. Think you can handle all that?"

"Damn straight," mimicked Graywood without hesitation. The best answer to give.

Yet Piper continued testing. "You doctors say you're always practicing medicine, right?"

"Yeah, we say that."

"That means you're always learnin' something, right?"

"Yes, we learn from our patients all the time."

"Well that's damn straight of you, Gary, 'cause you're always learnin' when you're flyin' too. That's how I see it and how I say it. You remember this ... every time you're up in the air, you're damn well learnin' something."

Piper called himself an old-school bush pilot, meaning he'd learned airborne skills by wits in all sorts of weather conditions without the aid of aeronautical charts, beacons, or cockpit radios. If pressed, he'd hint earning wings over unknown foreign terrains dodging unmapped mountains in some of the worse conditions nature ever inflicted.

Decades before the advent of GPS, he'd mastered the magnetic compass. For navigational landmarks, Piper memorized lakes, hill groups, and river sways. A few times each season, he'd uncouple the Beaver's GPS, dead reckoning the old way. It kept abilities sharp in a manner a seasoned engineer might calculate a construction project with a slide rule to avoid letting fundamentals lapse from only key-pressing the latest, brainless, hand-held marvel.

"One more thing, Gary."

"What's that?"

"You should know I'm what some people call dys-lectic."

Graywood leaned closer, unsure he'd heard right. "Did you say dyslexic?"

"Ahh yeah," replied Piper. "I guarantee I don't see things upside-down. Sometimes it's backwards seeing I get screwin' up a bit." Piper studied the fresh student to measure his resolve. "So you still think I'm not crazy?"

Graywood kept a pencil-thin smile and recalled the effusive recommendations given by two air traffic controllers at Merrill Field and a third stationed at the international airport. By them, Piper wasn't just a good pilot—he wrote the book on how it's done. They credited him with incredible talents, confirmed by the coolheaded ease he'd shoehorn seemingly impossible aero-evacuations through the most difficult weather systems on earth. On wheels, skis, floats, or the thirty-five-inch tundra tires needed for far north approaches, he'd take off and land any fixed-winged aircraft on surfaces a white-fronted goose passed up as too short or too steep.

Graywood locked eyes to Piper's. "I've already said you're not mad. But if I don't get my money's worth out of you, I'm the one who's damn straight crazy!"

Both heaped up laughing.

"Damn good idea, Gary, lettin' me help with that."

After Graywood had signed his pilot's license, he approached Piper for advice in buying an airplane. "I need a reliable aircraft and your recommendation on who'd maintain it."

"Best mechanic 'round is Tailwind Talbot over at Merrill Field," said Piper. "I use him for the Beaver's big overhauls. I do the routine stuff. I'll help you with that too."

"That's great."

"Ahhh … what kind of bird you thinkin' of?"

"I've no particular make in mind right now, except one I can change wheels over to floats or skis and back, depending on destination."

"That'd be my choice," agreed Piper. His hand rubbed nervously down his face and neck. "Ah, Gary, I'm meanin' to share somethin', and now's a good time."

"Okay."

"You know, I've too many customers to haul round who don't need all the space in the Beaver. So I need another plane, a smaller one, for a damn straight fit for my business."

Graywood remained silent, yet raised eyebrows to signal him on.

Piper cut to the proposal. "Gary, I'm looking for an equal partner to share a small bird, like a four-seater. Would you be interested?"

Flattered, the best pilot in Anchorage had invited Graywood into a business commitment. Piper trusted him enough to risk his livelihood. They'd have to become good friends and stay that way.

Perhaps the higher bond had been forged when Graywood had snapped in two a strut gliding the Cessna trainer onto Spencer Glacier. They had roped up and rappelled off the ice floe as a team on the day that had lasted forever. Alone, neither would have survived.

"How'd sharing the plane work?" said Graywood, probing.

"Let me know flyin' times you'll want to check your clinics. That'll be the scheduling priority. I'll fill the gaps with my smaller hauls or maintenance."

"How'd we split costs?"

"We each buy half the bird and split operation and maintenance by number of hours we each log every month."

"So you mean if I fly twenty and you forty, I'd pay a third of fuel, hangar rent, insurance, and maintenance, and you'd cough up the other two?"

Piper stopped to think the proportions—for him, thirds took longer to divide than halves. With an orb-to-orb grin, he answered, "Damn straight," yet wryly added, "but if one of us breaks something, he's gotta' fix it 100 percent."

For Graywood, it made sense both pilots leveraged the other's needs. "Any idea where to start looking for a plane?"

"So you're agreein', Gary?"

"Damn straight!"

They shook hands to seal the deal. Nothing more needed.

"So you're interested in a bird," cracked Tailwind Talbot, a wizened, grease-smelling, Vietnam veteran, who'd splice a workable aircraft together out of parts scrounged from ten planes, even cannibalized off choppers.

"Damn straight and blue, Tailbone," kidded Piper. He called Talbot "Tailbone" to his bearded face because the mechanic's hind vent stayed glued to the ground while Piper's preferred to crease the air flying. "You got something to look at?"

Tailwind stopped dirt-picking fingernails to point out a single-engine Maule at the bay's end. Its sole red stripe graced the sides on the exterior's dune-white.

"That STOL's in fine shape," gruffed Tailwind, "and heard the owner got a heart attack last Halloween. The widow bolted back California way. It's up for sale."

"Let's take a look," said Graywood.

The three men passed a disassembled Cessna Grand Caravan as Graywood recalled STOL meant short take-off and landing.

"It's been parked here since then," said Tailwind, dog-eyed. He ran a shrewd palm across the seventy-six-inch Hartzel propeller. "I've kept her in a good way. She's ready to go."

"A real gem," confirmed Graywood.

"The widow leave any papers?" asked Piper.

"Yep," spat back Tailwind. "Old invoice, operating and maintenance manuals. Got 'em back in the office."

"What about the pilot's log and registration certificate?" queried Piper.

"Got 'em too."

"Gary, head over with Tailbone and get 'em," directed Piper. "I'll start looking over the bird."

Piper circled the MX-7-180B Star Rocket model with 180 HP, Lycoming engine; length, twenty-four feet; wingspan, thirty-three feet. He estimated engine performance, when matched to wingspan, placed the stall speed around forty miles per hour in average weather. Configured with tail-dragger landing gear leading an oleo strut, she had fittings and mountings for wheels, skis, or amphibian floats for increased utility. The taupe-colored cabin fitted four seats with three-point shoulder harnesses. Cargo straps and tie-down rings lined the fuselage. The control panel displayed standard avionics for GPS, navigation, and communication.

"Piper, I've tabbed the specifications summary," boasted Graywood from excitement, returning from Tailwind's office.

"Let's take a look," said Piper, closing the left eye to limit dyslexia.

"Manufactured 1993, gross weight—2,500 pounds; empty weight—1,438 pounds; useful load—1,062 pounds. Takeoff distance, 300 to 1100 feet depending on load. Service ceiling, 15,000 feet. Best climbing speed, 90 mph. Two main fuel tanks plus two auxiliary, 73-gallon capacity. Fuel consumption at 65-percent power, 9 gallons per hour."

They skipped the faded illustrations to consume the maintenance instructions.

"I'm pretty interested," said Graywood, trying to dampen his enthusiasm to neutral.

"Let me show what I found," said Piper. "Then we'll talk Tailwind into letting us try her out."

They bought her as equal partners. Graywood named her *Seneca.* She'd become the woman who'd never fail him. She was not human like the others.

Piper dubbed her *Sky Woman.* Piper's women were another story …

At the end of the twentieth century, Piper stood forefront in the battle to move the state capital from Juneau to Willow. Politicians could not be trusted whenever holed up in a panhandle town one-tenth the size of Anchorage and inaccessible to the rest of the state unless one owned or rented a plane or boat.

Born in 1952, he mushroomed into a handsome charmer with an appetite for women, preferably rich. Baptized John Pierre Gunlock Jr., he'd have none of the Junior title once he'd mastered a Cessna 140 as a teenager on his uncle's thirteen-thousand-acre ranch south of Pueblo, Colorado.

Leaving home, he adopted "Piper" as his moniker. At six feet three inches, a loping stride complemented casual, deep-set eyes and receding, grey-brown hair on his Arctic weathered face. Afflicted by money anxieties and aging lust, Piper repackaged his obsessions for social justice and sex.

Piloting a de Havilland Beaver, he ferried groups of adventurers to remote cabins for hunting, fishing, and photography. The Beaver handled the bulkier air-taxi business. Piper leased smaller aircraft to transport one or two individuals or cargos weighing less than a quarter-ton. The subletting ceased after the joint purchase of *Seneca-Sky Woman.*

Quipping over the intercom to passengers, he joked about their current airborne status or *Sky Woman*'s overall condition. When approaching the airport, he might banter: "I once put my contact lenses in backwards, and you know what I saw?"

"No, tell us, Piper."

"I saw the back of my goddamn eyeballs, that's what. So I ran to my wife yellin' at the top of my lungs, 'It's goddamn amazin' to see the whole world backwards, and it's scramblin' up my brains.' And she got really huffy and yelled back, 'Piper you take those out right now 'cause I never want you looking at your brains like that again. It's too dangerous.' So I took them out to please her, but now I don't use contacts anymore … and it sure makes everything kinda blurry, 'specially when we're 'bout to land."

Whenever he flew toward the Alaskan panhandle, he lampooned Juneau: "Two brown bears caught a clown and started to eat him. After a couple of bites, the big bear asked the littler one, 'Don't he taste kinda funny?' And the little bear answered, 'Nah, I don't mind if you don't.' Then they caught a politician from Juneau and chewed him. Once each took a good sized bite, both spat him out, and the poor little bear cried,

'Don't he taste really icky to you?' And the big bear bellowed, 'Well, hell, he's damn straight plain putrid!"

Piper flew by his ears as much, if not more, than by his eyes. He sensed uncanny variations in atmospheric moisture and temperature from air movements over the wings.

He'd color-coded the Beaver's control panel to lessen proclivity to invert letters or read numbers backwards. To compensate for his dyslexia, he extracted better use than other pilots of terrain clues, airborne positional cues, and general balance perceptions, all of which combined in a survival advantage. With or without instrumentation, he cruised and breathed weather and read terrain as the famous bush pilots of old.

Piper never confirmed nor denied piloting missions for Air America, a CIA subsidiary that went dark after the fall of Saigon. He did admit, without qualms, to shuttling cargos for Wien Air Alaska when based in Seattle.

And there he'd married Elizabeth, his first wife. Yet when Wien Air went out of business in 1985, he relocated alone to Anchorage to operate his flying service. They'd divorced. Those who'd known them had said that Beth wouldn't leave Seattle for the harsh Alaskan climate. For other reasons, the marriage had failed much earlier.

Piper's airborne access to Alaska's diverse topography reawakened a drawing talent from boyhood. As an adolescent dreaming to get his wings, he'd copied airplanes, jets, and helicopters from magazines. Contrails, flaps, tail rudders, lift, drag, every detail got embellished in teenager doodling. Once he'd become a paid pilot, the artwork stopped but resumed after he beheld Alaska's vastness, molded by unique shades of light twisting through the four seasons. Sketching sharpened his deft eye to surface features, and minute shadows spoke volumes whenever choosing landing sites in rugged back country. A reinforcing loop continuously played: lining out detailed landscapes made Piper a better aviator; flying made him take grander strides as an artist.

After a decade tom-catting evanescent female tourists and bored women who resided in southern Alaska, Piper ardently wooed his second wife-to-be, Rachel Steeder. A native from Palmer, a town forty-four miles north of Anchorage, she worked public relations for the Anchorage Chamber of Commerce.

Rachel resisted Piper's predatory attentions out of cautious distrust until she'd perused a batch of his paintings at a chamber-sponsored showing for local talent. She swooned to all of his one-of-a-kind, raw acts of creation. Intrigued, she agreed to the umpteenth overture to soar to a scenic wonder where Piper sketched and photographed the unfolding vista multiple times in varying natural light. Each winter in his makeshift studio, he'd mature the sketch-photo combinations on canvas.

Piper and Rachel simmered in their first freeze-up together and reorganized his split-level cabin. They prepared the finest art pieces to show at the Snow City Café, located across from the Brady Building in downtown Anchorage.

The iconic diner served full lunches and "eggs as you like 'em" until closing. Walls daubed neon orange, lime green, flat yellow, and periwinkle blue demarcated table groupings. All year, skillet-sized snowflake cutouts hung from the ceiling with metallic blue, red, and green Christmas tree balls.

The café sponsored month-long solo exhibits of photos, paintings, or sculptures by regional artists. The displays changed monthly, the day before the business district's First Friday Gallery Walk. For the June 1996 program, twenty-nine of Piper's acrylic-on-canvas and watercolor landscapes supplanted a novice photographer's Ansell Adams-like pictures of the Alaskan Range.

Piper had dabbed each scene in colored band sequences to give impressions of layers veering toward the horizon. The directness of expression and paint handling created distinct harmonies between the clouds and trees and the reflections off water. They impressed local critics.

One year after the showing, Piper and Rachel's son, Cub, walked his first bold steps. Piper's annual work pattern condensed into remunerative summer aviation with spliced-in sketch sessions, followed by winter paint dressings and whatever flying commissions that presented.

A clique of admirers developed too. An artist might become a babe magnet like a pilot, but a man who donned both sets of talents and skills shimmered pure, unwholesome irresistibility. Rachel's lack of trust in Piper rekindled. Indiscretions poisoned their relationship, and they filed for divorce.

And as the bewildered moth, Piper ardently flamed into a Juneau woman, Sheila Klockridge, the gold-digger.

Women like Sheila will marry without love in their hearts. To her, marrying was a business. Tall with the classic hourglass figure, her most striking feature showcased pursed lips color-matched to shocks of auburn hair. She pursued successful men simply because that's where the money was. Taking cash through wedlock seemed nothing more than permanent loans from the community bank.

Meeting Piper at a Juneau political rally, she assessed a reliable man of means. He had boasted two cascading, income streams—air transport services and art—and therefore met the threshold qualification.

Not a complete fool, Piper knew the tendency for women to marry up. But adroit Sheila gushed and charmed. She twisted his awareness and appealed the lack of resources after ending a terrible relationship. Fearful for her physical security, she had no choice but to flee barehanded to Anchorage. She felt so safe with Piper yet calculated her seductive campaign to exploit his wealth.

Up front, Sheila only hinted at teetering above broke. With just enough to survive, she hoped for Piper's undying trust … and any help. Outwardly she professed how money shined pure evil and wished she didn't need it. Piper remained clueless to her meaning wealth was a vile sin only if she had none, and a woman without assets emerged simply more sinister than one who did.

Piper granted total confidence and deferred verifying her background of three failed marriages in the Lower Forty-eight before she'd skipped to Juneau to knot a commercial salmon fisherman. After two years, she'd gilled and discarded the gullible chump.

Graywood first cautioned Piper about her. He suspected Sheila close to hitting forty years, and unattached women that age loomed notorious for marrying for money, not love. Regardless if her professed love for Piper appeared genuine, Graywood argued Sheila's foremost feelings shined downright mercenary.

The men insulted each other and threatened to fight.

Raw and ballistic, Piper discounted Graywood's warning of Sheila pushing a price-tag partnership. He fired back how Graywood spoke out of jealousy and could never appreciate the devoted feelings the acclaimed bush pilot had for this gorgeous woman who believed only he was the world for her. Sheila could never be a sweetheart swindler.

Graywood pressed no further to back off the relationship, despite hearing Sheila needed more cash to rent an opulent apartment sporting a Cook Inlet view.

Once they signed their marriage license in August 2002, Sheila held to her divorce agenda as Piper's resources depleted. With her uncompromising lifestyle, his wallet would not remain fat and accessible forever.

Naïve or stupid, Piper believed their union would last. He relished the bliss she showered on him.

Her fifth marriage, Piper's third, did not make three years. Drained dry, how he felt mattered not. She had to look after herself and move on.

Piper sought his closest confidants, Graywood and Monroe Bearhead, to help purge her from his soul and bind the scars dredged by heartless talons. With the clarity from a forgotten number of beer nights, Graywood implied Sheila had acted predatory toward men of means as much as Piper had pursued women for physical appeal.

And Bearhead added Sheila might have come Piper's way to reveal how it felt pounced upon and coveted for one fleeting quality, such as money or sex. Bearhead even suggested their pairing was shaped by a spirit to force Piper to open his eyes.

Brusquely dismissing Bearhead's candor, Piper transposed Sheila's acts of profitable preying onto his nemesis—the jaded government in Juneau. The political scummers devoured Alaskans' fiscal independence and fashioned clever schemes to abscond every citizen's permanent fund money or hijack it to finance a new state-sponsored health-care plan. Piper compared the twin bitches, Sheila and Juneau, as zooming straight into twilight … and hoped they'd rot in Hell.

Bearhead and Graywood listened to the rant and wondered who'd be next in Piper's string of romances gone awry. Bearhead hoped a woman angelically sent. Piper's path needed remarkable repair to grow his spirit.

Graywood and Piper—reliable, predictable men, partners since ninety-eight—were also fathers.

Whenever the boys played at Piper's studio, young Bobby shared the most recent Rum Tum story with Cub and his dad. Out of kindness or curiosity, Piper sketched the mythical cat while keeping an eye on the boys. Graywood framed and nailed the feline's best portrait over Bobby's bed.

The fresh series of Rum Tum bedtime stories were created after Bobby lost interest in the standard canon for his preschool age. He wanted adventures set in Alaska, not fairy tales from a pretend faraway place. The common folklore sounded like television cartoons, and Bobby knew how they'd end. So Garywood conjured Rum Tum and tagged him, "Kayak Kitty of Unalaska."

The saga lasted a year but stopped the month after Brandy Belle because Bobby wanted no jealousy between the real feline and the make-believe one. Before the narrative ceased, however, Rum Tum had joined other characters: little Aleutian Girl, Oscar the Sea Otter, the stalwart Uncle Oo-otek and his floatplane, Aleutian Girl's unnamed mother and father, Sammy the Seal, Patty the Porpoise, the shed mice Papa Moe and Momma Lois and their eight tiny babies each named for a type of cheese, and the evil Baron White Gull who led the crafty minions stealing everybody's food. Sadly this assembled host, the fabled denizens of Unalaska, faded to oblivion. Years later, Graywood wished he'd recorded the nightly oral tradition.

Monroe Bearhead, Bobby's godfather, enjoyed snippets of the Rum Tum lore retold with great fanfare by Bobby whenever he visited the Graywoods on Snowline Drive. To encourage his godson's storytelling flair, he carved him a miniature Rum Tum from yellow cedar wood.

He left a different sort of memento with Bobby's dad. Monroe Bearhead's favorite saying meandered into Graywood's brain whenever he prepared a meal: "There're lots of philosophic tomes full of life's recipes and lots of cookbooks complete with life's wisdom. Together they boil down to four basic things: temperature, ingredients, amounts, and timing when to mix together." Graywood added a fifth—when to serve food and life to a hungry child.

Graywood and Bearhead taught back-to-back Wednesday lectures to the first-year medical students enrolled in Alaska's contingent of the regional medical school. Professor Monroe Bearhead, tenured in the Indian

Studies Program, covered Cultural Aspects of Medicine and Health, and Doctor Gharrett Graywood, Public Health Service officer, instructed Introductory Epidemiology and Disease Control.

Wyoming, Alaska, Montana, and Idaho lacked an intrinsic medical school to train future physicians. To correct the shortfall in the 1970s, the University of Washington medical school in Seattle created the WWAMI medical program—comprised of Washington, Wyoming, Alaska, Montana, and Idaho. Its cardinal mission centered on erasing the projected physician deficits within the region. The state governments, in turn, appropriated funds to leverage their shares of medical training costs, and the initial year of student instruction commenced at each respective state's university. Thereafter, the students transferred to the University of Washington to complete degrees. The Alaskan WWAMI students trained the first year at the University of Alaska Anchorage.

Graywood preceded Bearhead in lecture sequence, yet Bearhead often arrived early to listen to his colleague. Graywood rarely stayed to absorb Bearhead's cultural pearls. When he did, afterwards they'd share lunch. They became close friends.

"As Yogi Berra said, 'If I hadn't believed it, I wouldn't have seen it.'" That bit from a Bearhead class bubbled up whenever Graywood surveyed the refrigerator's leftovers.

The rest of the Bearhead-Berra musing often gonged in Graywood's head while jotting down a grocery list. "I'll expand Yogi's wit," interpreted Bearhead. "You see only what you believe, and you find only what you're looking for. These statements suggest how fundamental biases each one of us harbors are woven into our human perspectives of culture, science, and religion. I could soften Yogi's awareness down to this: in any culture, science, or religion, you will tend to see what you believe, and you'll tend to find what you're looking for. These tendencies are pernicious because the culture that we see conforms to our social group, and that heavily slants toward our tribal beliefs. That's why it's so hard for an individual to change and why it's so difficult for a neighborhood to grow past itself, unless pummeled by catastrophe. By inhibiting self-growth, these tendencies are indeed the signposts of a closed-in spirit, even worse, a spirit made smaller."

Monroe Bearhead, burly and balding with tawny skin, prodded and charmed the best out of people. His credo emphasized hospitality, happiness, hope, healing, and honor.

Born in a village longhouse near the confluence of the Copper and Chitina Rivers, Bearhead's ancestry bridged the northern Pacific. His Athabaskan mother, Annie, belonged to the Ahtena tribe, Tallchief clan; Samwon, his father, hailed from South Korea.

On a fishing trawler licensed out of Japan, Samwon harvested salmon, ocean perch, and pollock near the Copper River estuary beyond the continental twelve-mile limit. Leaving home in Taegu, he migrated across the ocean each year to nature's clock of salmon runs returning to natal streams to complete their cycles of life.

Near the end of the 1947 harvest, Samwon suffered abdominal pains that mandated emergency surgery. Taken to the Alaskan port, Valdez, his shipmates refused to wait and paid his cut of estimated profits. They promised to pick him up at the coming season's start.

The stranded wayfarer, once healed, learned broken English and native phrases to find part-time jobs. When he was dockside repairing yards of fractured fishing nets, the brother of his future wife befriended and introduced him to an Ahtenan potlatch. Details of the romance between Samwon and Annie Bearhead remained sparse and soft spoken. Tiny Monroe Bearhead entered within a year.

Samwon resumed the annual oscillation between the Korean and Alaskan coasts. In 1949, he held Monroe in his arms for the final time. Allied with soldiers sent by the United Nations to Korea, he perished fighting for his country.

Monroe roamed the river bluffs and woods beyond his mother's lodge with an inner sense of time and freedom not known to other American children. Annie's father stood as the leading elder of Chitina, and her brother, his right hand. Both men taught Roe the Ahtenan ancestral insights, village history, and traditions.

Roe showed uncommon intuition. He found the soul's true path, his spirit guide to hidden mysteries and wisdom, in the Raven atavism and chose to avoid the village males who hunted, drank at night, and practiced the common circles of abject subservience. Instead, Roe read with the greed and gusto of a wolf, devouring books and magazines, sucking up pages to his brain.

Bearhead became a comparative cultural anthropologist and Indian studies professor at the University of Alaska Anchorage. From a corner in the Social Sciences Building, his third floor office overlooked a collage of trees. The faculty and students regarded him a quiet leader, woven—by gentle, sagacious, and loving ways—into the native Alaskan community mosaic. Everyone recalled the parties at Bearhead's uncomplicated home: a miniature potlatch with shoulder-to-shoulder people eating the incredible cuisines he'd prepared. Thoughtful and deliberate, Bearhead championed the university and his international research.

Bearhead's Anchorage house possessed Asian influences to create a calming milieu. The carmine joists, wainscot, and protruding logs from the rafters incorporated the subtle contrast in the home's rounded arch design. Comfortable chairs absorbed worries and provided contemplation. Ceiling drapes emphasized quality over clutter. Not a prisoner to possessions or wealth, Bearhead's home exuded a sense of sanctuary and assisted in finding balance.

In a crook of the great room sat a glass-fronted cabinet in cherry wood, lined with ebony. Three shelves exhibited Bearhead's scrimshaw carvings from sperm whale teeth and the tusks of walruses or extinct wooly mammoths, the latter gathered secretly from eroded banks by the upper Chitina River.

During light-shortened winters, Bearhead's grandfather had taught him how to carve and dye patterns in the ivory. They'd scratched the designs with a jackknife and filled the traces with a black-soot and tobacco-juice mixture before drying the pieces by the fire.

The room's opposite corner held three Korean stoneware vases on a five-step, poplar-and-walnut *tansu* chest, flanked by portraits of willow branches etched on Sekishu. Each ceramic's opening flared from broad shoulders that tapered to a base with full curves displaying distinct, incised boughs or plum blossoms covered by a celadon glaze. A sitting jade Buddha and two pumice-stone Shiva statues dominated the top shelf.

An entrance off the kitchen led to the wood-carving studio where Bearhead sculpted birch, maple, yellow cedar, Sitka spruce, African mahogany, and Brazilian cherry. Two opposing lathes anchored the walls, both tucked under racks clenching hand tools of various sizes and ages, from penknives and scalpels to drawknives and chisels. The outside door opened on a fenced, pocket-sized yard, encircled by sentinel red cedars guarding a pedimented gate to the alley. Wind chimes hung at the entry to deter demons.

Myths and legends inspired Bearhead to liberate the enclosed stories from the blocks of wood. Sawdust and chip detritus scattered the tiled floor from the freed statues—an open-tailed peacock showing off to a peahen, a gray whale guiding her calf, twin zebras entwined, and something Bearhead called a mastodon in transition to mammoth to elephant. More figures populated the shelves between the lathes: whittled snow hares, eagles, owls, dogs of multiple species and sizes, an albatross, and three gulls squatting on a broken log. A four-foot, varnished monk seal curled on the floor beneath the room's square window. On a sideboard, a black lacquered disc anchored seven cranes, posed within rows of bent reeds. The central table supported an unfinished, man-sized, winged creature evolving out of a block of British Columbian yellow cedar.

Cooking was Bearhead's other great passion. A pot of Oolong tea forever brewed in the meticulous kitchen, the tannin scent making it as comfortable as an old lodge.

Bearhead had a gourmet chef's reputation, yet humbly inferred he'd learned culinary skills through observation when globe-hopping as a budding anthropologist. For him, kitchens remained the natural gathering places in all abodes around the world—how people cooked and carved made two excellent insights into their culture.

A year short from college graduation, Bearhead entered an arranged marriage with a Chitina woman of the Eagle matrilineal moiety. His grandfather maintained it not wise for a man to be alone, and a wife stood given unto a man only by the blessings of the ancestors. Ten years senior to Monroe, her name was Ume. Bearhead's uncle cautioned how she might not be perfect, but neither was Bearhead, and the ancestors knew best in bestowing their favors. Gleaming like a never-ending summer solstice, Ume radiated kindness in all ways, far beyond Bearhead's hopes.

Bearhead pursued his studies and deferred championship of domestic life to Ume. They kept a lodge in Chitina plus the house in Anchorage where Bearhead rose to tenured professorship. Their dinner table remained open to all visitors and friends. They boarded university students and welcomed travelers from the villages. Every August, they hosted a Chitina-wide potlatch where the rivers converged and invited guests from Anchorage to partake in the week-long celebration.

Ume and Monroe had one natural child, Sophie. They cherished her unlimited joy for two years until she passed away from bacterial meningitis. They grieved for her and the fragile nature of human happiness—the shaded gift from God, which confused more than blessed.

Thereafter, they unofficially adopted every child in the village. Auntie Ume and Uncle Roe assisted each girl and boy on individual spirit quests. Both sensed the ancestors pleased, and both understood all things on earth remained frail unto God's eyes.

Crow's feet distinguished Bearhead's middle-aged face. He called the skin lines hard wisdom gathered out of Raven's ever-reaching, splayed talons. And he breathed more deliberately from creeping emphysema made worse by smoking tobacco.

On an icy day in 1997, long after the bears had gone to den, Bearhead's beloved Ume passed on from liver cancer. Heartbroken, he took a year's leave to seclude himself along a line of fishing huts aside the Tebay tributary upstream from Chitina.

When the spirit path brought him back to the village healed, the ancestors evinced more kindness and provided another gift of union, actually, a double union to the Coldsnow sisters.

April and May Coldsnow were widowed twins whose husbands had succumbed within months of each other from cross-cultural excesses. From the study of Islam, Bearhead recalled how the prophet Muhammad instructed that a man might have as many as four wives, so long as he treated them equal. Fortunate Bearhead had only two. His joint commitment to April and May—not so much a formal, licensed marriage but a personal covenant with privileges—required the most perfected attempts to intertwine their mutual respect, trust, and compromise. For outsiders ignorant to the Herculean work required, it appeared he played the lucky bigamist.

Muslims revered Muhammad as the Perfect Man. Bearhead believed Muhammad had to be so, for indeed, he had treated four wives evenly, and no other man ever on earth shall again.

Yet Bearhead attempted with two. Bewildered, he pondered why the ancestors bestowed the mighty endeavor onto his spirit path. Then again, they knew what seemed best. They had sent Ume, and for her, he'd forever remain grateful.

Graywood co-lectured with Bearhead, learned to fly from Piper, and thanked God for Rachel and Cub.

Graywood believed Piper's biggest mistake stemmed out of forsaking Rachel for bimbo Sheila, the serpentine gold-digger. Rachel served as Bobby's de facto, full-time auntie and part-time mom. From last-second babysitting to afterschool latch-key supervision and emergency sleepovers too numerous to count, she bestowed gracious love. Rachel raised Bobby as much as his dad did.

Cub's given name was John Pierre Gunlock III. Born four years ahead of Bobby, he'd become the boy's surrogate older brother and best friend. Bullying or negative feelings never occurred. Indeed, each cultivated the other with wry touches of Piper sprinkled in whenever he got around them.

Piper had coached Cub in many skills. Once he'd told Graywood, "Boys need to go off and do some kind of pursuit 'stead of just sittin' in rooms. That's the way it's been for sons, gettin' them ready for life, and the way it's been for dads by their boys too."

Cub marked his quest in an identity distinct from Piper's—he mushed sled dogs. Ahead of glory derived from individual achievement, he grasped the happiness in a group's accomplishment. The charisma of dogsledding outshined everything.

Cub preferred solid ground to soaring over it, and Piper reluctantly acknowledged his son's diminished attachment for aviation. Out of respect, Cub learned to maneuver *Sky Woman* through the clouds, yet his main goal had bull's-eyed to become a champion sled-musher who, if required, could fly the back country as well.

Cub knew he'd never attain pilot status like his dad. He lacked his father's remarkable sky senses and never could be one with a plane. Rather, he apprehended the sublime unity with an adoring team of canines. Out of wages garnered from two part-time jobs, Cub fed, trained, and procured their equipment. At age fourteen, he'd mastered the skills expected in a first-rate musher and dreamed to race the Iditarod.

"Why not shoot to win?" encouraged Piper when Cub unharnessed the lead pair after a twenty-mile practice run.

"Dad, the Iditarod is THE toughest race. Only half the competitors complete it, and just a handful do it more than once." Cub coaxed the two crossbreeds into traveling kennels, and then he added, "More people summit Everest than see Nome's finish line."

Piper admired Cub's self-control. *Must have gotten that attribute from Rachel.*

"Dad, I always remember you saying to calculate risks when taking on Alaska," declared Cub, unhooking another canine duo to remove the booties protecting their paws from jagged ice. "It's the risks you don't calculate that'll get you."

Hearing that stellar bit of judgment, Piper corrected the proportions: Cub had received equal parts of self-control from his mom and dad.

A blue heeler and chow mix, Sable was Cub's lead dog and matriarch of the pack's huskies, malamutes, and crossbreeds. Other members were Slade, Raider, Houdina, Zeker, Smiley, Bud, and Zeus.

A mix of growls and moans acknowledged whoever entered Sable's territory. She'd issue warning barks if the trespasser hadn't made eye contact and called her name. More inclined to emit a calm or jovial presence, Sable kept her alpha role intact with snaps and bared teeth when needed. She and Cub commanded the team and told each other what to do.

Eight dogs created gargantuan winter deposits of frozen mire and rubble. With those light-shackled days, their care could exceed Cub's capacity when pitted against school and employment. Not able to add more now, when Cub raced the Iditarod, he'd augment the octet by co-training another eight canines borrowed from another kennel.

Bobby was the other human fully accepted by the pack. Cub and Sable had designated him the team's junior partner once he'd fulfilled the pissing stone initiation.

The receding glaciation twelve thousand years ago had deposited an obtuse, wheelbarrow-sized erratic at the east corner of Cub's backyard. On Valentine's Day, after a treat of orange soda and Rachel's homemade, pink-frosted cake, Cub blindfolded seven-year-old Bobby and led him to the granite mass. Cub rotated the novice three times in place before instructing him to unzip his pants and let loose. If Bobby's stream hit the boulder the first try, he passed. If missed, he'd wait for spring to try again.

Despite covered eyes, ungloved hands, opened fly, and fourteen degrees below zero, Bobby repositioned a quarter turn and shot over the megalith until the arching flow withered to splatter down its center. With quavery glee, Cub unbound Bobby's eyes and blasted his own urine above Bobby's. Sable wandered by, sniffed the double scent, and tinkled to make three. The rest of the pack followed suit.

Cub trained Bobby to place booties over Sable's paws for protection from injury on the longer runs. Petting her when done, Bobby read in Sable's head tilt the expression, "I'm so happy you're here." From then on, the three defended each other as one.

Cub raced the Copper Basin dogsled competition when he reached eighteen. Once Cub crossed the starting line, Piper ferried the sled's supplies ahead in *Sky Woman.*

They fought minus-thirty-degree temperatures and ferocious winds gusting fifty knots on the second day. Sizing up the conditions, Piper worried he'd be a hindrance to his son.

"Sweet Jesus Christ, boy, don't be a fool tryin' to out-native the natives! Hole up twelve hours and let the damn storm pass."

"Dad, I am a native."

"Ain't you tired?" Piper huffed. "Me and *Sky Woman*, we're 'bout out of gas."

"My dogs don't run out of gas."

With nature pushing them to the limit, Piper barely kept up. He'd not fail Cub. Frigid enough to grip *Sky Woman*'s engine tight yet not even close to icing the athletic hearts of the pack or the Gunlocks, they pressed ahead and almost won. And for the first time, father and son learned by the other what it meant to be equals. A worthy rivalry commenced.

CHAPTER THREE

JENNELLE

Overnight flurries had lowered the snowline to fifteen hundred feet with September's equinox two days away. Graywood surveyed the Chugach Mountains from the house deck and pondered Bobby's illness. Would passing out at his birthday affect returning to school? Would it interfere with his hockey, which started in a month?

The cellphone jingled as Graywood entered the kitchen to cook eggs on toast.

"Hi, Raych."

"Gary, how'd everything go with Bobby last night?" Rachel's caring cadence harbored subtle tones of guilt for what had happened.

Detecting it, Graywood reassured, "He's okay. Even beat me playing Wii bowling."

"Oh, good! I've been so worried."

"Raych, it's not your fault. The tests are all fine."

"I just feel bad for Bobby and you."

"He'll be all right. It's going back to school and telling friends what happened that worries me."

"You're taking him to school today?"

"Yeah, but he'll miss the first hour by the time we get there."

"Bobby's a good talker. Everybody loves him.

"You're right. He'll handle it."

"I'll have Cub bring him here after school. You can collect him after work."

"Rachel, you're wonderful as always."

"I just want to help you two."

"Thanks."

The complex rapport between Graywood, Bobby, Rachel, Cub, and Piper remained intimate and within boundaries. Like a home's gambrel joist, Rachel supported two cross-linked, father-son duets.

Graywood had met her once Piper and he'd purchased *Seneca-Sky Woman.* On the surface, Rachel and Graywood appeared close friends who co-parented both boys, although she mothered Bobby more than Graywood mentored Cub. There, Piper maintained the senior male role.

A deeper connection with Rachel didn't exist within Graywood, yet she wished it did. Graywood willed not to jeopardize the kinship that held the five of them together, but Rachel was willing.

And romance for Graywood came challenged—checkered by colossal failure with Bobby's mother and then compounded by Jennelle, a colleague. With Maren, he'd probed the dark waters of despair between a man and a woman in search for acceptance. Never finding it, they grappled into divorce.

But simmering rapture had intertwined him and Jennelle. It had commenced with her introduction five years earlier at the end of a WWAMI class. One of them had to change to stay in the relationship, yet neither Jen nor Graywood had done enough to make it work.

He loved Rachel, Maren, and Jen, but loved them differently. Missing Jen as Bobby dressed for school, Graywood thought of her …

She opened the classroom door with caution and observed a tall man with lush, dark blond hair, side-tinged in silver wearing an emerald-green sweater and trim khaki pants. He rocked back and forth before a whiteboard marking four, slate-blue letters—a, b, c, d—into a black square grid subdivided into four equal parts. In the left two quarters the *a* was penned above *c*, and the right column held *b* over *d*. Left of *a*, he wrote PREGNANT and left of *c*, NON-PREGNANT. He printed TEST RESULT

POSITIVE atop the *a-c* column and TEST RESULT NEGATIVE above *b-d*. At three large tables sat ten students: eight pecking laptops at various speeds, two scribbling notebooks.

She took a chair in the back next to a mixed-raced man with a high-domed forehead wearing clothes permeated by tobacco fumes. Muffling his mouth, he coughed and nodded her way.

The clock overhead read 11:04. She leaned toward him and asked, "The man teaching, is he Doctor Gharrett Graywood?"

"Yes," he replied.

Her pleasant face drew him in: she appeared thirty and owned searching brown eyes with enigmatic confidence adorned by rosewood hair, bow-braided in back with two ringlets hanging in front of the ears. Voided of studs, each bare earlobe possessed a single piercing. Nothing dangled from her slender neck ... and no finger rings. A white woman without jewelry, simply pure and elegant. Perhaps she had a hidden tattoo someplace. He was intrigued.

"I was told the lecture ended on the hour," she whispered, hoping for clarification.

"I teach next," he said. "I'm Monroe Bearhead, and Doctor Graywood asked to go fifteen minutes into my time."

"Thank you," she said and smiled. "I'm here to meet Doctor Graywood. My name's Jennelle Daniels."

Both refocused on the lecturer explaining diagnostic tests and meanings behind a medical result. "Hillary, our patient, presents to your clinic very concerned she's pregnant. She doesn't trust the self-pregnancy tests for home use sold at local pharmacies, so she's come to see you for help.

"Let's say you have a new diagnostic test for pregnancy. A positive test result indicates pregnancy and a negative test does not. Now I want to emphasize, however, that for any test in clinical medicine there are four possibilities, not just two. I've just given two of them which I'll explain in a more complete way: with possibility number one, Hillary's status is she's truly pregnant, and her test is positive. That's what we call in clinical medicine a true-positive result. With possibility number two, Hillary is not pregnant, and her test is negative. That's a true-negative. As I said before, there are four possibilities for every clinical test. What are the other two? Can anyone tell us?"

"A test result that's wrong for the patient's condition," volunteered the female student jotting in a notebook at the right front table.

"Correct," confirmed Graywood. "The test can give a false-positive result. By that I mean Hillary is truly not pregnant but the pregnancy test says she's so. The test is in error, and Hillary believes she'll have another baby and can't wait to tell her husband, Bill."

Many students laughed. When the rumbling settled, Graywood asked, "And what's the other example of a wrong test?"

"The test's a false-negative," replied the bearded student at the room's center with eyes flickering between the whiteboard and his laptop.

"Yes, it can be indeed," said Graywood. "You've been reading your assignments. A false-negative is a result that erroneously indicates Hillary is not pregnant when in fact she is."

Entertained by Graywood's selection of Hillary and Bill for the main characters to explain how clinical tests varied in reliability, validity, and yield, Jennelle leaned forward to better view his face. And Bearhead's peripheral eye confirmed no tattooed nape.

Graywood pointed to the divided, four-part square with the *a-b-c-d* and explained, "So every test has four possible results: *a* shall represent the true-positives, *b* the false-negatives, *c* false-positives, and *d* true-negatives."

Clearing his throat, he continued, "Let's take one thousand women of childbearing age and test them for pregnancy. Someone pick a number to represent the fraction truly pregnant."

"Five hundred," boasted the bearded student, triggering snickers from the class.

"That's way too high for a representative sample," replied Graywood, side-shaking his head. "Let's go with a hundred—a nice 10 percent of a thousand making it easy to calculate."

Graywood marked numbers in the squares. "So we've got one hundred pregnant women out of one thousand. Let's say the test correctly identifies eighty of one hundred pregnant women as positive, but incorrectly labels the other twenty as negative. So *a*, the true-positives, is 80, and *b*, the false-negatives, becomes 20. The sensitivity of the test is its ability to correctly identify women who are pregnant, and for our example, it's the ratio of true-positive results to the sum of the true-positive and false-negative results, or *a* over *a* plus *b*, which is 80 over 80 plus 20, and that makes 80 divided by 100, which is 80 percent."

Graywood paused to let laptop clicking diminish and then said, "We still have 900 women of the 1,000 who aren't pregnant. Let's say the test correctly identifies 890 as negative for pregnancy but erroneously labels ten non-pregnant women as being pregnant. So *c*, the false-positives, is the number 10, and *d*, the true-negatives, becomes 890. The specificity of this test is its ability to correctly identify individuals who are not pregnant, and in our example, it is the ratio of true-negatives to the sum of the true-negatives and false-positive results, or *d* over *d* plus *c*, which is 890 over 890 plus 10, or 890 divided by 900, which is almost 98.9 percent."

Graywood rotated to face the students and asked, "Is it possible in medicine to have a perfect test that's 100-percent sensitive and 100-percent specific?"

The students, on the whole, had decoded Graywood's instructing style, and several answered, "No."

"You certain about that?" Graywood egged them on, mining their mettle.

"Nothing is 100 percent, except birth, death, and taxes," intoned a thin student, squinting up from his notebook at the middle table. Horselaughs erupted to include Bearhead.

Graywood nodded, and said, "Births and deaths are called cardinal events, which means they only happen all the way or not at all. There're no half-births of quarter-deaths. You're either born or not. You're alive or dead, nothing in-between."

Graywood booted up from memory one of Piper's profaned, anti-tax rants against Juneau politicians, although a cleaned-up version. "As for taxes, that's a different story," he said. "Taxes are created in all shapes and sizes. There are no birth control pills or condoms to prevent a tax-baby creation, other than just saying no on referendums or voting politicians out of office who wanted them. Once a new tax baby gets born, it lives forever." Then emitting darker tones recognizable to Bearhead as coming straight from Piper's mouth, Graywood emphasized, "It will never die."

Bearhead and Jennelle chuckled with the students over Graywood's use of politics to embellish tenets of medical science.

"Let's wrap this up regarding medical tests," said Graywood. "There's no test that's both 100-percent sensitive and 100-percent specific. In medicine, our tests are primarily meant to sort patients into two groups: normal and abnormal cohorts. But we always must remember each patient is a complicated, biological open system and not a closed system as our physics colleagues like to study in their controlled experiments. So in health, we must modify our definitions of abnormality, based on the patient's age, sex, other concurrent medical conditions that he or she may have, all the drugs he or she takes, and so forth. And all that causes a peppered stew of overlaps between normal and abnormal whenever all these other parameters get evaluated holistically. Combined, they'll influence and confound the test results for groups of patients, just like our pregnancy example of one thousand women. Bottom line, if you can clinically verify that a test sorts out abnormal from normal with 80 percent or better sensitivity and 95 percent or better specificity, you've got a fairly decent test to use in clinical practice."

Graywood strolled over to the far side of the whiteboard and wrote PREVALENCE. "Next week we'll discuss how the prevalence of disease in a population affects the predictive value of a clinical test. Read chapters three and four on positive and negative predictive values. And one more thing … input this question for next week's discussion: which is better to have, a test that gives you fewer false positives or fewer false negatives?"

Finished, Graywood located Bearhead seated by an attractive woman. "Ten-minute break before Professor Bearhead starts," he declared, eyeing Bearhead for confirmation.

A female student from the right front table approached Graywood and said, "Doctor Graywood, I think it depends on which disease if it's better for a test to have fewer false-positives or false-negatives."

"That makes good sense, Caroline," said Graywood. She was one of the quicker students. "Right now, can you think of an example for each?"

After a protracted breath, she said, "When you screen for HIV infection, you'd want the least number of false-positives 'cause a false result would worry the patient needlessly, and then you'd have to do lots of extra testing to rule it out to reassure."

"Excellent. And fewest false-negatives?"

Tight-lipped, she stood bewildered.

Graywood answered, "Cancer."

Her eyes widened.

"You wouldn't want to miss a brewing cancer because of a false-negative result," he elaborated. "If a patient's screening test for any cancer, let's say colon cancer for example, is falsely negative when there truly exists a malignant polyp, then the cancer may become metastatic and incurable before it's detected at the next screening. A false-negative test is a terrible tragedy for a potentially curable condition. Sadly, it gives the patient a false reassurance but lurks like a death sentence."

"I see, Doctor Graywood." Her face unpuzzled, she returned to the table to tab notes.

Graywood hesitated about adding that doctors performed tests most of the time to rule out diseases, not find them. But she'd uncover that pearl once clerkships commenced in Seattle and the other WWAMI teaching sites.

"I enjoyed listening to the end of your class, Doctor Graywood," said the stunning woman, extending her hand. Graywood recognized her as the one who'd sat beside Bearhead. "I'm Doctor Jennelle Daniels."

"Gary Graywood," he replied, ratcheting down formality. He pumped her forearm once, yet lingered … captured by her black eyebrows and full lashes framing exquisite brown eyes. They hinted more than languid wells … a cerebral focus in pursuit of answers as persistent as a curse.

A month prior, he'd received her introductory letter from the Centers for Disease Control and Prevention in Atlanta, Georgia. It reviewed her background experience and the mission components underlying her posting to Anchorage.

"You're from the CDC," he said, letting go of her hand. "Glad to have you here. How'd I do explaining sensitivity and specificity to the students?" he asked, attempting to break the ice.

Jennelle appreciated his self-deprecation. Before leaving Georgia, she'd accessed his online curriculum vitae, bypassed the encryption and access firewalls, and studied his archived files in the Public Health Services Knowledge online site. All annual evaluations had rated him top-notch. Likewise, no negative entries existed in the Physician Data Bank.

"You were impressive," she replied and added in deepest voice, "Like taxes, sensitivity and specificity will never die."

Jennelle's wit pleased. After the divorce, it became Graywood's nature to compare every woman to Maren. Hands down, this fresh colleague loomed pleasant. "May I call you Jennelle?"

"Please do, Gary. And it's Jen."

Sharp, forthright, and approachable ... it had been eons since he'd felt comfortable this fast with a woman. "There's a Starbucks on the main floor near the Consortium Library, he said and motioned to exit. "Right now, I could do with a grande mocha. Will you join me, and we'll jump-start Alaskan liaison between CDC and PHS."

She accepted ... and ordered tea.

In 2006, the CDC assigned Doctor Jennelle Daniels to its Anchorage office as part of the national effort to detect deadly influenza strains spreading from Asia into Alaska by either migrating birds or contaminated passengers and crews aboard aircraft and ships. The international fear of an avian flu epidemic also had spurred the development of an effective vaccine. National prevention policies stationed key personnel at critical locations to rapidly assess and initiate immunization protocols wherever bird flu had been confirmed.

The viral H5N1 avian strain had most alarmed international public health authorities. It had exploded across parts of Asia and Russia in 2005 to infect tens of millions of birds and nearly one hundred people; almost half the exposed humans had died. If the virus pervaded more readily among humans, CDC officials feared a scourge similar to the 1918-1919 swine flu pandemic that killed over fifty million. Fortunately, an experimental inoculation provided protection against the current strain and appeared close to FDA certification. Doctor Daniels had been sent north to insure well-timed injections against the deadly agent if needed in Alaska.

The common, seasonal human influenza varieties—such as H1N1—often entered America from Asia first through Alaska. Doctor Daniels planned to sift out the cross-infected cases of bird flu hidden within the usual influenza victims. She'd coordinate surveillance with Alaskan state health officials, the Public Health Service, and the military—primarily the US Air Force at the Elmendorf Airbase north of Anchorage.

The Air Force Institute for Operational Health, or AFIOH, had stationed one of its global influenza surveillance sites at Elmendorf. Its principal objectives were the rapid discovery of novel influenza mutations and averting any potential pandemic affecting the homeland. AFIOH had monitoring sites across the world and coordinated its detection programs with the Department of Defense Global Emerging Infections Surveillance and Response System. DOD's year-round capability allowed receipt and testing of suspected influenza specimens for molecular subtyping and characterization. By mapping results in real time, any disease outbreak would be instantly disseminated to a wide spectrum of stakeholders, and they'd execute the rapid disbursement of resources for casualty prevention and management.

Doctor Daniels's CDC posting to Anchorage also embodied a second mission—she would watch for any terrorist release of biologic, chemical, or radiological weapons of mass destruction. Her advanced biological warfare training at Fort Detrick, Maryland, and chemical casualty management at Aberdeen Proving Ground made her one of CDC's valued WMD experts. She had extensive experience teaching the medical effects of ionizing radiation and management of radiological casualties to emergency-room doctors—a terrorist might detonate a dirty bomb at a high profile location, such as the oil pipeline terminus at Valdez. Doctor Daniels possessed the highest national security clearance.

Their Starbucks meeting lasted two hours.

She'd rowed crew in college and toned a sleek body with jogging, swimming, and cross-country skiing. Her silky congenial voice, never condescending, blossomed to astonishing gut laughs whenever Graywood joked about winter pitfalls and moose perils in Anchorage. Her comic ability to mock herself disarmed friends and co-workers, yet she attributed her coy self-confidence to her parents and four younger brothers. Regarding work, however, she effused intense seriousness.

Professionally, her depth of knowledge in bioscience and biotechnology impressed Graywood, but more so did her pristine standards toward conducting research. She explained at length how faking data had become easier to get away with: pictures deftly manipulated through computer programs—such as Photoshop—overly impressed scientific journal reviewers or made a point better than a boatload of narrative and got altered research published ahead of purer, competing ones.

She echoed the editors who warned how research misconduct had become their most increasing concern. This underbelly of science, which no one talked about, shaped in full force the publishing biases within the scientific literature. It had to be neutralized.

And she emphasized how fraud's belly prejudiced the process of awarding grants. Medical research had become highly competitive, and scientists coveted the limited, untainted funding from the National Institutes of Health and other government sources, rather than from the private industry doles with their inherent winks and nods. Getting published in a peer-reviewed journal improved a researcher's quest to hook a preferred federal grant. Jennelle stressed how temptation and fickleness were not foreign to scientists and how the well of knowledge had been poisoned with falsified data numerous times.

Utmost for Jennelle, fraud stood as the cardinal violation of research ethics and akin to smashing the Ten Commandments. False data created problems for other researchers who relied on them—spurious components and conclusions led to wrong directions and wasted valuable time and resources. One miniscule piece of sham could cripple one or more large follow-on investigations—what was derived out of falsehood, logically, was bogus as well.

She made the distinction, however, between promoting fabricated results and committing honest errors. Mistakes were expected and discovered whenever peers reviewed the methods and analytical sections in a research paper. But to knowingly and purposely hide or distort data and images deserved the harshest rebuke, condemnation, and expulsion.

When Graywood sipped the final swirl from a second mocha, he wanted her on his side in all confrontations.

As they parted, she handed her professional card. "Gary, please stop by my office anytime."

"Grace Hall … Alaska Pacific University," he read, out loud. "Have you met Cash Goodlette? He's got his office there, too."

"He's on the floor above me. Why?"

"Oh, a good friend of mine flies him around quite a bit. If you see him, please pass on I said hello."

Motionless, Bearhead gazed on the whiteboard after Jennelle and Graywood had vacated the lecture room for Starbucks. He mulled over Graywood's sensitivity and specificity presentation. The aspect of a test's ability to sort reality from fiction did not intellectually inspire. Rather, the method allowed one to observe four possible outcomes whenever two dualities were analyzed together. Might that be a swifter way to broaden one's worldview from solely thinking down to a pair of crude opposites, such as black and white, love and hate, or birth and death?

Buddha had envisioned the third way. To observe and hypothesize life and the afterlife from at least three paths had manifested an Axial Age hallmark and a beginning to higher levels in abstract thought. And now Graywood's four-square grids might define an exquisite tool to carve out extended, truer insights.

Bearhead worked through the mental progression. Most individuals viewed life merely as competing opposites in a world divided between day and night, good and bad, pride and humility, kindness and wrath, revenge and forgiveness, and so forth. Too many just lived at the extremes swinging from one end to the other out of circumstance, cultural preference, or prejudice. With thinking minds limited by such crass dualities, their polarized responses to internal and external burdens bore no more than a few hairs above baseline fights or flights.

Wiser souls sought smaller oscillations between the polar endpoints, or better yet, a third way like the Buddha, but that required revelation. Yet Graywood's four-square plots seemed sublime. They stretched insight four ways, not like compass points, but as psychic and social grids of four potential belief outcomes, similar to medicine's four-square grid matching test results and conditions with true existence or not.

Bearhead leaped into a thought experiment: he placed scientific and religious parameters to Graywood's four-square grid to create a belief comparison. He labeled the grid's roof "religion" and its left-handed side "science." Atop the left column, he marked a positive sign, and the right column, a negative. On the science side, he etched a plus by the upper left square and a minus by the lower. Then he filled the four squares—the upper left garnered two plus signs, the upper right one minus and a plus, the lower left one plus and a minus, and the lower right two negatives.

Next he humanized the grid: the upper left square represented individuals who believed in both science and religion, perhaps equally; the upper right held those not religious but confident in science; and the lower left possessed souls favoring religion over science. And the lower right quarter captured all who distained both science and religion for making sense of their worlds. Bearhead wondered what they'd employ instead—chaos, underworld myths, absurd trials by Kafka, or pieces of Nietzsche out of context? And what entities and voids existed in the fourth space? Much to ponder ...

"Professor Bearhead, the break's over, unless you need more time," interrupted Caroline, the bright student who occupied the front table on the right.

Jolted back, Bearhead thanked her and bounded to the lectern with a fresh tool to expand doublets of dull polarities into interfacing "quadralities." He drew the subdivided religion-science grid on the whiteboard but spoke nothing of it. This reasoning aid had to percolate in his skull. In time, he coined the critical method, "the bringing or crossing together of two selected dualities."

Once Graywood had heard it, he relabeled it social Bearhead-ian, bivariate analysis.

CHAPTER FOUR

Past Influences

Bobby suffered a prolonged blackout six days after returning to school. Video electroencephalographic monitoring at Providence Medical detected seizure-like activity.

Graywood catapulted through both past and present to defeat the agony a parent shares for a child unfairly struck by fate. Determined yet fearful, he restarted the search toward comprehending what had altered his son.

A seizure is a symptom. It is an abnormal, synchronized, repetitive firing of large clusters of cells, called neurons, within the brain's structure. These agitated neural cells discharge all at once from chemical imbalances or assaults on their integrity by such conditions as brain tumor, bleeding stroke, infection, or drug overdose.

Graywood and Doctor Timm reviewed Bobby's presentation to elucidate the episode's trigger. The boy's physical exam revealed no stroke signs. Encephalitis and meningitis—inflammatory brain processes leaving behind irritated scars—were excluded because Bobby never had suffered those infections. The CT scan the prior week had ruled out brain tumors. But several prescribed medications, such as extended-release Ritalin, could ignite a seizure in somebody prone to the malady. It was stopped.

Since clinical history, tests, and scans had ruled out these disorders, Doctor Timm diagnosed Bobby with a form of epilepsy. She cautioned

Graywood how its presentation varied from phasing out for a few seconds to total loss of consciousness with or without convulsions lasting beyond a minute.

Anti-convulsant prescriptions reduced the tendency to display seizure activity but had no effect on the underlying disorder. They only dampened excitability in the affected neurons trying to discharge all at once.

One or two medications in the majority of patients limited most occurrences. Yet over time, a minority would worsen to make the ailment more difficult to treat with drugs. Such aggressive seizures could be surgically cured by cutting out the inciting locus of tissue.

Shattered, Graywood second-guessed every detail.

Seeking anything, he replayed his son's childhood over and over to lessen the smoldering guilt. He backtracked to the adventures on Kauai and concluded Bobby then in total health—rambunctious and grasping the world like a normal, six-and-a-half-year-old boy. Peering through photograph albums from then to now, Graywood yearned for recollections, answers, or causes to the submerged truth.

At length, he paused on a picture of Bobby and Jennelle in front of a brown van …

"When will the real scientific community wake up and tell the damn politicians mankind is not the cause of global warming."

Cashel Goodlette entered Jennelle's office gusting on a cell phone. "It's 2007 we're living in, not the medieval world full of damn alchemists. We're wasting time and money on rotten thinking like that."

Jennelle cocked her trance from the computer screen to the towering geologist framed at the doorway. Lugging a licorice-colored rucksack, his sharp facial features, restrained pelt of white hair, and mature charcoal eyes presented the harsh image not to be messed with.

"I'll call you when back from Kaktovik." He flipped the phone shut against his chest.

"Can I help you, Cash?"

"I need a lift to the airport. Rita's pulled to some silly meeting at Gould Hall, and Taylor has to man the front desk." He holstered the phone into his belt. "You're the only one around right now, so can you break away?"

"Sure." She returned to the monitor. "Give me two minutes to shut down."

"You're a sweet one." He hauled the rucksack square on his back. "I'll wait by the van."

CDC's Atlanta office had transferred data files of the 2006-2007 Nigerian polio outbreak for Jennelle to review. Lacking an urgency to wade through the eighteen attachments, she saved them to her African folders and burned a backup disc. Besides, Cash was a kick to be around.

She stretched at the window while the info transfer whirled away. The birch trees by the beginning of August still possessed their full complement of leaves. As she'd discovered last year, they'd denude in less than a week at month's end, despite ample periods of sun. Seasons changed fast in Alaska.

She titled the CD, grabbed her jacket, and bounced down the stairs.

Cash had ear-molded his cell phone. He weight-shifted foot to foot and yelled, "Carping about mankind's industrial-age carbon emissions causing this round of climate change is like saying we've created higher tides that strike our shores out of the wakes of supertankers and cruise ships. It's damn nonsense!"

Piqued, he interrupted the unfortunate responder again and fired back, "You flaming idiot. The moon's gravity, foul weather, and seaquakes make tides and tsunamis." He shook his head. "Listen you snake-lipped jackal, my grant proposal's got more kick-ass merit to find what's going on with climate change than Ross's carp on human carbon footprints stinking up the oceans. You tell him to look at carbon dioxide emitted by dung beetles and termites because, shit damn, their worldwide carbon feet are a helluva lot bigger than man's." He noticed Jennelle listening yet refused to dampen the bluster. "Well, he's a shitheaded moron pushing that farce as a research question!" Cash snapped closed the phone, dismissively pointed to it, and said to Jennelle, "And he's an asshole too if he recommends that witless Ross proposal over mine."

Amused, she smiled pencil thin and asked, "Shall we go, Cash?"

"Sure."

"I thought oceanography was your primary field, not climate change," she remarked.

"Oceanography forces you to be a climatologist. It's the oceans, not man, that determine climate and weather. They're the crucibles where climate gets brewed up mostly by heat escaping the earth's core. Been that way through geologic time and always will. We've got to understand all of that first."

"Sounds impressive, Cash. Is it Merrill Field or Lake Hood this time?"

"Lake Hood, but take Bragaw to Tudor Road. I've got to drop off a groundwater report." Cash patted a thick folder on his lap.

Jennelle marveled at the hundreds of aircraft buoyed on Lake Hood and its neighbor, Lake Spenard. They made the largest seaplane base in the world. Tucked between Anchorage International Airport and the town of Spenard, the aviation zone effused the dynamic synergy of man, machine, and nature.

She waited in the brown van as Cash deposited the geological review at the Department of Public Works' front office. He strolled back punching numbers for yet another call.

"Cash, when I get to Lake Hood, should I turn on Aircraft Drive or Float Plane Drive?"

For more than a year Cash Goodlette had contracted Piper Gunlock for flights into remote research locations on the Bering Sea or Alaskan North Slope. If takeoff and approach required flotations, they'd rendezvous at Piper's buoy on Float Plane Drive. All other landing gear configurations departed from Piper's leased hangar.

"Aircraft Drive," replied Cash, lodging the cellphone at his ear.

Veering left on C Street, Jennelle heard him spit out, "All this horsebunk about limiting manmade global warming by capping greenhouse gases is a clever tax on everyone's carbon footprint. It's the biggest worldwide con job ever done to get money and shift it all around with the UN skimming the top as they did with Saddam's oil-for-food program."

Curious, Jennelle leaned toward him to hear more. Traffic thickened on International Airport Road.

Cash stayed true to form and bellowed, "They'll find a way to tax water vapor 'cause the dumbheads'll figure out it's the worse greenhouse gas of 'em all ... damn near a hundred times more able to trap heat than CO2."

And so it went the rest of the way.

Still kibitzing on the phone when they arrived at the hangar, Cash pulled the rucksack out of the van's cavernous back end—his flapping, open mouth a not-so-small replica of it.

Jennelle spied Graywood propped on a ladder adjusting the engine on the smaller of Piper's two aircraft. She approached in steps springing off the tarmac.

For the prior year, she'd encountered him often at his PHS office or Providence Medical Center. Their last face to face had been three months ago at the Egan Convention Center where they'd co-chaired the final statewide meeting for the 2006-07 influenza season. She admired his professional leadership, work ethic, and pear-blond hair with distinctive pearl fringe. His private life, however, had remained hard to pin down. Lacking a wedding band on his finger, she assumed he had a girlfriend and wondered what the hook-up might be like.

Graywood descended taking in Jennelle's broad smile. Her hair fell loose to the shoulders, and small riots exploded in his heart. "It hurts to look at you," he whispered. Since Kauai, he'd felt time's warning of passing years. Today it vanished as she closed the small gap.

"Are you flying Cash to Kaktovik?" she asked, dashed with a challenging lilt.

"No, Piper is." Helpless, he splashed about in her brilliant, doe-brown eyes.

After an awkward moment, she teased an eyebrow raise and asked, "So what're you doing with that wrench?"

Rapture popped, he answered, "Oh, ahhh … Piper asked me to finish a couple engine repairs, check the struts and tundra tires." He stroked a deft hand down the starboard tread. "Freeze-up is four, maybe five weeks away where they're going."

"You work as a mechanic too?"

"Enough to pilot this one when Piper's not."

"He lets you fly his plane?"

"Truth be told, we're partners. We each own half."

"Well, I'm impressed, Gary. You're a bush pilot too."

"Not anywhere like Piper, but I've survived ten years of landings and walked away every time." Graywood winced—*Oh, good God, you said that in such a stupid way, you dumb stud.* He attempted a rescue. "I save a lot of time flying out to clinics, and I love to get into back country and camp with my boy."

Instinctively, Jennelle stepped back on her heels and reinterpreted the signs received since exiting the van. So far he'd been charming to the degree his non-verbal cues confirmed a budding chemistry. Yet he'd never mentioned a child in the twelve months since they'd met.

"Gary, what's your son's name?"

"Robert, but he's really Bobby." *Oh please keep asking questions about him, about anything, and I'll figure out a way to tell you I'm divorced, his mother lives in New York, and you're spot on beautiful!*

Cash joined the duo. "Jen, they need the wheels back pronto at Grace Hall."

"Thanks, Cash." She hesitated, yet asked Graywood, "How old is Bobby?"

"Seven next month."

"Does he have brothers or sisters?"

"No, just him … and me."

"Well that's a good start," she said in a hush and strolled to the vehicle. Before opening the door, she bent around, and shouted, "Gary, tell him I said hello."

She wants to meet my boy. Graywood watched her disappear beyond the hangar rows.

In 2006, Cash contracted Piper to ferry him and three USGS personnel on a North Slope survey to evaluate the environmental impacts of mining and shipping natural gas deposits from there into US and Canadian markets. Discovered decades earlier, these reserves were estimated at thirty-five trillion cubic feet. Other accessible natural gas fields in North America had become depleted, and demand for the fossil fuel had lifted prices to levels where funneling it south through a new pipeline made business sense.

But today's week-long mission was solely Cash's: he'd check probes suspended deep in the vacated Arctic drilling sites that measured earth crust temperatures. The data collected over time would support or refute his theory on how heat cycles liberated from the earth's intense core were foremost in simmering the oceans and affecting their primary currents.

By Cash's reasoning, ocean warming derived from solar radiation played only a bit part in the planet's climate, compared to the immediacy of the earth's hot center.

Graywood met Piper and Cash on their return from Kaktovik, the hard-frozen hamlet tenaciously strung to the Beaufort Sea 160 nautical miles west from the Canadian border. In addition to retrieving results from the sensors in the abandoned wells, Cash had downloaded an automated, six-month record of underwater temperatures and ocean current speeds in Camden Bay. He planned to return the following year to Baxter Island where the US Air Force and Alaskan Air National Guard maintained a small landing strip. There he'd measure the discharged heat and resultant changes to flow velocities in Beaufort Lagoon employing unmanned, torpedo-shaped Seagliders.

Once Piper taxied to the hangar, a flurry of activity ensued to ready the Beaver come morning to haul a metric ton of construction materials to Youngstown Bend on the Yentna River. Cash offloaded gear from *Sky Woman* as Graywood and Piper fitted floats on the cargo plane before towing her to moor at the lake.

Jennelle arrived in the brown van. She made a point to greet Graywood before shuttling Cash and his equipment to Elmendorf Air Base where he leased storage for a dollar a month through an inter-departmental agreement between USGS and DOD.

By twilight, Graywood and Piper had the Beaver primed for tomorrow's shipment. Cash drove up alone and yelled out the window, "How about a drink or two to cap off a damn fine week?" His efforts had sparkled more than that. Cash believed he'd uncovered answers that would change every wrinkle on the biased faces purporting climate change was caused by mankind.

"What happened to Jennelle?" asked Graywood.

"Dumped her off at Grace Hall."

Cash got the "why, you jerk" look from Graywood, so he added, "She had a huge project to wrap up for Atlanta, and helping me stow stuff put her way behind."

Jennelle had brewed in Graywood's brain all week. The slow-forming fondness for her sprinkled over him from head to heel in sharp contrast to the downpours of affection and failure endured with Maren. With Jennelle, he'd take the risk for compatibility but not succumb to worship. The pedestal on which he'd placed Maren had warped to wavering mirages over cracked earth. Perhaps all lovers had erred this way in the beginning—good lovers wouldn't do it twice.

Don't blow it this time.

"I know a waterin' hole on the other side of the lake," said Piper, pointing toward Spenard.

A mile from Piper's buoy dwelled the bar he patronized after a backcountry stint. It avoided the sleazy, happy-hour circus, and once the ban on smoking in public places had gone into effect under Bush 43, one smelled only hints of tobacco mixed to overcooked trans-fat margarine fanning out the side kitchen. Above the main floor hugged a peripheral ring of flat-screen and standard-box televisions. Like battle flags, beer and football pennants descended from the ceiling. Opposite the entrance with an overhanging "Seattle Mariners Ave." road sign stood a pendulum clock.

At each of his regular bars, Piper savored a preferred drink: martinis at the Glacier Brewhouse in downtown Anchorage, lagers brewed onsite in the Talkeetna Roadhouse, and here, bittersweet Cuervo margaritas.

"Hey there, darlin' Colleen," greeted Piper to the bartender. "How's business been?" The three men took stools at the empty bar.

Piper had first known Colleen when conveying cargoes for Wien Air Alaska, and they'd shacked up after he'd relocated to Anchorage to open the air taxi service. Within a year, both had sought other lovers.

"Pretty light right now, blizzard face," she replied, smoothing her blouse front. "Most my regulars still flyin' heavy schedules. It'll pick up after freeze-up. Usual for you, Piper lad?"

"Yep," he answered and winked twice.

"What'll your friends be having?" She glanced past Graywood to focus on Cash.

"A beer; what've you got?" asked Cash.

"Try the Moose Drool," recommended Piper.

"That sounds good," added Graywood.

"Make it so," ordered Cash. He scratched an ear and strained to hear a news bite on sea ice melting off Greenland and the connection to burning fossil fuels. "Do you hear that bullcrap? Damn global ass warmers!" Cash's head shook negative at the television's association between man's carbon footprint and rising global temperatures. He wiped earwax off a pinkie on the opposite shirt sleeve. In calmer tones, he said, "They've got the inference backwards." He pulled out a cream-colored hankie to clear his nose. "It's rising global temperatures that cause carbon dioxide levels to go up … the exact opposite sequence to what Al Gore and his cronies promote. Those idiots got it back-asswards when harping about carbon emissions pushing up temperatures."

Colleen deposited two drafts in front of Cash and Graywood and crushed ice for Piper's drink.

"Gary," whispered Piper, sideways under his breath, "Cash can be a windbag, but I gotta listen to him just the same 'cause he's a steady, damn-straight paycheck." He broadened both eyes and nodded to implore Graywood to tolerate whatever Cash might say.

Graywood wondered what Jennelle thought of Cash as well. If he asked her out, a date icebreaker could be what it's like around Cash and other eccentrics working at Grace Hall. Willing to pad knowledge on the oceanographer for future use with Jennelle, Graywood picked up his beer and said, "Getting causality backwards happens all the time in science," and swished the Moose Drool over his tongue like wine.

"That shouldn't happen at all with good science," Cash replied and jerked his head from the offending screen. "One of my old profs hammered home two bad habits you see all the time with pseudoscientists like these assholes who advance their own little agendas."

"What's that?" asked Piper, licking lips waiting for Colleen's Cuervo.

Like a knife, Cash pointed to the TV commentator. "Whatever they can measure, they'll first speculate on improving, but then they'll make the stupid mistake of believing what they've measured they've actually caused."

"What? That's a load of shit," exhorted Piper.

Cash gulped brew and then said, "I know it sounds absurd, but it makes them feel important when they've measured something that's changing. Then they subconsciously overreach and think humans caused it."

"That sounds like a wacky psycho thing to me," grunted Piper. The margarita arrived.

"It's the pseudoscientist equivalent to your jackass politicians believing they can single-handedly affect the world's overall economy. So Piper, for all I care, you can lump those lackeys in with the whole lot of stupid pseudoscientists."

"What do you mean?" asked Piper, coldly aware of the adverse situations elected officials create and distort to stay in power.

"Try following this," said Cash. "We've been measuring worldwide temperatures and gas concentrations in the air for nigh six generations, and we've observed both temperatures and carbon dioxide amounts going up. Because we've measured them changing together, and because we're burning more fossil fuels, which create carbon dioxide, we've naturally connected the two and concluded we must have caused it. We're the gorillas who burn oil and natural gas and coal and wood, so we've rationalized inferences out of all that to explain climate change from our world-dominant view. And remember we tend to lump together things in the wrong order to satisfy our little egos just as Al Gore does. Gore's silly simplification of climate change condensed down to only his hand-picked emissions is overreaching, alarming, and damn-ass backwards."

"You fellas gonna order something to eat?" asked Colleen. She handed out bar menus and nodded toward the kitchen. She'd overheard tons of men spew over beer—mostly on sports, women, or work—but nothing like Cash Goodlette's high and mighty gale-force wind.

"Not for me," said Graywood, checking his wristwatch for when he must fetch Bobby from the sitter.

"I'll pass too," added Piper. He had to file tomorrow's flight plan for the Beaver with air traffic control prior to the evening deadline.

"How about you, big guy?" she said at Cash, laugh lines on her face duking it out with crow's feet.

"I guess none for me," answered Cash, not wishing to be different.

"So what's increasing the heat for us then?" she asked, gathering menus. "Unless you think it's pointless."

Eyebrows raised ajar, Cash leaned back. Her directness tripped him up.

Entertained by her forthright insertion into their conversation and provocative attention to Cash, Piper greased an introduction. "This is

Colleen Durrey. She owns this dive. Colleen, this is Cashel Goodlette, the scientist I fly round the North Slope."

"Cashel? Then you're Irish," she said, leaning across the bar to verify his features.

"That I am," he said, with reclaimed composure. Likewise, he slanted to her.

"Colleen's Irish too, from Belfast," blurted Piper. "Came over here round sixty-nine to work the pipeline when it started up."

She shot Piper the evil eye for chaining her to a year so long ago and then turned to Cash and whispered, "Thereabouts."

"To escape the Troubles?" asked Cash.

"My father and brothers stood IRA. Brits weren't kind to 'em." Her head drooped implying they'd been harmed.

"I'm sorry, Colleen … Ah, so you worked the pipeline," said Cash.

"I surveyed north o' Big Delta. But enough on me. If you're not gonna eat, you want a refill?"

"Sure, since you're serving."

"Fine. So tell me what's raising the heat, you big lug?" She stepped to the tap, bent over to highlight a trim, hand-grabbing tush, and drafted another pint for Cashel.

Stimulated, Cash recollected and said, "Ah … let me say we need a better theory about climate change than Al Gore's … much larger than his puny, industrial-age, carbon footprint to explain all the temperature fluctuations known to have occurred over millions of years of geologic time."

"You're saying," echoed Graywood, "a good theory on climate change has got to reasonably explain all the ice ages and the warming-ups in-between, not just the last couple of hundred years."

"Makes sense," said Cash, eyes admiring Colleen's alluring backside. "We've got to understand the processes of natural climate change first. Right now, we've only got theories. It's like what you do in medicine, Gary. You've got to understand a disease before you change its course. I'll tell you this for sure, going after carbon dioxide as the cause of global warming is a damn fool's errand."

Colleen wiped overflowing foam off Cash's mug. "Darlin', here's your order." She curtsied from her side of the bar, yet eyes mocked when she grabbed his empty glass. "Still waitin' to hear, dearie, what's causin' the heat."

Her sultry tone opened Cash's eyes to the size of eggs. Corralling her intent, he rolled his tongue to help shift focus back on Piper and Graywood. "There are four gases that retain most of the heat in the atmosphere," declared Cash. "Can you name them?"

"Ahh yeah, carbon dioxide's one I've heard." Piper stopped to slurp Cuervo, ignorant of the remaining three.

To rescue his partner, Graywood answered, "And methane, ozone, and water vapor."

"Which one holds in the most heat?" asked Cash.

Piper swallowed margarita again, so Graywood answered, "Water vapor. We've all felt a thousand times when cloudy nights trap in more heat than clear ones."

"Damn right," roared Cash. "Molecule for molecule, water vapor retains ninety times more heat in the air than carbon dioxide. If we're really serious about man-caused global warming, we better take action to reduce our foggy imprints on the environment before wiping away dirty human carbon footprints. But hell, it's in fashion to be against carbon, not clouds." With a finger tinging his drink like a clock chiming the hour, Cash innocently asked Piper, "So how much water vapor have you made today?"

"Don't know. Does pissin' in the air off the buoy count?"

"If you gotta whiz every hour," poked Graywood.

All smirked, yet Cash hardened to say, "If the politicians bite whole-hog into this carbon-dioxide folly, we're all damn fools. The ice sheets vanished because of natural climate warming. Does Al Gore seriously believe he can blame the half-dozen or so interglacial periods with higher temperatures that separate the ice ages on the tiny marching carbon footprints of stone-age humans and Neanderthals?"

"So the world has warmed up between the ice ages, and none of it's from us," summarized Graywood.

Rolling her eyes, Colleen asked, "Where you going with this, Cashel? Where's all the heat coming from?"

"There're just two natural sources of show-time level heat that I know … the sun and the earth's core."

"Ahh yeah, spurtin' volcanoes can get pretty damn hot when flyin' over them," agreed Piper. He signaled Colleen for a Cuervo repeat.

"Got that right," confirmed Cash. "It's chaos down in the earth's core. Condensed iron in its own ocean of liquid iron, and it's almost as hot as the sun's surface. All that molten stuff seething and roiling like pan water on a hot stove … even in whirlpools when the roiling gets in synch with the earth's rotation. All that inner chaos causes changes we detect on the earth's surface in a couple of ways … shifts in the magnetic poles and my research theory that the mantle under the earth's surface cooks our oceans way more than the sun does through the atmosphere."

"But how's that explain the ice ages and climate warmings in-between?" asked Graywood.

"Well, I propose the heat generated in the earth's core and mantle thermodynamically dissipates through the oceans and continents into the atmosphere and then outer space. Between the stars are the great universal heat sinks where all heat fluxes to. The earth's core generates and dissipates baseline heat cycles each year and, on the grander scale, in every epoch of geologic time. Granted, added or subtracted to the earth's surface and atmosphere are the seasonal and decadal variations of heat received from the sun because of the earth's wobbly axis and slightly eccentric orbit. But overall, I theorize that solar contributions to earth surface temperatures are minor league when compared to the heat rising up through the oceans from the core."

"You said a cycle of heat is generated over time from the earth's core," rephrased Graywood. "Does that explain the melting after each ice age?"

"No. The amount of heat generated in the core generally stays about the same. It's the cycles of heat emitted from the mantle that vary to give us warming and cooling periods on the Earth's surface."

"That's a pretty fancy idea you've got there, Cashel," said Colleen, serving Piper's tequila. She moved away humming a melody.

"I know that tune," said Cash. "What's it called?"

Ambling back, she gently cooed, "'The Wind That Shook the Corn,' darlin'."

"Where'd you hear it?"

"Oh, back in Belfast. You might find it in an old Irish Rover's album."

"Ahhh, Colleen," softened Cash to brogue, "me granddah sang eeht," and whistled a few hushed notes.

"In Ireland?" she asked.

"No, Australia." Folding his large hands, Cash sang a verse in mellow tones: "There I tend to wander still, sometimes at early morn/And with breakin' heart, sometimes I hear/The wind that shook the corn."

Surprised and touched, Colleen and the men waited for more.

"Granddah cared o' me whene'er be family troubles." Ashamed, Cash drew away …

Piper broke the silence. "Shit, Cash, I farted out on that word, thermo-whatever."

"Ah … okay," gruffed Cash, draining the schooner's contents empty to snap away from the kidnapped childhood remembrance. "Right … ah," he belched and returned to thesis mode, "the earth's surface is a series of gigantic slabs forty to sixty miles thick, called tectonic plates, which hold the continents and the ocean basins. The continents act like blankets unevenly directing the earth's heat out of the mantle at different rates with more dissipating into the oceans, less through land. As the continents drift apart, it's like pulling a blanket slowly off to expose a different piece of underlying mantle, which then emits greater heat. The ocean floor's constantly being remade. The freshly exposed areas allow more heat to pass than before, and the deep ocean currents correspondently alter direction."

Piper seemed perplexed, so Cash reloaded, "Think of it as hot water flowing in the grid pipes beneath a sauna's tiled floor and a hotter surge comes through to further warm things up. It's like a world-sized geothermal energy transfer trillions of times larger than what the Icelanders mine to heat their houses."

"Cash, I still don't see the connection to climate change other than shifting ocean currents," said Graywood.

"Oh, it gets better, Gary," said Cash, his face flushing alcohol red. "I speculate every cycle of heat emitted out of the mantle to the surface comes in a series of oscillations triggered by continental drift. Six or seven million years ago, enough drift between the continents had occurred to kick into play the initial mantle-to-surface heat oscillation."

"Why then?" asked Graywood.

"Well, let me back up a wee bit. The western continents had drifted far enough from Africa and Europe six and a half million years ago to create the initial magma oscillation. That made the heat transfer from the core through the mantle into the oceans different from what had happened before. But that change, in turn, altered the routes of the deep ocean currents and led to major global cooling that lasted over a million years. Eventually the Earth's crust and atmosphere equalized enough so the currents returned to flowing where they'd done earlier. That created a warming period, which melted the glaciers and shrunk the ice caps. But the continents continued to drift apart more and more, and that set up the next oscillation. I've always marveled at how the ice ages became more and more frequent during the Pleistocene, so I've attributed the increase to more frequent oscillations.

"The bottom line is this, Gary. If you're going to speculate or theorize today about climate change, you better be able to explain all the ice ages and interglacial warming periods too, not only the one we're in now. Otherwise you'll look damn idiotic."

"Magma heat oscillations," pondered Graywood. "I suppose they'd explain El Niño in the Pacific."

"Yeah, but I suspect El Niño is a tiny eddy off the main oscillation underneath the Pacific," clarified Cash.

"You kinda lost me at the tectonic plate stuff," said Piper, shrugging shoulders. "Don't think I understood much of it. Got good ol' Cuervo to thank for that." He licked the goblet's salted rim clean.

"Well, Piper, want to hear something funny about Venus then?" said Cash.

"Venus the planet or Venus the woman?"

"Planet."

"Sure, but if it ain't funny, you gotta buy me another margarita."

Colleen suspected Piper lining a deal to nab Cashel or Graywood into losing a sure bet. Which one might be Piper's sucker to pay for all the rounds?

"Okay," said Cash, firing back. "It's eight hundred degrees on the surface of Venus, and the air's 94-percent carbon dioxide. So Piper, who's been burning all the fossil fuels there to make its gigantic carbon footprint?"

"Bet Gore would love," inserted Graywood, "to take on the Venusians with cap and trade."

They guffawed and clinked beverages.

"You win that one, Cash," Piper said and gave a toast, "To Al Gore and his new mission to stop global warming on Venus!"

"Don't think Al and his Nobel buddies can explain that one," said Graywood half-joking, half in disgust.

"Can you, Cash?" asked Colleen.

"Well, try this on," offered Cash. "There can't be any carbon-based life on Venus at eight hundred degrees. So where did all that carbon dioxide come from?"

"From chemical processes other than carbon-based life," answered Graywood.

"Yep, an inorganic reaction or, more likely, a whole slew of them," said Cash. "When heating limestone here on earth, carbon dioxide gases off. And that confirms what I said after we came in the door."

"What's that again?" asked Piper. He circled a finger counterclockwise on his goblet's rim.

"Something about Gore being ass-ward?" said Colleen.

"As temperatures go up," repeated Cash, "atmospheric carbon dioxide levels follow and go up because of the temperature increase, the exact opposite of Gore's dribble."

"So what about carbon dioxide on Venus?" asked Piper, rotating his finger faster.

"Don't know about that; never been there!" kidded Cash. "There's no life there as we know it, and I know nothing about the limestone. So, Piper, should I ever get some grant money, you got a way to get me to Venus?"

"You've had too much Moose Drool, Cash." Piper picked him to be the chump but gauged he needed time to perfect the bet's scheme.

"Probably so," said Cash, "but I'm still miffed by Al and his cronies getting a Nobel for spewing out lazy armchair speculations about climate change."

"Give him credit for connin' the Swedes out of their money," said Piper. His rear swaggered on the bar stool to avoid springing the bet too soon.

"You mean the Norwegians," corrected Cash.

"Whatever," observed Graywood. "Gore keeps the illusion of being well-informed when he's not. Does a pretty good job buffaloing Swedes, Norwegians, and everybody else."

"Shit, Gore follows bad carbon di-OX-ide scents like a coon dog barkin' up the wrong tree at midnight," crowed Piper.

"Well double shit to that!" Cash bellowed and slapped Piper on the back.

"Agreed!" shouted Graywood and Colleen.

"Mother Nature's mightier than anything man can cause or build," Cash said and gulped the last trail of beer.

"There's an intellectual dishonesty with Al," added Graywood, "like spite going on in his head."

"Horsebunk, only arrogant politics," sneered Piper. He spotted Colleen and touched his upper lip—the old signal for backup.

"It's power," said Cash, "pure and simple. We humans want to control everything."

"Say guys, let's talk 'bout somethin' else," shifted Piper.

"Dear God, time someone did," said Colleen, relieved. "All this global malarkey's gotten way out of hand."

"I apologize," said Cash, bowing to her.

With mugs and margarita tumblers emptied, Piper commenced a new conversation. "A thing's been really botherin' me for some time. Maybe you two can help out."

"Wouldn't be the only time someone's covered your back," said Graywood.

"For sure," said Piper, rolling his eyes. "Last month I flew three Florida hunters to Kodiak, and on the way they got to arguin' on the Civil War and where the last battle was fought. Say, Gary, you know where?"

Graywood had heard the pitch when Piper pulled it years ago as Graywood's flight instructor. Playing along, he lied, "I think Petersburg, but that's something I don't know much about."

"Well one of them hunters said that. But another insisted a place in Texas, and the third argued Appomattox. They carried on something awful the whole damn time. It got really confusin'."

"It was Appomattox, Virginia," said Cash, in cool, pontific tones.

"You sure?" asked Piper. "The guy backin' Texas later sided with the Petersburg fella makin' two against one."

"Lee abandoned Richmond when Grant outflanked him at Petersburg. Sheridan's cavalry caught up at Appomattox and stopped Lee's retreat.

They tried to fight through, but once Grant and the Union infantry arrived, Lee gave up."

"You really sure that's how it happened, the last battle of the Civil War?" asked Piper, innocently.

"As sure as there's no God," Cash said.

"You wanna bet on that?"

"God or Appomattox?"

"Shit, Cash, we ain't got time to lock horns 'bout God existin'. I gotta get tomorrow's flight plan over to the tower."

"What's the bet?"

"If Appomattox's the last battle, I'll pay our bar tab. If not, you will."

They shook hands, and Piper motioned Colleen. "We're haggling 'bout where the last Civil War battle got fought."

Her eyes gleamed. "I heard. How long since you've hit with that one?

"Month or two."

"And you, Cashel, poor lad," she soothed, "you picked Virginia." She winked Piper's way and patted Cash's hand. "I'm sorry, dearie, but Virginia's wrong. The last fracas involved a rebel ship named *Shenandoah* sinking Yankee whalers off Alaska's coast."

Irked, Cash probed for collaborating evidence. "Tell some more, Colleen."

"It sailed around the Horn and attacked over thirty whaling ships a couple of months after Lee surrendered. They kept goin' on till the Brits cruised by and showed the *Shenandoah* some newspapers saying the war's over."

A slight arch of Cash's brow conveyed disapproval of his being duped. He opened his wallet.

"Darlin', you only pay for theirs," Colleen demurred. "Yours are on me."

CHAPTER FIVE

Tomorrow's Passion

Graywood groaned at the imposing sign with its misspelled Reserch. The painter must have owned a brush that stroked with a drawl.

Jennelle's office at Alaska Pacific University matched one floor below Cash's space in Grace Hall, an opaque white building with windows framed lime-green.

The structure's front placard listed the occupants top to bottom: USGS Water Resources Office, NIOSH, CDC, Alaska Geographic Science Office, Alaska Field Station—Division of Safety Reserch. Other US Geological Survey personnel inhabited the bulk of Gould Hall across the street.

He'd come to see Jennelle, but the secretary reported she'd gone to Providence Medical Center to coordinate 2007-08 influenza tests.

"She's expected back anytime, Doctor Graywood. I could text her to see."

"No need. I'll check on some work upstairs. I'll be back."

With a landline phone planted to his ear, Cash twisted his six-foot-six frame over a large table blanketed by topographic maps, corners pinned under glaciology texts.

Graywood rapped the opened doorway.

Cash motioned him in, held up one finger, and inaudibly mouthed, "Moment." Cash's candid eyes danced around and down in a way that accentuated his notched chin. He'd finalized the storage, docking, and loading of equipment and provisions needed for the next Bering Sea expedition with Nome's harbormaster. He felt as comfortable in a room full of suits or books as on a ship slipping past jagged Arctic ice.

By the entrance hung Cash's geological engineering degree from the Montana School of Mines. A doctorate diploma in oceanography from the University of Washington dressed the wall over a teakwood desk.

Waiting, Graywood scanned the old tomes crammed in the oak bookrack: Larry Laudan's *Progress and Its Problems*, Paul Feyerabend's *Against Method*, David Bloor's *Knowledge and Social Imagery*, and *Structure of Scientific Theories*, edited by Frederick Suppe. All published in the 1970s.

"Find anything interesting?" asked Cash, setting down the phone.

"These are pretty dense volumes on philosophy of science," observed Graywood. "You had to know all this stuff for your PhD?"

"I'll tell you a little secret, Gary," Cash said, joining him at the bookcase. "I take a couple of them whenever I'm at sea to help me sleep." They chuckled.

Out of curiosity, Graywood asked, "So which two are your favorites to take?"

Cash puffed up and extracted Frank Ramsey's *Truth and Probability*. "This lays a good deal of the foundation for a rigorous interpretation of probabilities as degrees of one's personal beliefs."

He fingered Helen Longino's *Science as Social Knowledge*. "I believe this is THE major work about social structure and our concepts of objectivity."

He tapped David Hull's *Science as a Process* and beamed. "I'm keen on this one because it examines such matters as our social reward systems linked to the social structures in science."

Rubbing the worn copy, *Philosophy and Scientific Realism*, he said, "In here J. J. C. Smart infers there are no laws in biology." Cash glanced at the oceanography sheepskin and added, "Smart's work marks the resurgence of scientific realism as it challenges our scientific fundamentals and absolutes."

He shelved the Ramsey text, pointed to *The Structure of Scientific Revolutions*, and summarized, "This by Thomas Kuhn lays out insight on how science is not an entirely rational enterprise and how its well-established paradigms are negated in non-logical, revolutionary processes."

Then he caressed Karl Popper's *The Logic of Scientific Discovery* and said, "This beauty, Gary, is my real favorite."

"Wasn't he controversial?" asked Graywood, examining the leather-bound spine.

"Damn straight," magnified Cash, emoting as if he'd adopted Piper's expression as his own. "Popper insisted on defining a line between the scientific claims that merited intellectual respect from the pseudoscientific contentions that weren't so entitled." With reverence, Cash pressed index and middle fingers on the volume perched at the shelf's center. "Popper made quite a stir when he created sharp distinctions between Einstein's theories and those of Marx, Freud, and Adler."

"Well, Cash, now you've upped my curiosity. But let me check if Jennelle's back yet." While Graywood called on his cellphone, Cash jotted manifest changes to the expedition's printout.

"Routed to voice mail; must be busy," Graywood said and took a window seat. "So tell me more about your idol, Popper."

Cash swiveled with a broad smile. "We researchers need a bit of Popper to keep us open-minded. At least I do." He interlaced fingers atop his chest. "In Popper's day, the theories of Einstein, Freud, Adler, and Marx were all considered genuinely scientific. Yet Popper argued Einstein's theory of relativity was more intellectually distinguished than Marx's suppositions on economic history or Freud's and Adler's psychological formulations because of Einstein's openness to criticism. He believed Freud's and Adler's patient case studies and Karl Marx's distorted views were akin to astrology … mere examples of pseudoscience chock full of carefully selected observations, reinterpreted into terms that supported only their personal assumptions."

Cash stepped to the room's coat closet and pulled two tomato-juice cans from a hidden refrigerator. "Would you like some, Gary? It's all I've got at the moment."

"No thanks."

"The pseudoscientist seeks everywhere to find just the confirming evidence for his hunches." Cash popped open a tin and returned to the map table. "It's the closed mentality that assures you'll find what you're looking for. And any apparent counter-evidence is turned aside or morphed into confirming evidence by clever arguments or manipulations, especially if one's professional self-esteem or livelihood is in jeopardy." Cash swigged half the container. "So the charlatan scientist works to negate evidence that falsifies his claims and usurps everything that confirms them."

"That's pathetic," said Graywood, but with agreeing tones. "It sounds similar to worker comp claims that've run amuck, where everyone involved with bogus disabilities consents to go along because loads of money exchanges hands making them all winners. They'll resist true attempts to disprove the claims and accept they're just a cost of doing business."

"I concur, Gary. The wagging tongues of pseudoscientists play the same old game of fitting the data as well as they can, especially data they've selected only for their biased presumptions. There was way too much of that sophistry back in Popper's day and is still too much going on now." Cash sipped his beverage. "So what's the mark of a good scientific theory, eh?"

Graywood sat clueless to where Cash was heading but punted with, "I'm sure Popper had something to say about good science."

"Damn straight," said Cash. "To Popper, a good theory should be surprising, even improbable, as well as informative. So in contrast to Freud and Marx, Einstein's theory on general relativity became an outstanding example of unbiased science because it survived a surprisingly severe test."

"What was that?"

"Einstein had predicted how much starlight would bend by the sun's gravitational field. So in 1919, prior to a solar eclipse, the physicist Arthur Eddington organized a worldwide expedition to falsify or prove Einstein's calculation. Eddington's teams verified light bending from the sun's gravitational pull and by the amount Einstein had forecasted."

"So Popper felt great about that one."

"Oh, you bet! Popper, like Eddington and the other observers, acknowledged the fit between Einstein's predictions and the fresh evidence, but what mattered even more was the theory had survived a stringent test. To Popper, the mark of a genuine scientific theory is falsifiability. Genuine science makes bold conjectures and then tries to falsify them. Pseudoscience, on the other hand, collects only the data it wants to support its molded suppositions needed for gaining the next giant research grant from the government. It discards or denigrates any contrary ideas or data."

"Or sells the next version of snake oil to the public," added Graywood. He refrained from giving examples of new drugs that lacked effectiveness yet still came into pharmacies as medical pseudoscience.

"That's right, Gary, pseudoscience is motivated by advertising and selling, even going so far as promoting fraud," huffed Cash. "Genuine science is motivated by truth and bases its conclusions and theories on well-established patterns, like glacial cycles spanning thousands of years or the constant speed of light, not the occasional anomaly. It looks past the noise in the records and finds the true signal."

Graywood's phone hummed in his pants. "Hi, Jen."

Cash returned to the shipping manifest.

"I'm upstairs. I'll be right down." Graywood stepped to the doorway and asked, "Where're you exploring this time?"

"Bering Sea—deep-water sampling, fisheries assessments, and whale counts."

"Not going to boldly verify your hypothesis on how climate change is all about continental drift and oscillating magma heat instead of human carbon feet?"

"Can't. Grant money for that hasn't come in," returned Cash, disappointed. "Einstein was lucky to see his theories meet Popper's test. My Popper test won't happen until the coming ice age."

Graywood realized Cash's theory on climate change—like Wegener's hypothesis for a primordial continent breaking apart or Darwin's proposals on natural selection—made too great a leap for his peers and the public. Out of the tendency to follow short-term trends, most of Cash's colleagues had been trained to believe mankind was the main cause for global warming. They'd simply assumed current directions inanely marched one way in perpetuity.

"At least, Cash, you're counting whales and not harpooning, like the Japanese."

"Yeah, what a drum of dung that is." Cash unfolded a timetable. "We know plenty on humpback and pilot whale reproduction and feeding patterns. By hiding behind science, they're tricking the world to cover up their commercial whaling. It's that bloody plain. Sometimes I think there's still that Pearl Harbor deceit flowing in them."

"There's deceit all over the world," mumbled Graywood and then voiced, "I hope Greenpeace intercepts those whalers midway and sticks it to them before they get to the whales."

"Thanks, Gary. I hope so too."

"Have a safe trip."

No longer determined to remain distant and safe, Graywood descended the staircase to Jennelle's office with muscle-knotted resolve. He wanted her. He'd go after her and succeed or fail.

He toughened his inner core to exude calmness, whether she accepted the invitation or not, although all within might freakishly contract and sever the ability to speak. Three strides short of her domain, he repeated tantric breathing exercises Bearhead taught to energize mind and body. Fortified, he rapped the opened portal.

"Well … hi, Gary," greeted Jennelle, tapping her Mac's keyboard. A faint smile unfolded as she faced him. He looked disengaged and consumed, like a teenaged brother.

"Jen," he projected in professional voice, neutral as possible, "I've read your summary for this year's flu monitoring and reporting procedures. It's good."

"Thanks." *That's nice to say. His office is five miles away, and he drove here for that? He could've called. Must be something else.* She stood and studied him for clues.

His throat getting drier by the second, Graywood cleared it and said, "Do you think this year there'll be any problems with surveillance reporting from the smaller hospitals?"

"You mean the outlying ones?" Jennelle clarified.

"Eh … ah, yeah, the outlying ones."

"I hope not," she reassured. *Well, well, Gary! The tips are coming in. You know your office has first crack to follow up tardy reporting. Second, you're rolling your lower lip to your mouth. Haven't seen that before. You're nervous. Why are you really here?*

Graywood rubbed the back of his neck to loosen tenseness and then said, "So, ah … what's it like in the same building with Cash?"

Jennelle tilted her head and surveyed his motives: *He's gone out of his way and now changed the subject to a co-worker?* "Well, Gary, Cash is a hoot to have around whenever he's here." *He's come to see me!* She sparkled.

"Oh, Jen, I bet he is," Graywood spoke too fast within a faked laugh. He swallowed to wet a parched Adam's apple and wished he'd drunk some of Cash's juice.

She stepped around an ordered desk and toyed between dishing banter and nudging him on the quest to her. Eyes flowering encouragement, she drew right to him.

He stood as granite.

Frustrated, she formed a half-truth. "Ah, last week at the hangar, I wanted to ask how old your son was, Gary, and I'm sorry, but I've confused his name." She staged the timid look-away-and-down. "It's either Robbie or Bobby, isn't it?

Graywood's diaphragm rebooted. Saliva flowed again. "It's Bobby, and … ah, actually it's Robert, but he goes by Bobby, well … I mean, I call him Bobby, you know."

Touching his arm she brightened before his eyes. "Oh, yes, thank you, Gary. I'm really fond of that name. I'd like to hear more about him." She brought her soft hand back. "You're divorced, you pilot an airplane, and are raising Bobby on your own, aren't you?"

"Uhmm, that'd be me," he confirmed with relief.

"Seems terribly hard."

"Yeah, flying can be difficult." *Oh, good God, Gary! You've just cracked the most stupid joke on earth!*

Bemused, Jennelle grinned at the verbal awkwardness.

He switched into serious. "I've been divorced six years."

"I thought so."

"Ah, how'd you know?"

"You don't wear a ring, and you love to talk about your boy," she said matter-of-factly, hoping it enough. He didn't need to know she'd web-checked his marital status days ago and reconfirmed it with Cash in the van yesterday.

Jennelle's cell phone buzzed. "Excuse me, Gary." Reading the texted message, she angled to the work station to forward several files. "Stay right there, please. This should only take a minute."

Thanking fate for the opportune derailment, Graywood exhaled deep and long a half-dozen times to strengthen composure. He gazed out the second story window at birch and dogwood still clothed in full summer leaf and recalled parts of Jennelle's family tree revealed a year ago when they'd ordered mochas and tea adjacent to the Consortium Library.

Jennelle's father taught archeology at the University of California and specialized in Aegean antiquities. Her mother was a Christian Lebanese and the youngest daughter in a wealthy family involved in the Middle Eastern import-export businesses with its hub in Beirut. An illuminate Beiruti, she had broken from the traditional female role preparing for marriage and family to become a cabaret singer. She performed a circuit of gigs, migrating between Istanbul, Ankara, Amman, and Nicosia, but never sang in her home city; the Lebanese civil war had torn it apart.

Jennelle's parents met after her father had excavated a major Cypress site. To celebrate shipping thirteen crated artifacts to museums, he took in her Nicosia nightclub show. For the succeeding fortnight, he seized the center front-row table every evening to watch her act. Smitten, they married. The first of five children, Jennelle was followed by four brothers, the youngest whom she most adored.

Data folders sent, Jennelle rejoined Graywood at the window. In the most engaging tone, she asked, "We were talking, Gary. It's not done, is it?"

He dared hope never. "Jen, would you like to go this Sunday to downtown's street festival with Bobby and me? The air force band from Elmendorf is playing a concert."

"I'd love to."

"Fantastic!"

Heart on trampoline springs, he jounced to the door but paused abruptly when something mental clicked on. "Jen, you asked me a week ago how old Bobby was. I said then he's almost seven."

"I know, Gary."

Graywood had arranged to meet Jennelle in front of the Egan Center prior to the concert. She was not at the entrance when he and Bobby arrived, but they sighted her opposite the building, seated at an outside Starbuck's table sipping tea among a group of hybrid animal-human statues.

"That's Jennelle," said Graywood, directing Bobby's head with his hands.

She recognized Graywood and rose.

"Look, Dad, she's with Bessie!" screamed Bobby, and he sprinted her way.

"Ooo … Are you Bobby Graywood?" she asked after he collided into her.

"Yes, I am." Brash arms hugged her waist.

Bobby reminded Jennelle of her baby brother—charming, precocious, and daring. Jennelle had rescued Kent from drowning off Ventura Beach when he'd turned eight years old. "My, you're strong," she gasped when Bobby's arms cinched tight. "I'm Jennelle. I work sometimes with your dad."

"I know. He told me."

She wondered what else Graywood had mentioned but tacked another direction once Bobby let go.

"What did you call it?" she asked, flipping a finger toward the grotesque.

"Bessie the Moose," Bobby replied. He jumped to high-five the creature's metal nose. It had human legs tucked in painted black trousers but resembled moose from the waist up.

"So how do you know it's a girl moose?" she kidded.

"No antlers."

"No antlers?"

"Yeah, girls don't got antlers."

"Oh, I should've known."

"Everybody knows that."

"I see," she responded with wiser shading.

"So you've met the Bobby express train," Graywood said, arriving at the statue.

"Yes, Gary, we're already very good friends." Jennelle wore a simple, loose-fitting shirtdress. Bare legs and free-flowing bohemian hair parted in the middle gave hint to a svelte, carefree side. Appealing dark eyes and lively brows invited Graywood even more, the opposite to Maren's glittering, hard stare, coifed by manes wired in gold.

Without arms linked or holding hands, they strolled, connected in the way of people meant to be together.

The temperature on the twelfth of August hovered at an ideal seventy-three degrees—a rare summer treat for Anchorage. Vendors' carts, portable stalls, and intricate personalities bubbled out festive street noises to fill the town's center like a crowded stage. Jennelle bought Bobby a purple, helium-filled balloon from a clown after they'd watched two jugglers toss knives and batons.

"I've never liked tiaras. Saw too many gaudy ones in Georgia," she mentioned as they passed an artisan's sidewalk spread of costume jewelry and polished stones. For her, they appeared sorry attempts to upgrade status.

"You hardly ever wear jewelry," observed Graywood.

"So you notice things like that."

"Well, yes."

"I wear some if I want to feel fluffy-like but didn't today." In deadpan, she added, "I do kinda enjoy some trashy stuff. Sometimes I'm a step up from the trailer park. So, Gary, what do you prefer?"

"You know already … flying, going back country. I cheer Bobby playing ice hockey in winter and read quite a bit."

"Like what?"

"History mostly."

"Which period?"

"Probably all of them, but I'm really fond of biographies."

"Who's your favorite?" she asked.

"Anything on Albert Schweitzer or Abraham Lincoln."

"So, what don't you like?"

"Well, it kicks my guts to see hunters with assault rifles, and I absolutely hate when they shoot down animals from aircraft. And you?"

"I'd hate those too, Gary. I don't care much for rap music and hard liquor or card games, except poker and blackjack."

"Say, Jen, I'm curious …"

"What?"

"Ah … how many pairs of shoes do you have?"

She gasped at the unexpected probe, trimmed with verve. "Well, I don't really count them but guess, oh, maybe thirty. For sure, there're three good pairs of back-country dirt-stompers."

Graywood smiled inwardly *A practical woman. Low maintenance and not anything like Maren and her four hundred pairs of whatever.*

He wished to ask whether she thought jazz vocalists who trilled out scat were singing in tongues, but Bobby eyed a vendor selling reindeer hotdogs and begged for one.

"Only a dab of mustard," cautioned Graywood. "Too much upsets his stomach," he explained to Jennelle.

Bobby wolfed the carnal delight held in his right hand and grasped the balloon's string with the left. With his two fists occupied, the trio sauntered past a pair of Fourth Street art houses featuring homegrown artists. The second gallery's window displayed a painting trove by Piper Gunlock. They paused long enough for the proprietor to step out and encourage a sale.

"I see you're interested in the Gunlocks," he observed. "I've got more in the back."

"They sell for much?" asked Graywood.

Too early to broach prices, the owner soothed a skillful pitch. "He's becoming one of our big sellers. Each week I get three or four customers asking for him."

"Really?" Impressed his partner had developed such a following, Graywood swayed between fascination and disbelief.

"Yes," said the owner. "Gunlock is one of our locals with quite an art history."

After Sheila, Piper's creativity transmuted from colored landscapes into thickened gradations of blackened hues. He'd apply thin ink layers to form the picture's core and spread a saturated cover to evoke a misty sense of moisture in the air. His renaissance from the dark period happened on the advent of Cash's distant relative, Mary Anne Tarf.

Cash and Mary were third cousins once removed. Out of economic necessity, most of Cash's Irish Protestant family emigrated to Canada while Mary's lineage, the Catholics, were forcibly replanted by English overlords to Australia. Tarf was short for Clontarf, the Irish victory over the Vikings near Dublin in 1014. Mary's namesake pedigree had advocated Irish independence from Great Britain one too many times.

Cash reestablished contact with Mary's side when preparing an Antarctic expedition with Australian oceanographers. The Tarfs operated several sheep stations and gained wealth from diversifying into international shipping after World War II.

Mary's proclivity for globetrotting brought her to Anchorage to visit Cash in 2006. A summer courtship ensued between her and the pilot-artist while they assisted Cash on treks into the tundra to monitor data collection sensors. She shared perceptions gathered after three decades of viewing the world's masterpieces and expressed methods on painting to make a profit.

Overwhelmed, Piper pulled her to him out of admiration … and other desires.

Erupting from the gloomy shades induced by Sheila, Piper captured the ever-changing tones launched beneath his newfound shining sun. Mary encouraged glowing gradations of trees and rocks and skylines and to seize the effect of light rather than the things. Piper's vivacious brushwork, blurred and loose, contrasted tints and shadows with slab-like, horizontal strokes, evenly applied to suggest calmer water and air given up by the spectrum's bountiful effects. In her most beloved painting, Piper revealed a row of receding trees swimming within filtered splashes of blue and white.

Mary's influence pushed beyond modern Alaskan impressionism and inspired Piper's expressive talents to spawn portraits of birds. His technique broadened from acrylic on canvas to acrylic on hardboard and oil on linen, and he employed complex layered caresses to capture novel forms out of his dyslexic eyes. The results produced colors both gorgeous and raw. Up close, each fowl had humanlike presence and personality that mixed comedy, symbolism, and bits of coarseness, which approximated their creator's mood. Through flocks becoming caricatures of people, Piper had captured an Everyman quality. And they sold very well.

"Is that one Piper's?" asked Jennelle. An avian outburst of two species—a murder of crows mixed to a siege of herons—interacted on gritty ground like a bunch of earthy guys. One rook winked to tilt the viewer toward the depicted comedy.

"Yes, one of my favorites," said the gallery's owner. "If you examine the blackbirds, there's one that's the artist's self-portrait."

Graywood spotted Piper in a heartbeat. "It's the jackdaw second from the right looking straight at you with its left eye shut." Piper closed that one to maximize concentration and limit inverting sightlines whenever landing the Beaver.

"Who's the heron with a woman's face next to him?" asked Jennelle.

"That's Mary Tarf," said Graywood.

"She's his wife?"

"Not yet; they're engaged. Been quite a while. She's Australian and wants to be sure Piper's interest lasts before relocating here for good."

"She's smart," concluded Jennelle.

"I've got more Gunlocks inside," coaxed the owner.

"Thanks, but we're heading for the concert," disclosed Graywood, "and want a good spot."

For the season's Sunday in the Park program, the US Air Force Band of the Pacific gave a free performance at Town Square Park. Halfway there, Bobby let go of the balloon by accident. Jennelle grasped his empty hand and promised to buy another if they found the clown.

Spilling out with the crowd to parked cars after the show, they meandered past Kobuk's Espresso & Bakery.

"This is one of my favorite places," declared Graywood. "Has great pastries in back. You ready for a treat, Bobby?"

"You betcha, Dad."

Kobuk's served daily a complimentary tea sample. Today's customers tasted Sri Lankan Mist. Jennelle scanned the aisles and sipped the sharp, green brew heavy in tannins while Bobby chewed brownies with Graywood at the espresso bar. She discovered the sitting room with dancing, yellow-rose flames in the porcelain fireplace and two cozy couches ready to suck patrons into rich comfort. When Graywood and Bobby entered, the mantel's fire-glow effervesced her natural beauty.

"We'll have to come back and browse the place for ourselves," Graywood whispered.

"I'd love that," she said in a hushed voice.

And Bobby's keen ears heard all.

Father and son escorted Jennelle to her Hyundai Santa Fe. Their date closed with embraces all around.

On the drive home, Bobby beamed.

"What are you so happy about?" Graywood asked.

"Is Jen your girlfriend?" Bobby pressed forward against the safety harness and insisted, "You like her, don't you, Dad?"

Buying time to assess the unanticipated query, Graywood punted, "That depends if you like her."

"Oh, I likes her lots and lots!"

"As much as Brandy Belle?" Graywood asked, hoping to derail into something else.

"I love Brandy Belle!" Bobby sat back. Wide-eyed openness inched into contemplation.

Mission accomplished. Graywood steered onto Seward Highway and planned the standard mac and cheese and peas for supper, sprinkled with some fresh, chopped chives.

Exiting onto O'Malley Road, they passed the pungent animal park whiffed up by the Zoo-Doo fertilizer machine filling emerald-blazoned compost buckets—confirmation another generation of growth would come. Bobby's nose didn't crinkle at the smell. Instead of rocking back and forth and rolling out constant observations and questions, he appeared more and more confused.

Near home it happened. "Dad, you love Jen?"

Graywood's mind lit like ignited flares in the night sky. How to answer the almost seven-year-old? Even more, what would he risk for all-out love again? Maren had shot too many arrows and abandoned Graywood as well as Bobby. Yet Jen was Jen, and he wanted to be with her.

"Yeah, I like her a lot."

"I really like the balloon she got me," trumped Bobby.

Anxious to greet Brandy Belle, the boy finger-drummed the seat and hummed his made-up Rum-Tum tune.

Relieved he'd dodged THE question, father led son from garage to kitchen.

While grating extra cheese on macaroni, Graywood resolved, carpe diem-like, to invite Jennelle home for dinner.

Jennelle hefted a sand-colored cloth satchel when he answered the front door. The evening light toasted her hair chestnut brown. Three-and-a-half-inch heels, the first he'd seen on her, matched her styled flip.

"Any trouble getting here?" greeted Graywood.

"What a lovely home," Jennelle gushed. "Your directions were perfect."

"You didn't have to bring anything."

"I wanted you and Bobby to have a little something. It goes in the kitchen."

Intrigued, Graywood led her down the hall to the hub of the house. The aroma of pesto sauce wafted off a mixing bowl on the counter, and Jennelle audibly inhaled the scent, reassured he knew how to cook.

"It's one of my favorites," Graywood said. He left out the protracted negotiations he'd endured with his son on what to prepare.

Bobby sensed the occasion being a big event. His dad had hosted holiday house parties for the staff from work, and he'd prepared a meal once for Piper and his third wife and often for Bearhead and the Coldsnow sisters, but never had he asked one person, a single woman, to sit at the fancy dining room table. Bobby wanted to make sure his dad got it right and championed the ideal dinner of spaghetti, foregoing the funny word his dad used for tomato sauce. And spaghetti should be washed down with cold lemonade and plenty of chocolate cake and ice cream.

Graywood argued for baked salmon coated in pesto, framed by asparagus spears sautéed in lemon juice. Since Bobby's ADHD diagnosis, Graywood had increased the amount of fish in their diet after reading credible evidence its oils increased concentration abilities.

But that didn't seem right to Bobby. For Jennelle's visit, he adamantly knew better—Jennelle would want spaghetti, not salmon.

To attain culinary harmony, Graywood prepared both and suggested Jennelle could choose how much from each she'd like. He deferred creating crème brûlée, agreeing to Bobby's dessert proclamation. There had to be chocolate offered sometime to her, so why not let her eat cake?

"Salmon and spaghetti, Gary?" wondered Jennelle out loud. "I've never had that combination."

"You get to choose from two homemade sauces for your pasta," boasted Graywood, "Bolognese or pesto."

"Which one does Bobby like?"

"Bolognese, but he calls it red stuff."

"I take that only pesto, not the red sauce, goes on the salmon?"

"For sure," Graywood said with a wide grin. Her clear eyes expressed she understood the household dynamics, however comical, of two males—father and son—living together alone.

"When I lived at home, my four younger brothers loved pastas my mom prepared from scratch. As teenagers, they couldn't get enough." Jennelle inhaled each one's competing bouquet. "I'd like a small portion of each when we sit down."

"She compromises like a diplomat," thought Graywood and then said, "Jen, what's in the bag?"

"Have you ever made homemade sourdough bread?"

"No."

"I brought you some starter in case you ever want to. Whole wheat flour and pineapple juice too." She prominently lifted a Mason jar with contents the color and consistency of thick yogurt.

"What's the juice for?"

"It tarts up the starter with a little zing," she replied. Graywood's frown needed more wooing to the wonders of sourdough. "Gary, do you cook pancakes for Bobby?"

"Yeah, he really goes for them."

"How do you make them?"

"I blend flour, eggs, milk, sugar, and butter with some baking powder."

Delighted he created from scratch rather than out of a package, she recommended, "You must try whole wheat sourdough pancakes using my starter. I know Bobby and you'll relish the tangy fullness they'll have."

Her voice effused magical as she rotated the jar of paste. "Anyone who savors cooking has to have a bit of this in the fridge because everything tastes better spread on sourdough."

She listed the sourdough boules and the baguettes concocted in college at San Francisco to energize crewmates before they rowed the Russian River. Keeping the mysterious culture of wild yeast and lactobacilli required scant effort and could become a cool science project for Bobby.

Graywood acquiesced. Jennelle explained how to feed the starter to ripen it the night before its use. "Do you add vanilla extract to your pancake batter?" she asked, checking the boiling pasta and simmering Bolognese in neighboring pots.

"No, never have." He marveled at how comfortable she felt in his kitchen. Maren never would have done this.

"Try half a teaspoon. And I've got another trick."

"Please tell." Graywood opened the oven and stroked olive-green pesto over the sockeye as she stirred bubbling pots.

"Drop in a dribble or two of maple syrup."

Awed, Graywood connected her to another plane—with Bearhead whenever he recommended chef hints. They'd talk food all night. But hungry Bobby would soon beeline for the kitchen.

"I'll have to get your recipe," Graywood said. "Where should I store the starter?"

"I'm so glad you've stepped up to the world of sourdough." She placed the jar by the refrigerator and pulled out two three-by-five cards. "This is for bread, and this one's my pancakes."

Graywood read the latter—preparation and ingredients in longhand. Nutritional facts printed at the bottom: 1 pancake, 104 calories; 3 grams protein; 17 grams carbohydrates; 1 gram fiber; 3 grams fat; 1 gram saturated fat; 36 milligrams cholesterol; 249 milligrams sodium. He wondered what she'd fashion if teamed up with Bearhead—they might catalogue the entire cuisine universe.

"Fabulous. I'll try it out tomorrow."

Satisfied by Graywood's conversion, she asked, "May I help with anything?"

"Open the fridge. There's spinach salad in a green bowl. Please divide it on salad plates." Thankfully, he'd cleaned off weeks of chilled scuzz-crud the day before.

Lining up dinner plates for salmon, pasta, and asparagus, he considered giving Jennelle a house tour to acclimate her with the messes ensconced behind all the doors. Conceiving a better idea, he exited to the bannister and yelled, "Bobby, Jen's here, and I need your help right now!" He returned and found her manning the stove, three neat salads dished.

In slow pirouette, she smiled at him admiring her. Softly she cooed, "This all smells super. I can't wait to taste." She looked adoring and beautiful.

Graywood's heart cinched up. He wanted to kiss but couldn't close the short space to her lips.

Be careful, Gary, don't press too fast … Revel in her by the stove praising your cooking.

The tableau shattered when Bobby blew past straight into Jennelle.

"Ah," she gulped, "hello there."

Bobby bear hugged Jennelle's waist. "I've waited all day for you," he declared and then let go.

"I think he misses you," Graywood said, yearning feelings onto his son's catch and release.

"I missed you too, young man," she said with the broadest smile.

"Bobby, help me out and show Jen around the house while I finish up here."

"You betcha, Dad." He grabbed her hand and triumphantly led away.

"Start in the living room with the view downtown," guided Graywood. He checked the salmon … three minutes to perfection.

If she's anyway serious about us, she's got to see how we live.

He brushed pesto the final time. *Hide nothing, no surprises. Bobby will make sure of that.*

"No, thank you," declined Jennelle to a second piece of cake. "I love chocolate, but too full for more." She stretched by the dining room window. A noble blue spruce dominated the backyard's center. "Gary, you're a fantastic chef."

"Thank you."

She swayed from the glass and sighed, "Once we clear the table, may I take another tour of your beautiful home?"

"Bobby didn't show you everything?" half-kidded Graywood. He knew that effort came fraught with distractions.

"He was fabulous. I saw the living room and Brandy Belle and his upstairs bedroom."

"Anything else?"

"Oh, Bobby's very proud of Brandy. She's loving and attentive, but I'd like to see more."

"Well then, we'll start over. I'll clear the table later."

Compelled to peek further into this man's background, Jennelle mustered willpower not to appear obvious. For kitchen skills, Graywood had passed with highest honors. Now she wished to uncover the character of his home office, bathroom, and bedroom … accomplish the first two tonight, the third at another time of choosing.

Graywood guided to the den. Western twilight off the deck tinted the room. A roll-top desk was buttressed between the computer work station and a metal bookcase crammed with medical texts. Attached right-angled to the shelves was a walnut cabinet holding eight photograph scrapbooks—five filling the bottom ledge with three more on the leaf above leaving two empty upper shelves. Each album's spine, except one, had a year stenciled from 2001 to 2007. Side by side atop the desk hung two enlarged photos.

"You take scads of pictures, Gary," said Jennelle, stroking a hand over the walnut's smooth grain.

"They're all of Bobby," said Graywood, "and I plan a lot more." He left out that the eighth binder, lacking a year mark, contained snapshots of Maren.

Jennelle slanted around to the blown-up print of two red-faced boys, bundled in parkas aside a dog sled over tracked snow. "The smaller one is Bobby, right?"

"Yep," confirmed Graywood. "The other's his best friend, Cub. Taken six months ago at the end of a five-mile run. Bobby's the substitute cargo, and Cub's the musher."

"His name's Cub?" asked Jennelle, pointing to the taller child.

"Yeah. He's Piper's boy," explained Graywood. "He's putting a team together to race."

"Pretty ambitious," said Jennelle.

"He wants to take on the Iditarod when he's eighteen."

"He looks thirteen."

"Eleven," said Graywood. "Already a go-getter and absolutely as absorbed with dogs as Piper is with planes. Puts his mind to task and sees it through. Shows all the first-class signs for doing that race."

Jennelle sensed in Graywood's voice hints of admiration and envy for Piper and his son.

Clearing his throat, Graywood said, "Cub's kinda like Bobby's big brother. Just a really great kid. I hope some of him rubs off."

"I'm sure he will," echoed Jennelle, remembering her four brothers growing up.

The companion picture depicted a toned, younger Graywood leaning against an aircraft propeller.

"That's you in front of your plane," said Jennelle.

"Yep. Her name's *Seneca-Sky Woman*."

"Really?"

"You betcha. Piper and I kinda fight over her. He calls her *Sky Woman*; I call her *Seneca*."

"Why those?"

"Old Indian legend … Sky Woman is a Seneca Indian maiden who helped unite the sky and ground together."

Jennelle peered at the photo's staging and remarked, "I suppose she could do that with a decent pilot," and stepped back bright-eyed. "She's a fine looking machine, Gary, and you look very proud and handsome."

Graywood swallowed resolute at the opening she'd just broadcasted. "Would you like to go up with me?"

"Well, that depends," she teased through pretend pouted lips.

"On what?"

"On how good the pilot is."

"Jen, a good pilot's someone who's got the same number of landings as takeoffs and can talk about 'em all." He extended opened arms and palms up confident. "I've done that."

Her eyes and mouth flirted back. "That gets you to first base."

"I've flown ten years in all kinds of weather."

"Could you say that another ten years from now, Gary?"

"For sure."

"Perhaps you're halfway to second."

"How do I get round to home?"

"Tell how you became a certified pilot."

Graywood started with the gamut of emotions experienced each time he went aloft: the sudden rush that hits when disconnected from the ground, the excitement of defying gravity, the intense challenge of blending into whatever nature throws in *Seneca*'s path, and the satisfaction at journey's end.

Tying to Jennelle's penchant for details, he described the mastery of basics on a Cessna 152 and flight instrument training in a 185. He recounted the mechanics of steep turns, control stalls, and airspeed descents at both cruising and minimum control velocities. He explained cross-country aviator skills, course plotting, tower approaches, radar communications, ground reference maneuver routines, and the correct use of navigational equipment and terrain guides.

"If GPS fails, we revert to triangulation to determine position."

"How hard's that?" she asked.

"With time, it's second nature, like thinking in three vectors all at once."

Mentally, Jennelle detoured to the nickname the WWAMI students used behind his back—Doctor Triangle. His lectures often outlined triads: epidemiology—diseases spread by agents, hosts, and environments; health-care delivery systems—parameters anchored on cost, quality, and access; and so forth.

She refocused when he itemized his preflight checklist yet divided her attention between repeated glances at the two grand pictures above the desk. Outwardly, she absorbed his precautions against harsh storms bowling out of Siberia and how they differed from the weather systems percolating up the Gulf of Alaska. Inwardly, she steered into the realm of joining him and Bobby to create an instant family of three—another triangle for the good doctor. Half of her lingered there. The other half heard about Piper's bizarre methods of wind sensing and wing-lift perceptions aiding aircraft speed, control, and the safest runway approach.

"Safe landings are preferred, aren't they, Gary?" she asked, batting her eyelids.

Not derailed, he boasted, "Piper told me I took to airplanes like baby moose to walking. That's when we switched over to floats for water takeoffs on Lake Hood."

"Sounds like you've put all the required skills together," summarized Jennelle, faking a disappointed nuance.

Graywood nonchalantly opened the mahogany desk's upper left drawer and pulled out his pilot's license and copy of the Federal Aviation Administration's Practical Test Standards.

"These, Jen, are dry pieces of paper," he proclaimed. "It's the experiences in the air that count. I've logged over three thousand hours, day and night, in all sorts of weather all over Alaska. I've done it, Jen, and done it well." He slammed them down on the roll-top's edge.

She welcomed the confident bravado and scanned the den for more of his personal history. Bobby's haphazard tour had revealed no ex-wife portraits, and no apparent signs of her were glued in the room here. Locking her eyes onto his cornflower blues, she announced, "Well, Gary, I'll just have to try you out."

He wanted to kiss her hard but held back. "Jen, next week Bobby and I are flying my friend, Monroe Bearhead, to Chitina for the potlatch he has every summer. It's really an event and a chance to see one of the villages I support. I'd like you to come."

"I'd love to." Winging off into back country by the third date was a first for her.

Both dwelled in the other's windows to the soul … the moment twitched in the air, entry to richer connections … and danger. Hesitant and awkward, should he tuck her in embrace; should her hand smooth his hair? Might the kiss cascade or prevent perishing in full fathom five? Bending to her, he brushed the desk. The thick FAA manual splatted the floor and snapped their lures in two.

"Ah … Gary, should we clear the table and see what Bobby's up to?" Most of her didn't mean it.

"Yeah … I suppose; he's too quiet."

Don't press too fast.

CHAPTER SIX

Going Home to Potlatch

"Where's Monroe?" asked Jennelle, squinting against the morning sun. She ignored the asphalt odor leaching off the resurfaced taxiway in front of Seneca's hangar. Her maroon silk scarf flowed with the welcome breeze.

"He's smoking by the canteen," said Graywood. "He's not fond of flying." Graywood stroked the firmness of the spring steel wheels changed over from floats the day before.

Jennelle shined in the beige, oversized oxford shirt and snug, navy-blue pants. Pelt-like, on a shoulder draped a safari jacket. Her passion for adventure had fueled wardrobe choices toward practical garments that felt like a second skin.

Gooey-eyed, Graywood embraced her but flicked into pre-flight instructions once a side glance detected Bobby watching.

Jennelle interrupted Graywood's serious spiel on passenger responsibilities with lighthearted questions she already knew answers to. And Graywood enjoyed playing along.

Too young to recognize boundary testing that doubled for flirting, Bobby listened to the adults banter as they waited for Bearhead to bolster courage with nicotine.

Once pilot and three passengers had crammed *Seneca* with travel bags and dozens of wood carvings, Graywood radioed for clearance. Airborne, they arced across Turnagain Arm to Whittier and followed the Alaskan Marine Highway over Prince William Sound to Valdez. For ground guides, Graywood opted on Richardson Highway and the Trans-Alaska Pipeline. Beyond Thompson Pass, he banked east to the Tiekel valley where it joined the Copper River and followed the salmon-choked waterway north to Chitina.

One of Bearhead's younger cousins, Theo Nowell, met them at the rutted landing strip with a pickup truck, weathered and degraded to twice its age.

"I'm here to take you home," said Theo in menaced revolver staccato.

"How are your children?" came back Bearhead, his standard opening to every father.

"They grow well," answered Theo, meaning the family had a fair year so far jumbling dual lives of village subsistence with the white world's encroachments and benefits.

"You remember Doctor Gharrett Graywood and his son, Robert," introduced Bearhead.

"I remember you well from last year's potlatch," replied Theo in a more gratified tone. He looked over Bobby and added, "You got in bad trouble with my boy, Frankie."

"Uh huh," sheepishly confirmed Bobby. The children were the same age.

At the gathering a year ago, unaware of any danger, Bobby and Frankie had wandered the waterway onto a sand bar. Nine days of heavy rain on the surrounding watershed had swollen the Copper and Chitina confluence. The locals knew holms and sediments shifted treacherously or disappeared after runoff surges—lethal to foolish explorers. Robin, Frankie's older sister, was sent to find the boys at the start of the potlatch and discovered their peril as the thin isthmus on which they stood was about to wash away.

She rushed back to alert the adults. Theo, Graywood, and a third man, Wayne Sekorr, jumped in the latter's dinghy. Lacking gas to refill the empty outboard motor, Theo and Wayne rowed against precarious strong currents to within six feet of the rapidly shrinking island. The tallest, Graywood, waded the malignant swirls fighting the rest of the way strapped in a life vest tethered to the boat. Bone-chilling water rolled over with every misstep. Once he'd reached firmer footing beyond eroding silt, Theo tossed ropes and jackets and reeled in each boy like a line-caught fish.

Manning oars, Wayne joked the boys were the biggest king salmon ever caught from the river, yet to Theo and Graywood, they were the most precious. When pulling in Graywood, the boat's hull dipped too far, and torrents poured in, threatening to capsize them. With fury, Theo and the boys bailed as Wayne repositioned the jeopardized bow. The excitement warmed everyone's blood. Once stable, Theo yanked Graywood over the stern, and Wayne crowed he'd just harpooned a great grey whale. Wet and shivering, Graywood draped each child's head with dry parts of dinghy covers. Stripping off their clothes, he wrung every ounce of water as Wayne and Theo stroked toward the village like galley slaves. The families met them at the dock with blankets, and the fire in Bearhead's lodge warmed and dried all.

"Have you learned to swim in cold water?" asked Theo.

"I can swim but don't like cold water," returned Bobby, half embarrassed, half defiant.

"And this is Doctor Jennelle Daniels," shifted Bearhead. "She's from Georgia but works in Anchorage. I wished her to see our village."

"We're glad you're here," said Theo, admiring her figure. He wondered if she was a replacement sawbones at the Indian Health Service's clinic in Glennallen sixty-three miles away. An IHS physician visited Chitina once a month to review the rotating nurse practitioner's care plans implemented by the onsite health aide. Regrettably, after becoming familiar with the people of the village, the doc left because the assignment turned over every one to two years. Bearhead always accompanied the newcomer on the initial visit to help with orientation.

Doctor Daniels appeared wiser to Theo than the usual pill pusher. Out of respect, he unloaded *Seneca* and waited for Bearhead to add more about her background.

"Living your third way looks good for you," Theo said to Bearhead, arms bulked up with the elder cousin's presents.

Defending Buddha and white man's Anchorage to Theo had become lost causes. Bearhead simply deferred, saying, "I'm in my village now."

"Chitina welcomes all who stay quiet on certain things," Theo warned, a putdown that shielded smoldering contempt. He dropped the load in the truck's bed and pounded fists so loud on the hood that all heads turned and Bobby jumped. Theo's eyes peeled everyone like hoisted, gill-net fish. Smirking, he returned to the *Seneca* for more cargo.

"I'll try not to jar you too much," Theo said to Jennelle. The over-stuffed four-door rig thumped the broken highway.

"He doesn't get along well with roads," Bearhead explained. "They scar the land forever."

She raised an eyebrow catching the inherent irony of road, truck, land, and man in clashes to wound each other.

Four miles of potholes were interlaced with accountings on the welfare of eight Chitina families. Elder and younger cousin would have discussed more, but the route ran out at Bearhead's lodge—the post-and-beam meeting place for the village. The one-story longhouse's roof arched over stout sides of planked spruce and red cedar, trimmed in cottonwood. Natural contours deemphasized the structure's grander proportions.

A sentinel totem forty feet high guarded the front. Carved figures with intense expressions extended the length of the pole to herald Bearhead's lineage. Graywood pointed out to Jennelle a crouching bear, a man holding a fish, and a brown bear biting a killer whale's flukes. All marveled at the giant thunderbird perched atop extending wings.

"Inside we'll have potlatch when low twilight," decreed Bearhead.

Gift giving unified the First Peoples' social life. At its zenith, the tradition known as potlatch encompassed the tribal groups in central and southeastern Alaska, Canada's British Columbia, and the continental United States' Pacific Northwest. Potlatches redistributed wealth to solidify trading relationships and maintain harmony. The custom existed long before the Hudson's Bay and the Russian-American trading companies arrived to dominate the First Peoples' commerce. Prior to the Russian fort constructed at Chitina in 1819 to protect the czar's developing network, Bearhead's Ahtena tribe had bartered with Eyaks to the south and the Yakutat and Klukwan Tlingits living southeast. Their contacts among each other diminished after the Russians arrived with cloth, beads, iron, and guns to exchange for pelts.

To the First Peoples' great despair, both Canadian and United States governments prohibited potlatches in the late nineteenth century. Forbidding this vital ceremony equated to outlawing Christmas for Christians. Fortunately in 1934, Congress passed the Indian Reorganization Act that allowed the ritual's legal resumption within the United States and its territories. Canada followed in 1951.

Throughout the denial of potlatch, Bearhead's Tallchief clan led Ahtenan defiance against the federal government's destructive threats to strip away all tribal identity. Bearhead's ancestors pushed back the white man's ordinances and recognized or assimilated versions of intertribal traditions, such as the Raven-Eagle moiety delineation practiced by their Tlingit neighbors. And before Congress rescinded the potlatch ban, Bearhead's grandfather and uncle openly advocated Ahtenan dialects and ceremonies to strengthen and preserve their heritage. Combined, these southeastern Alaskan adaptations matured to the degree comparable to the Plains Indians collective embrace of the Ghost Dance ceremonies decades earlier upon the bison's near-extinction at the end of the devastating Indian Wars.

The individual who hosted potlatch bestowed most of his material wealth to the rest of the tribe to show goodwill and maintain social status. In earlier gatherings, the giveaways often included blankets, tools, weapons, drums, furs, even canoes. By mid-twentieth century, gifts had evolved to jewelry, appliances, and money.

When Bearhead made potlatch, he dispensed wood carvings and cash envelops. His art was coveted. His reputation held respect. If a family suffered financial crisis, the Bearhead carving often remained the final possession pawned or sold.

Copious consumption of the late-spawning Copper River king salmon accompanied the celebration. Caught early in morning on lines instead of nets, the fish were iced immediately to preserve the firm flesh, clear eyes, and sparkling sheen. To confirm he had the best parts to prepare, Bearhead examined for red oil coating the fingers of the women who knifed the fillets. Since they oozed such pureness, he'd sear the pieces without butter on a cast-iron skillet with meager touches of salt and pepper and finish them in a two-hundred-degree oven. He'd wrap each in foil to slowly seethe by an alder-wood fire until eaten.

Bearhead's longhouse enclosed an expansive great room for village meetings and ceremonies. A stone-ringed fire pit commanded the center with wooden bench rows on three sides. Decades of smoke wafting toward the yearly jury-rigged roof baffle had soot-coated the ceiling joists. The Dlam—a magnificent, interior cedar post—greeted Jennelle, Graywood, and Bobby once they entered the front portal. It showcased a black and silver raven clutching a sphere.

"Did you carve this one?" asked Jennelle.

"That I only helped a little," replied Bearhead. "My grandfather and uncle shaped it when I was Bobby's age." He pressed three reverent fingers to the top of the bird's beak. "Dlam is a place of respect … where guests are announced for the potlatch feast."

"What does it symbolize?" asked Jennelle.

"Raven stealing the moon."

"Stealing?" questioned Bobby. He knew about Uncle Roe's Raven super-clan, but stealing by Raven seemed out of place.

"Why's a raven stealing the moon?" asked Jennelle. "Was there a greater purpose, Monroe?" Stealing linked to the custom of potlatch and giving tripped her up too.

Grasping the confusion, Bearhead beckoned them further inside and spun a modern version of Raven's drama once they'd settled at the fire pit:

"Let me tell you a story. Long ago, the First Peoples did not have the moon to mark the night sky, not like the sun that embraced the day. Too dark were the night heavens, and it was out of balance with the day. The First Peoples feared the sun might never reappear if the lack of balance went on. And great Raven, our First Elder, felt their distress.

"Raven knew of a shiny circle called moon, hidden by the gods of misery. These gods hid moon like a great jewel, and it was coveted by them. These terrible gods did not believe the First Peoples worthy to see moon's gentle light or have it shine down on them. The gods wanted moon only for themselves. They hoarded it and locked moon far away to the north behind the great mountains.

"Yet Raven believed everything should be shared and nothing hoarded, and he flew to the far north. He tricked the gods of misery with a dazzling display, conjured out of the Northern Lights, making the whole night sky into ribbons pulled out of many, many rainbows. And while they watched with delight, Raven snatched the moon from behind the great mountains and brought it to our world's night for all of us to see its beauty.

"That's why the Dlam displays Raven stealing the moon to give it to the First Peoples. Potlatch is a tradition of giving, not hoarding like the gods of misery. And we're grateful to Raven for making the first potlatch."

"Monroe, I'm curious. How does Raven account for the phases of the moon?" asked Jennelle, straining her eyes to see in the great room's sparse light.

Bearhead paused. Over thirty Raven moon myths existed across the northern Pacific, from the Oregon coast to Japan's Kurile Islands. With Bobby present, Bearhead spliced together a story shaped for the boy's age.

"The gods of misery were furious when they discovered Raven had stolen their jewel and given it to the First Peoples. They threatened to hide the sun if moon was not returned. And without the sun, there would be no warmth and life for the animals and the trees and the First Peoples. Raven gathered all the chiefs and won them over to let him talk to the gods of misery. Yet as they talked, behind Raven's back, the gods cheated and captured the sun."

Bearhead stopped the saga. A glow, ushered from the great room's rear door, carried the blessings of baked carrot muffins. Two women approached.

Bearhead brightened. "Jennelle, let me introduce my wives, April and May Coldsnow." All stood and focused on the channeled course of radiance.

They were twins, seventeen years junior to Bearhead. April assisted her sibling's halting steps.

Bearhead reached and held May. After steadying her, he then embraced April and kissed her on the lips.

Upon release, April said, "Welcome to our lodge." Four inches more in height than Bearhead, her jet-black hair framed high cheekbones and nut-brown eyes. "Are you Bobby?" she joshed. "You're much bigger than the little boy who came here last year."

"I've grown a lot."

"You've grown more than I've imagined. You'll be taller than your dad," she said with nurturing reassurance.

Incomprehensible sounds pealed from May. Thinner than April, most notably around the throat, May's height topped no more than her sister's chin. Under a beaded skirt protruded hard plastic braces. May touched Bobby's blond hair with an outstretched hand that revealed an intention tremor. Jennelle also detected vertical head oscillations—May's marginal neck muscles struggled to support her skull. More garbled sounds followed.

"She says you have wonderful hair like our sun," interpreted April.

"Dad, she said that last year," moaned Bobby, embarrassed.

"It's wonderful to see you both again," said Graywood. "I'd like to introduce my good friend, Doctor Jennelle Daniels."

Graywood recalled the episode when he'd met the twins after Bearhead's first wife, Ume, had died. He'd asked why their given names were April and May and expected an insightful reason.

Bearhead replied matter-of-factly, "They're twins. April was born before May."

Searching for a shred of meaning, Graywood followed with, "So their births happened in spring?"

"No, January," Bearhead said, annoyed.

Graywood wanted to tell Jennelle this past little comedy but had to wait as another unfolded.

"You are welcomed in our lodge," April said to Jennelle. To Graywood she remarked, "On all your visits, you never brought a woman."

In the great room's half-light, the three dark-haired women assessed in silence—Jennelle and April scrutinized each other in the adult way while May observed Graywood's companion more as a child would.

May vocalized again, and both April and Bearhead grinned. "She asks if you're Gary's girlfriend," translated April.

Surprised, neither Jennelle nor Graywood answered.

"Dad loves her!" volunteered Bobby triumphantly.

Jennelle caught her breath with Graywood's embarrassed sidelong glance.

"Well, Gary," she cooed, "I'm honored to be the only woman you've brought to Chitina," and added a coy wink.

On the frigid winter night when the village midwife delivered April, a partial placental detachment ensued once April's tiny head crowned her mother's vaginal opening. Although May came out seven minutes later, the placenta's premature abruption had diminished the critical oxygen transfer long enough between laboring mother and unborn second twin to cause the anoxic effects of cerebral palsy.

The proximal muscles in May's arms, legs, and neck remained sparse and compromised as they grew. She endured successive stages of braces and physical conditioning exercises necessary to strengthen the ability to walk and hold upright her head.

May's impaired speech resulted from tongue and pharynx incoordination that therapy could not correct. Fortunately, the gag reflex and swallowing nerves functioned well enough to direct food and liquids to her stomach and not the lungs, as often happened with cerebral palsy. Globally, she possessed the intelligence and innocence of an eight-year-old.

After their mother died, April became May's guardian at age sixteen. Their father, an army draftee, had been lost at Tet during Vietnam.

April bloomed into the beloved one pursued by the village's sons. Yet her devotion to May exceeded all marriage proposals and entreaties to separate from her twin. Bearhead suspected she harbored never-ending guilt for being first born and spared the crippling anoxia May suffered.

By fathomless remorse, April shaped her life's duty to care for her sibling. Or did an incomprehensible spiritual bond, shared only by twins out of the same womb, exist—a connection single-wombed individuals never fully understood?

In time, April agreed to marry Johnny Toofish. From the village's Orca clan, he'd pledged Ahtena-Tlingit ancestral oaths to be kind and equal to May and let her live with them.

In a childlike yet serious manner, May pretended Johnny had a twin brother, Guy, and when April married Johnny, May wedded Guy. Close family members played along with the fantasy, but with passing years, May gradually let Guy go. At the 1998 Klondike Centennial celebrations, she announced he'd mysteriously passed on.

Like most men in the village, Johnny Toofish worked summers crabbing the Bering Sea or netting salmon out of the Gulf of Alaska. The rest of the year, they subsisted stretching out three checks from the Alaskan Permanent Fund.

In 1995, Johnny injured his spine in a lashing ocean storm and thereafter collected disability. His demeanor turned brusque, detached, and critical. From an excess of something unforeseen and never talked about, he died within a year of May's make-believe Guy.

A widower, Bearhead had known the sisters' plight. Five months after Johnny's death, they accepted Bearhead's invitation to take to his lodge. He deciphered May's unique speech patterns and became as good as April in understanding May.

Bearhead's actions had illuminated his grandfather's greater will. Destiny had fashioned a new life circle: Bearhead had become provider and protector and was both husband to April and father to May. The elders had given April to replace Ume and had blessed him with May to watch over as he'd done for precious little Sophia.

"Uncle Roe, how did Raven save the moon?" asked Bobby, pushing for the story's ending.

"Where was I?" asked Bearhead, scratching his skull.

Jennelle answered, "Raven was going to fly to the angry gods who'd taken the sun 'cause the moon was missing."

Even in sparse light, Graywood appeared blushed when he sat by Jennelle. She pressed a shoulder to his and worked to flatten a wide grin.

With Bobby and May seated before Bearhead, April excused herself and prepared tea and juice.

Bearhead focused upwards to the central support beam and spoke, "It was agreed by the chiefs that Raven would talk with the angry gods and make treaty over moon and sun. The gods of misery had taken the sun, and all stood dark, even in the middle of the day. The gods wanted Raven to accept a very hard bargain. Only that would soften their wrath."

Bearhead eyed the Dlam and lowered his chin. "But clever Raven brewed a treaty even these gods could not refuse. No one knows what he said, but the sun's full roundness returned to shine each day, and every night the prideful gods of misery were allowed to borrow the sun to keep and admire in their special place far away to the south—we must remember how much the gods of misery always wished to possess the sun. Raven's bargain to share the sun this way saved the First Peoples, it preserved the animals, and allowed the trees and bushes and the grasses to grow strong.

"In return, the First Peoples could borrow the moon to adore at night, but the gods decreed part of it must be held as ransom because Raven had stolen it once. Raven agreed to give up a part at dusk, but he shrewdly offered if the moon was permitted to shine fully on the First Peoples once a month, then for a different night every month there'd be no need to have the moon at all, and the gods could keep it all to themselves. All agreed to the trade."

Bearhead raised his right hand, palm forward, and peered at the rafters. In reverent timbre, he said, "Raven had created a new balance in the heavens. But the gods of misery were powerful and capable of changing the treaty anytime. That's why the sun sometimes is quickly blackened in the day and at night the moon gets blotted out. It means Raven and the angry gods are talking again on how long the sun and the moon will dance in the sky and how long they'll remain hidden. The gods of misery are very wary of Raven, so they begin each treaty parley by hiding part or all the sun, or part or all the moon, to gain advantage. Raven must stop whatever he's doing and bargain again. So far, he's returned the sun and the moon back to the First Peoples in less than a day or a night, making their fears go away. He's very good and clever."

"Who'd like hot tea or cold berry juice?" asked April. She carried an ample tray with wooden mugs, two porcelain pots, and a basket of carrot muffins. Bearhead's favorite was marsh tea simmered from wild rosemary. The chilled beverage had been squeezed from ground-hugging blueberries and crowberry.

Bobby stuffed half of a warm roll in his mouth.

"What a beautiful basket," praised Jennelle.

"She made it," said Bearhead, with pride. "April is keeper of teaching the basket."

"Bobby, please take this and carefully give it to May," said April, turning a deaf ear to her husband.

Employing both hands, Bobby transferred the drink and returned for his own.

"What's the basket made from?" asked Jennelle.

"Spruce root weft and maidenhair woven with cedar strips," answered April.

"I love the wonderful triangle patterns," said Jennelle. "What else do you weave baskets from?"

"Alder bark, bear grass, and cedar root."

"She's the talent in our family," said Bearhead.

"Your storytelling is wonderful too, Monroe. You're both very talented," Jennelle said and selected tea. "I've never heard that rendition on the phases of the moon. You even explained solar and lunar eclipses."

"Across the seas, our ancestors somehow had to make sense for the phases in the moon, and by creating stories, they made the mystery less. That's the way we are," reflected Bearhead. "It sounds similar to the Greek myths, which explain the seasons of the year, don't you think?"

"You mean where Persephone was kidnapped and confined in Hell by her Uncle Hades until Demeter demanded her release?" replied Jennelle, searching for clarification. "That's about seasonal growing cycles, summer to winter and back to summer, not the phases of the moon. I don't understand, Monroe."

"All cultures developed explanations for the moon and sun's existence and why we have the seasons. The three are tied together," amplified Bearhead. "I told only of Raven stealing the moon to give to the First Peoples and the treaty that followed. Can you imagine the circumstances forcing Raven to bargain with the gods to explain the cycle of seasons for the First Peoples? Now that's a grander folktale."

"Monroe Bearhead," interrupted April, "you can't tell stories all day. You're not in class in Anchorage. Prepare the fish. Tala and Snowbird have boned them since morning. Go now."

Rubbing his neck, Bearhead cat-footed away.

"Bobby, please carry this tray to the kitchen for me," said April. She helped May to rise.

"You think Cash would want to hear about Raven and the moon?" asked Graywood, half in jest to Jennelle as he assisted April with May.

"I'll tell him the saga when we return," replied Jennelle.

"Have I met Cash?" called Bearhead from the Dlam.

"I don't think so. He's a geologist morphed into an oceanographer," said Graywood.

"Tell me about him."

"He works on ocean food chains and climatic impacts on them. Piper flies him all around the Arctic."

"His office is above mine at Grace Hall," added Jennelle.

"He sounds interesting," said Bearhead, reversing steps. "I wonder what certainties and speculations a scientist like him might have on global warming. I'd like to meet your Cash."

"Oh, he's a fine character for sure," said Jennelle, assessing her colleague out loud, "and he rails against those wrapping political agendas around science—says too many twist their research and science into myths and religions only to get more grant money."

"Does he challenge this?" asked Bearhead.

"All the time but believes it's futile," she replied.

Clanking noises and cautious words popped from the kitchen. April and Bobby had stacked plates and platters for placement on folding tables.

On the gathering room's opposite side, a swelling of radiance engulfed the portal to the Dlam.

Bearhead's breathing slowed. His eyes, clear as brook water, molded impenetrably black as if searching a giant sea. Fingers entwined, he said, "Science and religion and mythology are our vain attempts to make sense of the world and its question of purpose beyond ... making sense from life and why we even exist. We don't know which of the three is best to believe, so we choose some of each, and from there see directions to take our lives."

Targeting Jennelle, Bearhead said, "I'd like to know how your friend sees the world." With a ginger laugh, he added, "But now I must see to fish and make sense of them."

"It's fun, Dad. Everyone gets gifts!" gushed Bobby's voice. "It's like a really big birthday party."

April and Bearhead had bedecked long buffet tables with foods and desserts. When announced at the Dlam, each Chitina family received a wood carving and an envelope with several fifty-dollar bills.

The Graywoods were given an eleven-inch, yellow cedar statuette of Brandy Belle. Bearhead had etched into the wood her blotchy fur pattern with paws encased in short hewn socks. When he handed it to his godson,

Bearhead recounted to Jennelle the episode on Christmas Eve three years earlier when Bobby had laid out four stockings for the little feline, one for each foot for Santa to fill.

Touched by the story, Jennelle asked, "Did Bobby actually do that, Gary?"

"Oh, it was something," said Graywood, "our very first Christmas with Brandy. Piper's boy had given her to Bobby as a kind of birthday present." Graywood repositioned so only Jennelle heard. "He gets embarrassed when I tell it."

Waiting in line for salmon and trimmings, Graywood didn't need to be discreet—Bobby had disengaged to the whittled cat and stroked the arched back with curled tail. From the fire's glow, he caught each angle's awesomeness.

Leaning in, Graywood whispered, "He'd asked for one of my hiking socks to hang on the fireplace for himself because his were too small, and he'd been really good so he thought Santa should bring him extra presents. So I went upstairs to get one, and when I came down, four of his little socks were in a row beneath where he wanted to hang my big white one. These were two pairs I'd bought him earlier for preschool. He'd unwrapped and positioned them just like treasure chests on a pirate ship's deck. I asked why all the extra socks, and he got real serious about how they were meant for Santa to leave presents for Brandy. He was worried she'd get nothing, so when he got the two new pairs, he'd saved them just for Brandy and Santa. Then he looked at me as if I was stupid and said, 'You know, she's got four feet.' I'll never forget his determination to make sure I understood how things had changed after we'd brought her home."

The dimness only enhanced the sparkling of Jennelle's eyes from the story. "When I grew up with my younger brothers," she said, "it seemed the only thing they thought about after Halloween was Christmas. Is it the same with Bobby?"

"Yeah, pretty much."

"Did he place out four socks the next Christmas?" she asked in a hushed voice.

"No, just that time. Ever since, we've hung only one stocking for Brandy. But you know what I'll do this Christmas?" Graywood pointed to Bobby, spellbound by the gift. "I'll find those four little socks and fill 'em with cat goodies and put 'em under Brandy's sock with the carving he got tonight."

Jennelle fought hard not to giggle when Graywood mimicked Bobby's serious tone, "It's the first Christmas for the cat statue, and Santa can't forget her. You know she's got four feet."

A joyful tear rolled down her cheek—Graywood was some special dad. She squeezed his hand.

"So, Jen, what's it like growing up with four brothers?"

"Normal."

The simple answer caught him off guard, not by its shortness but by how it confirmed the ache he'd harbored for family. As an only child, he'd felt his life had passed outside the norm. Like him, Maren had no brothers or sisters. Neither of them was "normal" in this sense, and maybe that had caused their marriage to fail. Yet Graywood knew divorce happened as often to couples who each had siblings as to those where each lacked them.

He rubbed Jennelle's fingers back and forth once.

Four brothers ... she's so lucky.

Over a hundred villagers flowed around the great room's fire and food tables and brought it all to life—kids running, noise, endless eating, and fun. Resin-filled smokes from burned alder and spruce vented the roof's soot-blackened baffle. Unclosed kitchen windows and the Dlam portal drafted fresher air to feed the flames. Once Theo Nowell covered the openings with massive woolen blankets to shield away the twilight, the inside perimeter contracted into new-moon murk. All appeared ready for silhouettes and shadows to merge in ceremony, dancing, and storytelling.

Donned in distinct garments, the four elders of Chitina processed in single file around the flickering stone hearth to reach the cardinal compass points. The leader wore a spruce wood hat. His clan crest, an orca whale, splayed the robe's back. Each hand held a round rattle chipped to the shape of a gull.

The second chief poled the earth with an eight-foot, brown bear staff of spruce, abalone shell, opercula, and human hair. A headdress and frontlet made from maple wood, ermine, baleen, and sea lion whiskers cloaked his skull.

The third displayed a manlike face mask of alder and cedar bark, trimmed with mountain goat hide. He gripped a whalebone war club.

Bearhead, clothed in a black-and-silver raven vestment over a woolen shirt with bear-hide collar, squared the quartet. Glass beads and pearl buttons embellished the front and sleeves. A helmet of spruce, opercula, abalone shell, red paint, and bear teeth clad his bald crown. Close to the heart, he grasped the talking stick.

Following opening ritual chants, the honored serving dishes—opercula shells wedged in cedar wood—were presented heaped with salmon to the elders. And the rest of the village also partook more food.

The blazing pit consumed split logs twice over, and at the third stoking, children huddled in front of a narrow platform three feet above ground. Adults reversed on benches or rotated chairs to favor better views, and Bobby went to sit with Frankie. Once torches brightened the sides of the mini-stage, Bearhead stood and announced, "Who will win the Talking Stick?"

A corridor formed for him to step to the podium. "Now we tell stories so our human face may reach above and touch its spirit face," he declared.

Each spring the Alaska Native Studies program at the University of Alaska Anchorage participated in the annual Alaskan Native Oratory competition, and Bearhead judged the finals. College students vied to win the Talking Stick in five speech categories: oratory, declamation, native languages, traditional introductions, and storytelling.

Bearhead searched for raw talent among Chitina's school children to groom for the contest. The annual potlatch might uncover a future state winner, and he fashioned a Talking Stick award for the village champion.

He evaluated stories on delivery and content. Foremost, a good rendition not only adhered to tradition but also tried to teach its listeners to see the world from two sides, and if so, all should be richer for hearing it. If two viewpoints were good, three seemed even better by Bearhead's preference, but then that edged too close to philosophy or preaching. The longhouse gathering was meant more for custom and entertainment. This evening, two were enough.

Four high school students had rehearsed for tonight's honor. The first, a boy of fourteen, cleverly mixed the emoted sounds of Raven and a mountain goat who together warned a sea bear wishing to paw a frog. He lacked a flowing storyline.

A fifteen-year-old girl followed but rushed the rendition of a maiden swallowed into a chinook's belly and then popping from the fish's gills with supernatural powers to sustain abundant Copper River salmon runs.

She'd memorized the drama well but lacked voice inflections and patience to pace its heart.

By the second story's end, Bobby returned wearing a let-down face and said to the floor, "Dad's Rum Tum stories were way lots better."

"What?" inquired Jennelle. "What're they, Bobby?"

"When I was littler, Dad told all about Rum Tum."

Her face shifted to Graywood for details.

"They're bedtime stories," he confided, "from when he was four years old about a cat named Rum Tum searching for home in Dutch Harbor."

"Dutch Harbor, in the Aleutian chain?" she asked.

"Yeah." Graywood wished not to say more because others might believe them rude to the competing talkers.

After the final two narrators, Bearhead returned to the stand, thanked the foursome, and announced, "Before I award the Talking Stick, I wish to introduce my guests from Anchorage. Many of you know Doctor Gary Graywood and his young son, Robert."

Bearhead pointed them out and added, "The Graywoods and I've invited our friend, Doctor Jennelle Daniels, too."

"I met them at Gary's plane," interrupted Theo Nowell. "Say Monroe, what's their connection?"

"Phht. This village," muttered Graywood. "Everyone damn gossips."

"Doctor Graywood and Doctor Daniels work in health care," explained Bearhead, as comments among the crowd flowed under, over, and around his. "You know he's from Public Health Service. And she's with the Centers for Disease Control."

"There's much more between them," April Coldsnow piped out. Curious vocal bedlam ensued. Bearhead raised the Talking Stick to dampen the cacophony and asked, "To be fair, Gary, you wish to tell your story about you and Jennelle?"

Put on the spot, Graywood stood and said, "I'm not a good storyteller."

"I disagree," teased April. "You must tell your story." She cheered everyone into unison with "Story, story, story …"

To quell them, Bearhead lifted the staff horizontal above his helmet and said, "Gary, you must come up and speak."

Embarrassed, Graywood looked to Jennelle for help. Serene, she emitted a gleaming smile to encourage him to the platform. Bereft, he cast to Bobby who gave the idea to save him: "Dad, tell 'em a Rum Tum story."

That's it! If they want a tale out of me, I'll tell them all about Rum Tum.

Graywood bent to Jennelle and said, "You're in for a surprise." He wasn't sure if her eyebrows shot up from delight or cautious awe. With purpose, he swaggered forward bolstered by applause.

"You've got the stage," said Bearhead, stepping down. He itched to warn Graywood to ditch his stodgy lecture style and go with the heartfelt energy from these people whom he so loved. Once he saw close up Graywood's confidence, it wasn't necessary.

"You've asked for a story, so I'll tell you one I know," opened Graywood. "This is a saga not about Doctor Daniels and me but about a cat in search for a home."

Rum Tum, Aleutian Girl, and Oscar the Sea Otter became noble fixtures in the minds of the Chitina villagers. After the initial fable, they wanted another, and Graywood divulged Rum Tum's adventures with Sammy the Seal and Patty the Porpoise and how the three had aligned against the crafty Baron White Gull and his infamous minions. Yet Chitina still craved more, so he narrated Rum Tum and Aleutian Girl's thrilling quest to find her father …

"I'm talked out. Please, I can't go on," pleaded Graywood. They jumped to their feet and clapped in swells. He'd spoken well in their tradition. More important, he'd shown respect, instead of blowing them off as other whites had done.

Impressed, Bearhead joined Graywood. "Gary, you're a great storyteller. I shall make you a Talking Stick too." The assemblage nodded approval, and Graywood received repeated ovations as he joined Jennelle and Bobby.

"Dad, you're it! You're the best!"

"Wow," whispered Jennelle. "Simply wow."

He kissed and hugged them.

The potlatch phased into Raven and Eagle song chants and dances.

Graywood forgot which student Bearhead awarded the Talking Stick. Like Rum Tum in Dutch Harbor, Graywood had found home and family with Bobby and Jennelle.

CHAPTER SEVEN

Transitions

"When tonight?" questioned Bearhead's guarded voice over the phone.

"After midnight between one and two is best," persuaded Graywood.

Bobby entered second grade accompanied by the rare celestial phenomenon of the earth eclipsing the full moon. Graywood had read the pending event in the morning paper and planned to treat Bobby with watching it. To make it doubly exciting, he'd keep it a secret and invited Bearhead.

"After you wake him up," said Bearhead, "can you get him back to sleep? Didn't school start today?"

"He'll be fine. It'll give him something to brag about tomorrow," reassured Graywood.

"Well, I love seeing my godson even at one in the morning. When do I show up?"

"It's a surprise, Roe, so come around midnight and help set up the telescope."

"Will Jen be there?"

"Nah, she's in Atlanta presenting at a conference."

"Mmmh, too bad …" Yet Bearhead sensed an opportunity to do something else Bobby might brag about even more at school. "You know, Gary, I'll have to call out an ancient chant or two with the disappearing moon," warned Bearhead.

"Bobby's awed whenever you do that stuff, Roe. Just don't wake the neighbors, okay?"

"What if I brought my drums?" said Bearhead, testing.

"How many drums?" asked Graywood, warily biting his lower lip.

"I think … ah … four."

"Four? Why so many?"

"One for each of us and one for the ancestors."

Graywood exhaled like a balloon with an untied tail and cautioned, "Promise me you'll play quietly, especially the ancestors' drum."

"The ancestors and I shall bang no louder than Bobby," quipped Bearhead. "Gary, I've got two students in my office. So see you tonight."

In raising Bobby, Graywood tried for the middle ground: he didn't pamper and he didn't ignore. Some parents might believe tonight's surprise excessive, but to Graywood an eclipse of this magnitude appeared worth it. A forever memory created.

Watching over Bobby and his wonderment for the world recaptured Graywood's youthful, untroubled heart. Bobby charged ahead pell-mell, and Graywood set the goals to guide the boy's direction half the time, to contain most of the collateral damage, and to always emphasize safety. Often Graywood relived what he'd done when Bobby's age. To see the little guy discover special orbs of pearls through adapting, conjuring, and coping—what joy will it be today, this hour, this minute?—was a father's blessed marvel.

And he wished Jennelle were here to observe the lunar eclipse … love might come full circle with shimmering possibilities. He'd unshackle, risk bursts of expression, and inhale the intoxicating madness.

But it also seemed wiser not to zoom in adoration too fast. He'd pursued Maren blinded to warning signs of incompatibility. One thing he had learned from his failed marriage: never forego caution with women. He resolved to keep his wits, remain steady, and deploy time as an ardent ally since there appeared plenty.

Ten minutes before midnight, Bearhead parked in the driveway's circle. Two roundtrips were needed to carry all the drums to the house.

"There're five of them," said Graywood.

"I forgot Raven's drum," replied Bearhead.

Bearhead and Graywood were Ravens in the Ahtena-Tlingit tradition. Graywood never understood how Bearhead determined he possessed this spirit sign but gladly accepted the privilege. By Bearhead's custom, whenever a drum ceremony with two or more Ravens took place, the sign-drum must sound rhythms to honor the spirit ones.

Bearhead arranged them on the kitchen floor in the ritual order they'd be struck underneath the vanishing moon. "Bobby will be surprised, won't he, Gary?"

"Well, not quite," Graywood said, starting to brew tea. "His teacher told his class about the eclipse this morning. When I picked him up from Rachel's after work, he begged to watch it." Graywood filled the copper kettle with tap water and placed it on the front burner. "I told him we would, but only if dinner chores got done, Brandy got fed and combed, and he went straight to bed so I could wake him at the right time to see it." Graywood scooped Earl Grey in the ceramic pot. "But I didn't say you'd be here," he added, with a wink.

"Where's the best spot to watch?" said Bearhead, dabbing seal oil on the drum skins.

"Southwest from the front porch." Graywood retrieved mugs from the dishwasher. "We'll need ground covers to sit on."

Bearhead rotated and inspected the Raven drum and nodded approval. "Where's the telescope?"

"I put it in the den to clean after Bobby fell asleep," Graywood said and left to find blankets.

Bearhead ambled into the room holding the old-fashioned Tasco refractor: the black-and-white 25.5-inch metal tube encased a coated, 75-power lens. He swiveled the cylinder on the equatorial tripod and imagined Graywood's father presenting it to Gary when he was a young boy.

"It's not heavy," Graywood said, entering with three quilts. "I remember it a lot larger. Take these, Roe, and please catch the front door for me." Graywood hoisted the tube from its mount.

The two Ravens hopped about the house and yard to set the scene for Bobby. Bearhead rolled the barbecue from the patio and ignited scrap wood to roast marshmallows and tell stories. Graywood diluted frozen juice concentrate and mixed chocolate into steamed milk.

The earth's shadow pinches the moon's face," said Bearhead. "It's time to wake him."

"Stay here, I'll get him."

Bearhead gazed on Graywood entering the house to spring the surprise. He recalled the Gary he'd known with Maren and compared then to now. Bobby pulled hard on his dad to live a complete life, and Graywood needed that. Day by day, father and son enriched the other's spirit.

"Bobby boy, it's time to get up." Graywood nudged the child's shoulder.

"Do I hafta take my pill now?" he yawned, eyes shut.

"No, later," Graywood whispered and stroked Brandy Belle's back to coax her off the bed. "It's time for the marvelous heavenly eclipse."

Bobby's blues sprung open like springs. Off flew the feather comforter.

"Put on your jacket and slippers Auntie April made 'cause Uncle Roe's here too," Graywood said, heart bouncing in tandem with his son's. "Go out the front door," he yelled, as Bobby raced down the stairs carrying a shoe, leaving behind the other.

The stars brightened with the progressive lunar covering in the crisp, clear night. Graywood and Bobby identified constellations and traded telescope turns. Bearhead, ever the comparative cultural anthropologist, told legends of the ancestors who'd lived along the northern Pacific Rim and what they'd have done ten thousand years ago had they beheld the moon shift to blood. Four minutes before two o'clock, the red-orange shading had blushed full. Challenging them, Bearhead pushed the Raven drum toward Graywood and Bobby.

"Whoever chants and pleases the old ones will bring the silver moon back and be proclaimed a medicine man. He slid the instrument to Bobby.

"This drum has much power," Bearhead said in a respectful low voice. "Godson, you have first honor to bring moon back as Raven did."

With pupils as large as the full moon, Bobby encased the drum with his thighs.

"Use this special drumming stick," Bearhead declared and cast a lionized stare. "Be brave in heart, full with spirit."

Awestruck, Bobby pressed the wad-tipped wood between prayerful palms. Spotting Ursa Minor overhead, he struck taut caribou hide six even times. Eyes veering to the shrouded orb, he beat a tempo to match his heart. Center stage, Bobby's alto emitted a languid, two-pitched, "AH-aye … ah-ayh … AH-aye … ah-ayh."

Graywood picked the moose skin drum and thumped supporting strokes. Bearhead likewise percussed his drum and layered resonating, crescendo-decrescendo sequences.

Graywood stopped his part in the trance-like interlude to stoke the ebbing flames in the barbecue's basin. Rolling, the wood unyoked skyward an intense column of sparks.

On they went, and the moon returned.

"I did it!" shouted Bobby and lifted the Raven drum to his chest. "Oh, Dad, I really did it."

"Wow. You did," said proud Graywood.

"You led like a young chief in training, Bobby," observed Bearhead. "When you're ready, I shall show you more on our drum."

"Show me now," Bobby pleaded, "please, Uncle Roe."

Bearhead held up an opened hand to refrain the entreaty. "You're too young. You must prove patient and grow and learn everything you can in school and, most of all, listen to your father. If you do this for three years, you'll be worthy, and I'll pass the secrets of the drumhead, which very few know, to you."

Enthralled, Bobby lowered the instrument as if setting Brandy Belle on his bed.

Graywood gaped at Bearhead's charm on uncomplicated minds yet perceived the need to rescue his child from further pulses of bravado. "It's time to roast marshmallows, sip hot chocolate, and tell a story or two before going to bed."

Bobby skewered three marshmallows, burned two black and one cinnamon brown. He heard Dad and Godfather pretend what might have happened with the ice-age hunters, chasing wooly mammoths from Siberia across the Bering land bridge to Alaska, when they'd viewed an orange-red moon such as tonight's spectacle.

And only God knew Bobby's dreams once Graywood carried him back to bed.

"You deviated from your ceremony," said Graywood, loading the drums into Bearhead's Land Rover.

"I wanted Bobby to feel important, so I went Hollywood white on him," replied Bearhead. "When we carried out the telescope and blankets, you mentioned he'd started Ritalin."

"Roe, you're the most considerate man I know," said Graywood. "I dreaded him going back to school with that label stuck to him."

Pulling out car keys, Bearhead asked, "How long has he taken it?"

"Started the week after potlatch. Didn't use it last year when the first-grade teacher implied he wasn't doing well in reading. I'd hoped he'd pick that up with my extra help at home, but it didn't work."

"We've three children in Chitina treated for ADHD," sympathized Bearhead, granting the subtle family failure attached with the disorder.

"You know, Roe, I've got to agree with Bobby's principal that to make it in today's workforce you need at least an associate's degree. They preach how Ritalin will help him concentrate and read better so he's got a chance. And I found last year's primer and plan having him read two pages after dinner to Brandy Belle and me on school nights."

Bearhead looked at the silhouette of Graywood's house. "How's he adjusting in school?"

"Fine after one day, I suppose. Better than when beginning first grade, and I had to rush around to get a chicken pox booster. They wouldn't let him come to O'Malley without it. That's my fault. I'd put it off … he's a terror getting shots."

"Does he like school?"

"For sure after they flood the basketball courts outside to make a hockey rink. That's his element."

The two Ravens wedged the five instruments so as not to roll inside the vehicle. They paused to follow the remade moon as it skirted behind incoming clouds.

"Guess we'll see how Ritalin helps this year," said Graywood.

Bearhead patted the father's shoulder, saying, "Don't worry, you're doing great," and drove home.

CHAPTER EIGHT

Duty

Two months into fiscal year 2008, Jennelle received relocation instructions to join CDC's investigation on what had caused the international AIDS vaccine failure. The immunization provided no protection against HIV. Worse, preliminary field data coordinated by the World Health Organization had implied it may have harmed recipients and hastened the deadly infection's acquisition. Senior CDC leaders had hand-picked Jennelle for their primary team, based on her stellar expertise and past performance.

The covert reason behind the Atlanta reassignment was an acute federal fund shortage. A mandate to meet the congressional FY 2008 discretionary spending target at $933 billion forced the health organization to reduce and consolidate personnel costs. CDC had taken an immense hit.

Deflated, Graywood willed to accept her departure. Stoic, he explained to Bobby how she had a duty to go where the government reasoned it best for the country, and she'd come back to work in Anchorage or at least visit. They helped pack and clean her apartment. Graywood arranged a small send-off party at the Glacier Brewhouse.

"Where you leavin' for again?" asked Piper, sitting at the bar without a drink.

"Jen's moving to Atlanta," said Graywood.

"Christ, Atlanta's a hot beast; nothing like here," Piper said and hand-signaled a dry martini. "So why you movin' back?"

"CDC's short on operating funds," said Jennelle, handing Graywood her coat.

"She got a promotion," injected Graywood.

"Ah, well, so congratulations," praised Piper. "What'd you do for it?"

"Oh, presented conclusions on some data I'd worked on."

"She won a commendation for spotting problems buried in the field data on a polio outbreak in Nigeria," clarified Graywood. "She advocated checking on the vaccine itself as the cause."

"Nigeria? Thought you handled only stuff happenin' here," said Piper.

"I do. Nigeria was on my own time."

"She'd figured it all out. That's why she got the award," lauded Graywood. He gently stroked her shoulder and asked, "What would you like to have?"

"What are you thinking of?"

"A mug of Beam. GB brews its house ale in Jim Beam barrels."

"I'll try what you're having, dear," she said, "only a pint." Eyes absorbed on Graywood, she asked Piper, sideways, "Where's Mary tonight?"

"Puttin' things to right down in Sydney. Should finish come thaw, and then she'll stay put here."

Jennelle had concurred on Mary's cautious approach to Piper's hither-thither ardor when hearing his checkered past. A sophisticated woman of means, Mary must have delved into Piper's background as a Lothario before accepting his proposal.

Cashel Goodlette entered as the waitress announced the table ready.

"I'll miss you, Cash," remarked Jennelle, grinning while they relocated, "and your world views. I've enjoyed driving to the airport and hearing your take on global warming."

"You oughta hear his rakin' when flyin' eight thousand feet," added Piper, sucking a martini olive dry. "And 'bout brown-nosed scientists playin' patsies to politicians and Hollywood whackos …"

"Or the UN with their pseudo-environmentalists," completed Jennelle, "conspiring to use global warming to shift gobs of money to the developing world as they skim some off the top."

A wry look crossed Cash's face. He decided against biting the bait. It was Jennelle's party tonight, not his soapbox. "What beer you trying, Gary?" he asked.

"The Beam." Graywood pointed at Jennelle's glass. "I had them open a fresh barrel for Jen."

"Looks pretty good." Cash caught the waitress's eye, pointed to Jennelle's beverage and then himself.

Jennelle's knee tapped Graywood's to tip him off to the conversation she wanted with the geologist. "I must confess, Cash," she said, setting him up, "I overheard you rail yesterday about ocean tides and global warming. I didn't hear it all but hoped you'd repeat it for me, if you don't mind."

Astonished, Cash took a prolonged breath. "You want me to blabber here at your party?"

"Please, Cash, just one more time. I don't know when I'll get back to hear you." She leaned toward him. "I'm really curious."

Cash surveyed the table with the attention focused on him. He glanced at the bartender and yearned for beer. Giving in, he said, "I think what you heard was my comparison on manmade global warming being as improbable to climate change as mankind causing the tides going out and coming in."

"Well, that's certainly cashing in on a new Cash-ism," croaked Piper to guffaws.

"Now I remember how you spoke it," said Jennelle. Dervishly swinging arms, she dropped into contralto: "Man controls climate change as much as he controls the tides."

Cash shook off a smile as the rest snarked at Jennelle's impersonation. "Actually," he corrected, "I said man *causes* global warming as much as he *causes* the tides to change."

The waitress brought Cash's Beam. After a long swallow, he observed, "This tastes like what's served up Talkeetna way. Damn good stuff."

"It's probably shipped from here to there," said Piper. "I'd love to have that contract."

"Makes sense," said Cash. Fortified, he continued, "Anyway, to change the tides, you'd have to change the moon's orbit or suffer a gargantuan seaquake. To end climate change, you'd have to stop the continents from drifting apart. Can we do that?" He mocked, "Can mankind push the western hemisphere back to Europe and Africa?"

Cash appeared ready to launch into the misdirected politics behind global warming, but Bearhead arrived with Rita and Taylor, the young secretaries employed at Grace Hall.

Spotting them, Graywood yelled, "Hey; Roe, over here." Bearhead never went to a party it without two women.

"Say there, Roe," kidded Graywood, winking to Jennelle, "you think April and May might say something about you coming here with them?"

Jennelle and Piper caught the Coldsnow sister reference, yet the ribbing about two months of the year perplexed the others—likely an inside joke.

"I stopped at Grace Hall to confirm tonight's festivity and these lovely ladies insisted on bringing me," Bearhead replied, fostering the most innocent face.

"Guess you don't like phoning for information," said Graywood.

"Guess not," deflected Bearhead.

Graywood introduced Monroe Bearhead to Cashel Goodlette. Despite Bearhead being a foot shorter than Cash and having half his massive frame, both sensed they were world explorers and intellectual equals. Jennelle embellished admiration for each.

"Cashel is your given name," repeated Bearhead. "When I first heard it, I thought it was your surname."

Cash smoothed to brogue. "I be named after ah faah-mous spot een Erie, the Rock o' Cashel."

The others leaned in and warmed to this rare facet of Cash's demeanor.

"As legend be, the Rock was where Saint Paddy baptized the Irish king, but tell ye sure, I dinnah believe none o' that crap."

"Guess there's no baptismal record to verify the event," Graywood interceded, attempting to mitigate Cashel's religious disbelief in front of Bearhead. "No doubt it passed down as legend through the centuries."

"No, lad, I be atheist. And ye know how nature and the whole ooniverse bein' soooo huge," Cash un-brogued, "for any human god to let it expand and expand forever. What kind of god designs a damn runaway universe like that?"

Shaking her head, Jennelle nudged an elbow to Graywood's side not to answer. She'd witnessed Cash ramble a dozen times on the monotheistic God not caring for his creation enough that he'd allow the world to spiral into a swollen red sun in four billion years: "If we're destined to be cooked asunder in a grand solar furnace, how could a god do that to us, even if we don't kill ourselves all off first? God wouldn't, so he doesn't exist."

Jennelle hoped Cash would belt down his godless tongue. Thankfully, Piper downshifted the shaky encounter with offers to relieve Bearhead of his two companions.

Jennelle coaxed Cash to sit across from Bearhead. Gallant Piper pulled out chairs for the young women. "What can I get you ladies from the bar?" he asked.

"A Lemon Drop," requested Taylor.

"I'll have a Peach Mojito," said Rita, coy and half as loud.

"One Lemon Drop and one Mojito," repeated Piper, moving away. "Say, Roe, you want Saketini as usual?"

"Yes, thanks." Bearhead switched to Jennelle. "Gary told me you've been called back to Atlanta on short notice."

"Yes, it's unexpected." She side-glanced at Graywood with regret. "I was getting used to being Alaskan and looking forward to my second winter."

"What's in Atlanta?"

Ticking off countries with her fingers, Jennelle explained, "I won the lottery for uncountable trips to eighteen cities in the Lower Forty-eight and Canada and overseas to Brazil, Peru, Haiti, Jamaica, South Africa, and Australia."

Jennelle outlined the CDC team's mission: microbiologists, epidemiologists, and medical researchers would attempt to determine what went awry with the highly touted, worldwide AIDS vaccine trial. Inoculation volunteers had become more, not less, likely to contract HIV disease.

Piper returned bearing social lubricants for his ladies.

The party of seven divided by subject matter and motive into two groups: the quartet of Jennelle, Graywood, Cash, and Bearhead tended toward social philosophy; the trio of Piper, Rita, and Taylor effervesced into the arts of painting and aviation. The quartet's goal sought to broaden their intellectual intimacy. His fiancée away in Sydney, Piper targeted bedding one or both women.

Bearhead selected the calamari from the menu. "The best I've ever tasted," he said. "Tender, consistency of butter, not the least bit rubbery."

Jennelle adopted his recommendation. Others ordered salmon, halibut, or crab entrees, and Piper and Cash added a cut of beef to their brain food to complete a surf and turf. The table discussion covered general health and family summaries as they shared appetizers: Piper's trio dipped a three-cheese fondue, and the quartet divided the antipasti of Kumamoto oysters, king crab cakes, pancetta-wrapped sea scallops, and salmon-fin sushi.

After mixed salads, the intellectual side of the conversation broadened to the debacle of mismatched health-care funding between urban and rural districts and the perceived cultural, economic, and social barriers to accessible health care overall. Interspersed within the serious talk, Bearhead impressed the others with details about how GB's chef—once his pupil—had prepared each main course. Bearhead connected every platter's protein, starch, and sides to a particular culture that made sense as only he could.

With dessert and another beverage round, the table talk drifted back to Cash's cynicism for the current state of science and its frank domination by those doling out grant money to further political agendas, instead of pursuing truth. Despite Cash's gruff tone, Bearhead—like Graywood and Jennelle—found the geologist-oceanographer fascinating.

"It's a damn fantasy to believe mankind can change the world's climate on the global scale," disparaged Cash. "We should thank Hollywood, Hiroshima, and Neil Armstrong for that."

"Neil Armstrong?" questioned Piper, shifting attention from the two secretaries. "He's the first to walk on the moon. What's he got to do with Hollywood whackoheads and Hiroshima?"

"Start with Hiroshima," responded Cash. "The worst one-day environmental disaster caused by man was that nuclear explosion at the end of World War II ..."

"And repeated at Nagasaki," interjected Bearhead.

"Yeah, Monroe, that too. But let's stick to Hiroshima," replied Cash. "That man-caused devastation, horrific as it was, pales when compared to Krakatoa's explosion."

Listening too, Rita and Taylor shrugged, confused.

Cash noticed and said, "Krakatoa was an Indonesian volcano. It exploded to pieces in 1883 and created a towering tidal wave that submerged a good chunk of Java. That blast packed the power of over thirteen thousand Hiroshima nuclear warheads." He sipped water to allow the natural disaster's magnitude to register. "You have Mount St. Helens in Washington State blowing up in 1980, and every year there are hurricanes and cyclones packing hundreds or thousands times more destructive power than Hiroshima."

"So you're saying nature's the eight-hundred-pound gorilla, and we're just itty-bitty mosquitoes when it comes to climate change," joked Piper, in light-hearted baritone.

"That's the simple idea," said Cash.

"So what's the Hollywood connection?" asked Taylor.

"I'll get to that in a minute, but I want to make a point. In Hiroshima's aftermath, people believed and feared the tremendous power at their fingertips, and they mistook manmade nuclear power being greater than nature's, but on the whole it's miniscule compared to the energy unleased within the earth's inner core."

"And Hollywood?" reminded Taylor.

"Hollywood magnifies that ego power trip with film fantasies like *Star Wars* and *Star Trek* where funny-dressed people and humanoid creatures warp across the galaxy at a thousand times the speed of light and teleport to planets as scrambled up atoms reassembled without a single flaw."

"Those are entertainments, Cash," retorted Piper, turning back to Rita. "People don't take 'em seriously."

"Perhaps," said Bearhead, "but many believe movies set in outer space explain more of our world than what's catalogued in libraries or on the Internet."

"Monroe's right," agreed Cash. "Look at it this way. There're three days almost every boomer alive remembers where he or she was and what he or she was doing."

"Okay, so what were they?" asked Piper.

"Kennedy getting shot in Dallas, the day Neil Armstrong walked on the moon, and New York's Nine-Eleven."

"A few in my village don't believe we walked on the moon," said Bearhead. "There're many in the world today denying we ever did."

"If it's not mankind's greatest achievement," emphasized Cash, "landing on the moon should be second on everybody's list. You'd have called me a crazy coot back in 1903, if after watching the Wright brothers at Kitty Hawk fly just a hundred yards, I'd then predicted we'd walk on the moon sixty-some years later. Any boy standing beside us would've believed me, but his father would've called me nuts or worse."

"So you've got Hiroshima and our lunar landings inflating anyone's head that we're the most powerful masters in the universe," rephrased Graywood.

"And reinforced by Hollywood space flicks," added Piper.

"Yet we're capable of extraordinary and terrible events," said Bearhead.

"But we'll never go faster than the speed of light," concluded Cash. "And we're a gnat to nature's gorilla regarding climate change," he emphasized, broadening both arms over the table, confident he'd tied a bow on the argument's package.

"So, Cash," probed Bearhead, "what's your take on Hollywood getting involved with manmade climate change?"

"They're absurd money-grubbers like everybody else. At least they're smart enough to set the *Star Wars* and *Star Trek* actions two centuries ahead, long after we're dead. Remember, these are people who refute Einstein and routinely daydream one can travel at multiple speeds of light. Is there any wonder they voted Al Gore an Oscar? What planet do they really live on? They're greedy fantasy wonks led by the fanaticized."

"Well, Cash," countered Bearhead, "maybe aging boomers are afraid of their approaching mortality. Perhaps they wish to relive their youth and believe in something greater than themselves, as the landing on the moon years ago did for them. So their egos manufacture the thinking for manmade controls over global warming."

"I'll accept that, Monroe," said Cash. "But it is sad people survive the harsh world through the whimsy created in films and jackass awards like the Oscars."

"Say, Cash, what's your stand on the UN conference now going in Bali?" prompted Jennelle, tired of hearing about Hollywood.

"Bali?" asked Piper.

"The United Nations conference on manmade global warming in Bali, Indonesia," clarified Cash, popping his knuckles. "So, those Bali people behave like tweeners wanting their allowances increased. I always say follow the money trail. The main reason people do things is for money's power. That's what Bali's all about … taxing and redistributing wealth under the guise of human-caused global warming. Of course we can change an island's ecosystem, dam the Yangtze River, or attempt to wipe out the American bison and Alaskan sea otters, but we'll never go faster than the speed of light." Cash repeated his digit popping to release his internal stress. "And we can't stop continents from drifting apart. That's the real cause for global climate change."

"The continents separating," said Graywood, "that's hard for people to grasp, and they don't know your theory based on it."

"Crap, of course not! The witless wonders in Washington won't select me for grant money. Beyond this table, no one will ever hear it."

Bearhead lifted a hand for calm and said, "I'm interested in science taken over by agendas for profit instead of truth. Yet I'm sure we'll agree, for the most part, science and technology so far have made life better for everybody."

"Sure, there're antibiotics, immunizations, higher yielding crops," listed Graywood.

"Air conditioning," added Jennelle. "Without it, the south would fritter away half the year from heat."

"And flight," championed Piper.

"The good examples are legion," said Bearhead. "But to what Cash cautions, I'll throw in two shameful instances where people invoked science to hide their real agendas.

"Only two, Roe?" teased Graywood, his head swiveling in mock disbelief because Bearhead could rattle off twenty anytime.

The scoff made Bearhead smile. More than two felt redundant, and the evening shouldn't allow a second lecture similar to Cash's.

"For you, Gary, I'll mention just a pair of what I call agenda science examples, and in fairness I'll indicate two where faith was condensed to the same sad end."

"Please, Roe," pleaded Graywood, "don't bring up the Spanish Inquisition or the Taliban destroying those giant Buddhas in Afghanistan. I've heard them a hundred times."

"You can skip the religious paradigm," intoned Cash. "By my thinking, all religion is shameful. If there's a god, I don't know him. I study nature. It's the purest thing I know."

"Nature's part of God," spoke Bearhead.

"That's your belief, not mine."

Bearhead paused to assess Cash in a different intellectual light ... an Irish skeptic as a traditional acolyte illuminating the parishes of classical and modern science yet lacking the structures of faith. Why had he chosen to forego that vast part of humanity? To make sense of the world, Cash limited his spirit to strict rationalities. Why did he void religion to move his reasoning forward? Why had he allowed science to become his straightjacket on The Path instead a path?

How and why people inhabited disbelief realms enthralled Bearhead. But tonight he deferred these thoughts to accommodate Cash's atheism. Besides, the dessert course had heard too much philosophical blood-letting, and the others might find it tedious. It was Jennelle's going-away party, not a debate.

"Yes, there's shame in many aspects of human religion, historical and present," compromised Bearhead. "I'll leave it at that. So my two shame samples in science are the eugenics theory fostered a century ago in western culture and today's commercial whaling by Norway and Japan under the camouflage of scientific research."

"I like your choices, Monroe," complimented Cash.

Bearhead outlined early twentieth century eugenics and the perceived horror within certain influential circles over the deterioration of the human gene pool because society's best people bred less than so-called inferior races. He ticked off twelve famous individuals from all professions—President Woodrow Wilson, Supreme Court Justice Oliver Wendell Holmes, playwright George Bernard Shaw included—who supported identifying third-rate groups for sterilization or isolation in institutions to cease their reproduction. Bearhead reviewed how the American Medical Association and the National Academy of Sciences had championed research efforts to deal with the impious crisis, and that twenty-nine states had passed laws to allow sterilizations of imbeciles—with the most done in California.

Bearhead asked his table mates who society deemed, at that time, to be imbeciles. Jennelle and Graywood correctly identified foreigners, immigrants, Jews, African-Americans, and all other cultural degenerates.

"Monroe, I think we'll agree your second science shame, where Japan harvests whales for research, is a total crock of dung, too" injected Cash. "We know it's done for profit."

"Fine," said Bearhead. "I yield the floor to you."

"Monroe's examples and my critique against manmade global warming show what happens if we politicize and pollute science with pseudoscience," said Cash. "It's damn dangerous."

"And social politics," declared Bearhead, "are most about creating and protecting hierarchies. The ones unfortunate to be labeled the lowest are often shunned or killed."

"It's done because of money," gruffed Cash. "Mankind seeks resources, and that drives the world's actions. Everything, including scientific truth, is warped by the dollar. The global warming debate is the latest instance. Look at this folly in Bali … the damn UN has already pronounced the debate over."

Cash's fist smacked the table. "According to them, only civilized peoples within the past hundred fifty years have caused the bulk of climate change, and the richer countries contributed the most. Whoever says otherwise gets denied access to their forum. It's the UN's show, and no one shall rain on their parade …"

Jennelle touched Graywood's wrist. She'd tuned out the Cash-Bearhead session. Into Graywood's ear, she whispered, "I'm sorry they're digging so deep. It's becoming a downer."

"Who knew they'd take off this way at your party?" mumbled Graywood, biting his tongue yet twisting to dwell in her expressive brown eyes.

"It's my fault, dear," she said, caressing his hand. "I started them whanging away." Her exquisite brows arched to an oncoming loneliness. "Gary, I'll miss you," muffled her pained mouth.

Graywood's sad dogface conveyed inner torment wanting her to stay against morning's obligation to depart.

"I've got to hogtie my tears to leave you," she said.

Likewise, Piper and Rita had shifted into intimate undertones. Left alone, helpless Taylor listened to Cashel the atheist and Bearhead the spiritualist agree to man's minor place on the planet.

Finally, the party closed.

"Roe, I've offered to see Taylor and Rita safely home," said Piper.

"Oh … ah … yeah, okay," uttered Bearhead. His eyes sparkled when he addressed the secretaries. "In the air and on ground, Piper's an excellent pilot. I'm told he's very reliable and dedicated to task, if hard or not."

"I owe you, Roe," Piper smirked, tongue wetting lips. He retrieved the women's winter coats.

As Bearhead pushed back his chair to go, Cash said, "Monroe, except for the god issue, you and I've got much in common."

"You don't have to believe, Cash, and that's fine. But please believe that I do," requested Bearhead. "You and I should talk more."

Cash nodded assent.

Bearhead bade everyone goodnight.

"I like your friend, Monroe," Cash said to Jennelle and Graywood. "I usually don't with social intellectuals," he commented through sips from a third decaf. "He's a wise man without ideas of intrigue. I like how he folded eugenics and whaling masquerading as research as biased pseudoscience and pinned them on human ego and greed instead of truth."

Side by side, Jennelle and Graywood faced carnally and heard none of Cash's rambling.

"I'll have to try the eugenics angle on those grant maniacs in Washington," said Cash, staring at the doorway Bearhead had egressed. "That might get funds sent my way and some good science done."

Graywood placed a hand over Jennelle's. She blushed and pressed back.

Impervious, Cash reflected out loud, "It's rare to find an intellectual who improves a complex discussion like Monroe." He set down the empty cup and noticed his companions' mirrored entrancement. "I'm finished," he boomed. "Time to go."

On the sidewalk outside GB, Cash extended his farewell. "Jennelle, I'm not happy you're leaving," he chattered. Cook Inlet's frigid air gnawed his exposed face. "All the same, I wish you good hunting on finding truth. Remember, follow the money."

"Thanks, Cash. I'll miss you too."

He plodded up Fifth Street.

The couple wrapped arms and trudged the opposite direction, fending off penetrating cold so severe it cracked moans out of the frozen spruce.

By the hotel room in the hallway, Jennelle stroked Graywood's cheek. Teeth unclenched, parted lips waited. They focused on kissing, and …

Bobby had a fortunate sleepover with Cub and Rachel.

Lovers don't mind dawn held back by December.

Graywood fetched his child and returned to the Sheraton to pick up Jennelle. Bobby gabbed non-stop about what had happened with Sable and her young at Cub's.

Graywood registered few bits from the recitation. Navigating icy streets on autopilot, he replayed the long night with Jennelle and how she'd eyeballed him don wild-flung clothes come daybreak.

Since Chitina, they'd had unions. Now she had to leave. He ached. He understood.

Jennelle waited in the lobby. She wished to remember the twelfth-floor corner room as only theirs.

Ejecting out of the Subaru, Bobby sprinted her way emitting unconditional affections to her soul's delight. "Did you have a good time last night?" she asked once they embraced.

"Oh, the best, Jen! Cub's got five new puppies, and we petted 'em and brushed 'em and fed 'em, and they licked us, and Cub's gonna get some more and race 'em, and I'm gonna help, and—"

"Wow, Bobby, slow down a little, sweetheart," she interrupted. "Before you go on, tell me if your dad's with you, or did you come here by yourself to take me to the airport?"

Thrilled a grown-up considered him so capable, he blurted with pride, "We both come for you."

"Well, that makes me very happy." She peered beyond the foyer and saw Graywood striding to the lobby's entrance. "I wouldn't ever want to miss saying good-bye to your dad."

"Oh no, he loves you lots and lots," Bobby confirmed.

She tried not to laugh at his innocence.

"Have you been greeted properly?" asked Graywood.

Bobby watched in stunned silence—without hesitation his father and Jennelle lip-pressed in public and way too long! Whenever adults did such on television or the movies, Bobby shielded his face and let loose distasteful noises. But this time, he jelled into egg-eyed paralysis, mouth ajar.

Jennelle released Graywood's lips but clasped his nape and cooed, "Bobby did a fine job greeting me." She pulled harder. "I'm not sure about you yet." They kissed open-mouthed.

The boy wasn't sure what he saw, but it had to be a good thing.

As Bobby sat in the Subaru's back seat on the way to Stevens International Airport, his skin detected the glowing from the adults in front. His dad managed the treacherous, snowplowed roads with just the left hand on the steering wheel. He'd never done that before.

Entering the terminal, Graywood walked between Jennelle and his son. In front of security, Jennelle hugged Bobby up off the toes and planted a smooch on his forehead. "I'll miss you terribly, dear."

"Please come back?" he pleaded, sobbing trickles.

"I'll try very soon." Her fingers stroked the child's hair. "I promise to write until I do."

Surrounded by travelers, Graywood and Jennelle unpacked one fleeting kiss. "I'll write you too," she murmured when they broke. Her left palm flattened on his heart. Motionless, he couldn't breathe. "I'm sorry to go, Gary," she quavered, wet eyes darting back and forth on his blues. Dutiful, she turned and walked away.

Crestfallen, numb, Graywood remained mute.

Clearing the guards, she about-faced and waved good-bye.

Furious limb flapping erupted from Bobby.

Graywood's insides pranced. Pool-eyed, he attempted to blow a kiss but couldn't muster mouth or arms.

Claimed by overlapping crowds, she disappeared.

"Dad, why'd she go away?"

Graywood scanned the concourse and imagined where she'd be now, tonight, in a week, and beyond.

"Dad, why'd she go?"

"Something went wrong with a new shot meant to help people all over the world," escaped out of Graywood. "She's gotta go and figure out why." Sensation returned to his legs when Bobby's grieving shoulders pressed into them.

"Is it kinda what you do, Dad?"

"Yeah, like what I do."

"I hate shots! I hate 'em and hate 'em!"

"I know."

Jennelle's unfolding world stretched so distant from Alaska … so much might happen whenever pursuing answers to a medical mystery.

"Let's go home, Bobby," he said with a tender lilt. "Maybe we'll find a Christmas tree and can decorate some, huh?"

"I can't wait!"

He embraced his son and beheld in the child's eyes how great a dad he'd become.

And Graywood thanked God for giving him the boy.

Jennelle wrote Graywood and Bobby. Punctual, she called on their birthdays and mailed Bobby the largest-sized postcards from every country she investigated.

With his father's encouragement, Bobby returned handwritten, half-page letters in broken sentences about Brandy Belle, school, and *Seneca.*

She read them in-between overseas missions and copious data analyses, correlated with her international colleagues.

Her correspondences to Graywood blended equal parts personal life and work. And for some time, the enchanting Alaskan memories held their own against the mounting number of adventures into varied hinterlands and cities of the Caribbean, Brazil, and Africa.

In short order, she confided the HIV debacle had grown incredibly complex. Federal and WHO bioscientists had realized within six weeks they did not understand why the HIV injection had failed or how other HIV inoculations in development might interact with the human immune system, even at the most basic level, to diminish or eradicate HIV from infected blood.

Fundamental research facts were not known, such as what immune reactions played primary roles in preventing or clearing an established HIV infection. Authorities conceded they had to begin anew, one step at a time, and reconstruct the knowledge for how a fresh candidate vaccine would lower HIV particle load in the circulation and through which immune systems.

Jennelle also revealed anguish and disappointment by how the government had pursued a crapshoot mentality to this point in AIDS immunization development and the best scientists had relied, in essence, on biological chance for its success. And she seethed against longstanding preferences that condoned chancy inoculation trials starting on the planet's poorer peoples and having only token recruitments from first-world countries to provide a modicum of moral cover. Brazen legal convenience had outright trumped humanity's ethics.

To regenerate professional faith in the CDC's overall mission, Jennelle felt obligated to assist colleagues and set right the immense professional gaffs. It would take longer to return to Alaska than she had originally expected.

She encouraged Graywood's acceptance.

CHAPTER NINE

Eden's Womb

At June's solstice, Graywood anchored Seneca to the northern shore on an unnamed lake nestled in a mountain curl, the Seven Sisters. A narrow river entered the tarn eighty yards eastward.

For the six months since Jennelle had departed for Atlanta, his heart remained as sharply cleaved as the moment she'd waved goodbye at the airport.

Binoculars and hiking boots strung around the neck, Graywood plowed the clear lake in hip waders to the sandy gravel beach and its thick whine of insects. He slathered on DEET juice, switched footwear, and surveyed the hidden discovery.

It grasped the soul … a craved paradise to arch a man's life … an Alaskan refuge to strengthen and keep one's center whole.

Shaded spats of forget-me-nots clung to the ground. Five sky-blue petals ringed the flower's inner circles of white on yellow to declare a miniature sun, laced within clouds enveloped by day's expanse.

Sitka spruce hid ridges that buttressed the natural reservoir's western and northern contours. Crystalized water provided rainbow trout and sockeye salmon home. Aromatic forest bouquets vanquished the pungent bug repellent.

Massive rock gardens, sprouting west to south, sputtered outcrops tied by hardy saxifrages, roseroot, and cinquefoil. Alder clustered the northeastern riparian zone with scratches of purple lupine and dwarf fireweed. Graywood made a mental note to return at summer's end and harvest the bright magenta blooms for Bearhead to toss into one of his specialty salads.

He scanned with binoculars the opened range farther eastward. More than a mile of Barclay's willow, pink wintergreen, and yarrow flower had dispersed among the thatch to merge on mixed backgrounds of cottonwood, birch, and spruce.

A female brown bear probed the tree boundary while minding two sub-adult cubs. The threesome gorged on grasses and bunchberries. Soon the sow would pick up Graywood's scent. If she'd never smelled human—one smothered in anti-bug goo, no less—she'd no doubt investigate. To avoid the encounter, Graywood trekked north prior to circling back toward the airplane.

Conifer fragrances filled the lungs as he dodged branch-hanging witch's hair to reach the ridge's crest.

Ascending beyond eight hundred feet, the tree line yielded to the alpine world. Two hoary marmots munched on acres of flower-field salad made from Cooley's buttercup, azalea, mountain harebell, and white heather. A cluster of American pipits exploded from a seep warning others of the human interloper.

Graywood traversed the most western Seven Sister where aphotic tangles of elfin-wood and dwarf hemlock bolstered trunks against frigid storms too heavy in snow. He studied the granite crag—a moderate-level climb to summit—made worse by relentless, freezing wind slapping the face. He deferred the physical indulgence and descended to a haphazard grove splayed on alder thickets holding currants and salmonberries—two bear favorites. The direct route back to *Seneca* dropped off too steeply, demarcated by trees crippled from uncountable winters of titanic snowpacks. He chose the subalpine meadow with its cascaded declines in wide inviting loops. Passing patches of deer cabbage and northern geranium, interspersed with chocolate lily and narcissus, he nudged upon a melted snow bed sprouting sedges, mountain marsh marigold, and false hellebore—a poisonous plant he'd warn Bobby to avoid. Not quite the Eden here as by the shore. Then again, there was the bear family uplake as well.

He crossed woodland and cut to the water flow that drained the basin to Cook Inlet. The air condensed in adhesive aromas of dying fish. Sockeye salmon flashed their abundant colored flesh, ready to spawn in natal side streams. Easy to pick out, the thrashing females dug redds into the gravel beds under pooled eddies. Breeding males dorsally protected them and quivered their humped vertebrae and elongated kypes back and forth.

Bearhead called them redbacks for the brilliant rouge on their spines and sides. Pasting a secret spice concoction on them, Monroe cooked them in a distinct way from Copper River kings.

Come September, the water conduit would provide passage for their steelhead cousins. The trout could be caught until the channel froze over.

Graywood maneuvered upriver around light-dabbled trees to where the sweet, pervasive marsh and wet wood odors announced the estuary's border to the tarn. Creamy white blossoms of cow parsnip, clustered on seven-foot stalks, dotted the greened-up valley. Bearhead called them, "pootschki." Graywood noted the locations to avoid the toxic flowers that blistered skin on contact … another piece of Eden off limits.

Halfway through the outlet, Graywood discovered moose prints hoofed fresh in the receiving earth. He rotated counterclockwise to locate the giant, but cracking from broken tree branches iced all motion. He'd pivoted face to face into his new neighbor—a grand-racked bull with wood snarls in his horns. He guarded the willow clumps abutting a pond. Insects buzzed eyes and nose to feed on moist mucous membranes. He'd stopped munching on sedges and stared with up-pointed ears. A bellicose charge—signaled by lip smacking, raised neck hair, and ears cocked back—appeared not imminent, yet might come anytime if stressed.

Flushed and sweating, Graywood inched backwards. His only weapons were wits and a can of pepper spray. He'd never maced a moose, only a black bear lumbering into his fishing hole south of Bethel on the Kuskokwim River a decade ago.

Distance lessened mutual alarm. Holding eye contact with the beast, Graywood retreated into a strip of devil's club—the spiny, wicked shrub that sported palm-sized leaves with prickly undersides for protection. Trapped, he stood stone still and let the encounter's momentum shift moose-ward. Not threatened, the animal remained curious with ears skyward.

An eagle looming for a meal above the lake squawked bemusement at the face-off below. It circled twice and then lost interest in the farce.

Perhaps the giant simply had accepted Graywood's presence as an odd-smelling, deformed bear ready to shed its strange hide of colored pieces. Antlers dipped, he grazed on bog moss.

The devil's club grooved Graywood's exposed forearms. Piece by piece, he dislodged the plant's defenses. Navigating a wide berth from Mister Moose, he skirted brambles and downed trees to reach lakeshore and *Seneca.*

Graywood planned to retire from the PHS in three years and imagined—detailed down to the canoe swooshing across the silkened water's face—future summertimes spent here. Underneath limpid air enriched by forest purity, the cloaked terrain emerged ideal. He'd call it "Campsite."

And he'd triple the time devoted to help his child. Here he'd teach Bobby archery, fishing, and kayaking. Mastering fresh abilities would jump-kick the boy's brain to change. The new skills would increase concentration and improve sporting finesse on O'Malley's hockey team. And effort and adroitness could spill over to augment Bobby's scholastic attention. Brain cells that fired together wired together. Learning additional aptitudes might mitigate his distracting impulses and allow higher levels of function equal to that obtained with Ritalin. Then Graywood could stop the pills.

For *Seneca* to ferry the state-of-the-art, hybrid kayak-canoe to Campsite, Graywood asked Piper for expertise on flying what's called an external load. At best, carrying freight outside the fuselage bent Federal Aviation regulations. Pilots who fudged the rules and strapped cargo to landing floats had to maintain edge-of-performance skills. If not correctly calculated and balanced, the added weight and air drag from an outside mass—lumber, satellite TV dishes, dressed moose carcasses, construction lockers, or whatever not fitted inside the cabin—could stall the aircraft.

Piper flew external loads all the time and was one of the few intrepid pilots who'd hauled a complete Super Cub fuselage on a de Havilland Beaver's right-side float over open water from Spenard to Valdez.

"How heavy's this brand-new canoe of yours?" asked Piper.

"Close to ninety pounds."

"Ah, Gary, piece of cake. FAA will certify if secured properly on the starboard float," he said matter-of-factly. "So where you takin' it?"

"Out to a secret place near Kamishak Bay," replied Graywood.

"You gonna bring it back?"

"Leave it. I'll make a storage hut out of some spruce."

"Anyone else know 'bout this special place of yours?"

"Don't think so. Just you, Roe, and Bobby."

"Guess no bastard could steal it and get far unless he flew it out like you're gonna take it in." Piper ran a hand, chin to throat, whenever he shifted gears talking. "Gary, remember your Spencer Glacier approach where you broke the training Cessna's strut?"

"Only time I damaged a plane," Graywood muttered.

"So far," chided Piper. The old pupil-instructor relationship resurfaced. Pointing up an index finger, Piper downloaded some coaching. "Don't touch the water the least bit tilted, or you'll cartwheel *Sky Woman* and sink 'er with your canoe."

"You think I'm crazy? That's the last thing I want," Graywood defended.

"Me too," smirked Piper. "I haven't gotten my money's worth from her yet."

Keeping a straight face, Graywood recalled the jest years ago of getting full teaching value out of Piper when he'd started as a flight student. "Tell me, can I strap my old beige canoe to the other float and take both at the same time?"

"What's its weight?" asked Piper.

"About the same as the ky-canoe."

Piper methodically tapped his chin and calculated the added bulk. "Shouldn't be a problem. You've got the external load evenly split on the floats. There'll be a helluva drag but less than two hundred added weight … like having one less big person. *Sky Woman*'s got plenty of lift. How many passengers you takin'?"

"Just me."

"Must be some damn fine place you flyin' off to nowhere alone with two canoes."

"When I get it ready, I'll show you."

"Who's the main pilot when we go?"

"Whoever's done the best in *Seneca* ... and the canoes."

Laughing, they scurried for beer and martinis at the Glacier Brewhouse and troubleshot the pending flight plus other issues that constricted their world.

Exuding soothing calm, Campsite invited Graywood in rather than pushed. The location duplicated the growth potential he and his son had experienced on Kauai.

Graywood constantly read about ADHD and devised a plan to increase Bobby's concentration abilities by mastering outdoor skills. Mental development continued throughout life, driven by learning and adaptations that never ceased, so long as the brain's owner sought them out.

The organ's standardized structure with its defined locations for critical processes—such as speech, memory, and sight—had been challenged by the evidence collected from advanced imaging techniques. Spectograms and PET scans had updated the rigid cortex maps for where a particular function was harbored: at one time, vision cues carried on the optic nerves, for example, were believed to be interpreted only in the occipital lobe; recent evidence confirmed they also could be deciphered and understood at a different site within the gray matter. Bottom line, at any age, the brain could rewire itself to improve survival.

And new theory had usurped old dogma: it became more accurate to interpret a function or proficiency as a population of brain cells, called neurons, firing off together. For the most part these areas were located where the older neural maps had portrayed them, yet not for every individual, like victims who had recovered from severe brain damage and displayed no outward deficits.

Another exquisite concept also motivated Graywood: neurons discharging together over and over eventually wired together to represent a novel adeptness. Bobby took a pill to increase attention span. Might recently learned physical abilities equally increase overall mindfulness? Could kayak and archery prowess—which require flawless concentration to properly execute—cross over and augment the focusing power necessary for reading? Would fostering the inhibitory neural circuits needed to rein in impulsiveness in order to achieve success in either of these outdoor sports spill over to Bobby's scholastic work? In Kauai, the child showed he could snorkel ... If he trained his brain to properly maneuver a kayak and shoot bull's-eyes with arrows, perhaps he'd do better in school without the drug.

Graywood had chosen kayaking and archery to round out Bobby's desire for ice hockey. Combined, the three activities represented a spectrum of mental and physical control similar to the aptitudes necessary to master expressive dance by studying first ballet, ballroom, and gymnastics. Solo kayaking and archery molded one's acute attention and concentration. Hockey emphasized melding the individual into team achievement, and two-person kayaking reinforced the linkage. Together these endeavors of effort would multiply pristine neuronal connections to mature Bobby's brain and launch him onto higher plateaus of function. But would Graywood's strategy become as effective as Ritalin?

"Hey there, Bobby boy, come look at this map with me."

"Okay, Dad."

Bobby left the great room's big screen and spurted to the den. An atlas of Alaska covered Graywood's mahogany desk.

"This is our state when looking down from fifty miles up in the sky," said Graywood

"Can *Seneca* fly that high?"

"Oh, no. Too dangerous." Graywood pointed to Unalaska and Dutch Harbor. "See this string of islands?"

"Yeah."

"That's where Rum Tum and Aleutian girl have their home."

Close to eight years old, Bobby ignored his dad's reference to old bedtime stories and asked, "Where do we live?"

Graywood flipped a dog-eared page, saying, "Over here on Cook Inlet. Remember when we soared over the mountains on our way to Hope last year?"

"Oooh, yeah! Can we do it again, Dad, please?"

"That's what I want to show you."

"What?"

"Where we're flying to next."

Bobby's eyes widened like fat walnuts.

Graywood's finger dropped on Augustine Island. "We'll have to skirt around this huge volcano to get to a special campsite I've found right over here."

"A volcano?"

"Yep, we'll have to be really careful, and we're gonna land on this lake stuck in the middle of these mountains.

"When can we go?"

"In a week. First we've got to buy you and me a bow-and-arrow set."

"Wow!"

"And we'll take Uncle Roe so he can teach you how to shoot."

"Yeehhh! I love Uncle Roe."

"So let's go shop around."

"Well sure, Gary," crowed Bearhead into the phone, "let's spend a good week out at this Campsite and take home some wisdom."

"I'd like to leave Friday and stay nine days. That all right with you?"

"Just get me to the wild. No cellphones, emails, to-do lists. None of it."

"Then we'll pick you up Friday morning, say eight, okay?"

"You bet."

Graywood and Bobby loaded *Seneca* as Bearhead dosed his nerves with nicotine.

Whenever Bobby sat co-pilot, he acted settled yet unfurled poignant, make-believe wings. The oncoming high panoramas often overwhelmed his inherent restlessness to fill his senses with a calm wonder.

Graywood assisted his son's engrossment by playing object identification games. As *Seneca* zoomed over the Alaskan peninsula, they named mountains, watched out for lofting volcano smokes, or identified vessels sailing the Cook Inlet. The first to score twenty on naming watercraft won. Easy-to-spot barges or cruise ships counted a point, tugs or salmon gill-netters got two, house-forward tenders or purse seiners earned three, a halibut schooner collected five, a crabber house-aft pulled in six, and the rare power scow tallied eight.

Bobby won the initial game and led the second when *Seneca* banked from Augustine Island toward the Sisters. On the approach to the sharp valley between the crags, Graywood uploaded and toggled to the headsets the *William Tell Overture* finale and shouted, "Hi ho, *Seneca*, away!"

Juiced with *The Lone Ranger* theme song, they swooped down the mountains and executed a pitch and roll before setting on the placid lake.

"Ohhhh, Dad, you're the best-est pilot in the world!"

"I need a smoke," blustered Bearhead lighting up, forehead furrowed and sweat-soaked.

Graywood waded to shore and paddled back the beige canoe. Three roundtrips deposited Bearhead, Bobby, and all the gear. Bearhead selected the alpha arboreal to pitch the tent by and slung the metal food bin from the stoutest branch of a nearby great spruce. Graywood tethered *Seneca* and completed the post-flight checklist. Bobby hunted down the target tree for bow-and-arrow lessons.

A nonchalant family of pintail ducks floated across in front.

Clearing his lungs with the cool air draped in forest mulch, Bearhead beat out an acceptance chant on the Raven drum. "Gary, this is good refuge," he assessed. "There are bears about. We must be careful with trash."

"At nightfall, I'll hoist the junk can high in the big spruce *Seneca*'s roped to," answered Graywood.

"Dad, I found the tree for my target."

"Show me."

An alder rooted aside a muddy beach swath sixty yards beyond the aircraft sparkled under the sun. It beckoned, and Bearhead approved, saying, "We'll take the lower limbs. They're green and make good smoke, keeps the skeeters down."

"Come evening, the breeze off the big Sister should zap away the bugs too," said Graywood, uncasing a hatchet. Methodically he lopped off branches.

Before departing Lake Hood, Bearhead and Graywood split who'd teach what skills in this non-consequential environment: kayaking and canoeing went to Graywood; Uncle Roe drew fishing and archery. Together they'd develop Bobby's responsibility, accountability, discipline, and natural spirit.

"Bobby, let's have a try with the essence of the bow," intoned Bearhead. He measured the horizon's light with an outstretched hand to blot the sun, paced thirty feet, and plucked a score of granite stones into a circle measuring a yard in diameter. Threading back, he whittled a sharp point on a three-foot alder bough with a bone knife to craft a short spear.

"Aim the wood's center to hit inside the circle," he instructed Bobby. "When you get six times in a row, we'll string your bow and hang the target."

"Bearhead's a great coach," thought Graywood. "He'll make archery non-intimidating and shape inherent impediments into opportunities to transform the bowstring into a clever extension of Bobby's arm. Over and over, they'll practice drawing stances and delivery sequences until both become an ethos. In some things, uncles are the better teachers for boys."

Before leaving Bethel, Alaska, Graywood had kayaked the Kuskokwim River to photograph waterfowl, mammals, and terrain, as well as discover secluded fishing spots. Upon relocating to Anchorage, he'd explored the islands dotted on the Knik River. He felt like a bowling pin jammed into the little round hole making the boat's hatch, and as the years passed, the cramping claustrophobic numbness he felt seemed to come faster to thighs and feet. Graywood gave the vintage watercraft away after he bought the navy-blue, hybrid kayak-canoe for Campsite.

Bobby, like his dad, called it ky-canoe. Twelve feet long and three feet wide at the waterline, it resembled a short, flattened sea kayak. Less bulky than the old box Graywood had lugged, it weighed forty kilograms. Its broader beam required a few extra strokes to glide along the surface, but the permanent bottom skeg allowed it to readily track and made maneuvers less difficult. The extra beam width gave an all-wheel-drive stability, even when Graywood freely moved pelvis and legs to avoid muscles tightening up. Its inset modular attachment allowed either one or two occupants. Padded sling cushions strapped onto the seat platforms placed the pullers a good foot above the water. Even a small motor could be attached aft to troll. Its flexibility had enticed Graywood the most.

Swooshing the Kuskokwim River in the old kayak had needed more problem-solving skills than innate talent. The prime objective was avoiding flipping over. Alaskan waters remained unbearably cold despite wearing a neoprene suit for hypothermia protection. Wet entries and exits were expected, even with the best technique employed to control the vessel's tip-over nature.

The ky-canoe's inherent balance negated that curse.

Graywood and Bobby coursed the lake in the beige canoe first. The aluminum double-bladed paddles seemed eager to feather glassy water. With or against a southwestern zephyr, father and son practiced until Bobby's strokes attained power and purpose.

On the second day with Bearhead, the young archer-to-be advanced from stubby spear to junior-sized woodland bow. A full-arm draw pulled fifty-eight pounds. Striking any part of the target from thirty feet with the bowstring half tensed became this summer's goal. Next year when Bobby would be stronger, Bearhead would coach three-quarter draws for forty- and fifty-foot ranges. By age eleven or twelve, sporting greater triceps and shoulder muscles hewn from hours in the ky-canoe, the boy could, Graywood hoped, manage adult equipment and ranges—senior woodland or English longbows with their standard arrows.

Modeling for the student, Bearhead stepped forty yards from the target and uncased his woodland bow from the quiver, meticulously beaded in leather, that his uncle had given him. Demonstrating the fluid motion inherent in a master bowman half his age, he let fly one steel-tipped shaft. It hit the bull's-eye.

The archery sessions gave way to an afternoon of learning hooks and catching dinner from the canoe.

With Bobby and Bearhead engaged, Graywood ky-canoed to where the unnamed river opened the tarn to Cook Inlet. Frothing water cascaded parapets of boulders before it languished in the downstream estuary—prime habitat for migrating juvenile salmon to rest, eat, and hide from predators prior to venturing out to sea.

Forgoing a misted, whitewater adventure, Graywood zigzagged the lake's southern edge and startled fourteen herons as the sun tucked beyond the tallest Sister to dampen the sky into a resplendent palette of greys. Normal grey and whitish grey fingered the distant west. Arsenic grey to true grey wandered the east where the herons hunted hard, spearing fish. Bluish and dark grey receded northward as the boat swept the flat water past a flotilla of green-winged teals. Maren would have had a name for every grey. Graywood wondered if Jen might too … and missed her.

Evening created inky shadows and enhanced the outlines of stones and fallen trees guarding the water's rim. The dark vaults of forest gloom with their broken needle scents, where bear and moose and man stole to streams to drink below the mountain snows, gratified his soul—Alaska, so generous its beauty; so severe the means to living.

He angled back to the encampment lying in its own ribbon of emerald-grey. Maren would have had a precise name for that color too.

Powerful camp coffee greeted Graywood gliding to shelter. There was Bearhead, his elder, munching dried zucchini chips dipped in hummus, one hand holding a lit smoke. And Bobby, the bull's-eye of Graywood's heart, stood nearby waving.

"We've got rainbow trout ready to grill for supper," shouted Bearhead.

"Who caught the most?" yelled Graywood, knowing Bearhead's uncanny skill to read the water and see the fish.

"Bobby landed one. He'll catch more tomorrow when he lets the line arch like Brandy Belle's back when she stretches in the sun."

"Hurry, Dad. I'm hungry!"

"Can you wait and help me tie up the ky-canoe for the night?"

"It's so hard, Dad."

Midnight rain.

Summer languidness broken.

Moisture beading tent.

A sleeping-bag womb.

Carefree and dry, Bobby slept safe between Dad and Uncle Roe.

Emerging to the morning whine of insects, Graywood inhaled chilled air flavored by moss, spruce, and soggy brambles. Waterfowl crowded the lake. He planned the ky-canoe exploits for Bobby's day.

Bearhead joined wearing a water-repellent poncho, its workable hood tugged atop the ball cap sent by Cashel Goodlette touting a logo for the NOAA vessel, *Miller Freeman* R-223. "Gary, I'll start breakfast once I'm settled," promised Bearhead, hands delving side pockets underneath his fishing vest in search for tobacco and paper.

After devouring biscuits and leftover smoke-fried trout, Graywood and Bobby rehearsed kayak safety maneuvers: they smartly swung legs to prevent tip overs entering the craft, practiced wet emergency exits, and polished shallow-water turns to remain upright for two pullers compared to one.

With a team's confidence, they crossed the tarn's gossamer face. Shaggy trees danced in and out of the shore fog wisps while the basin's center speckled in glitters of light.

By noon, the calculated program to enhance Bobby's concentration appeared to have modestly worked. Graywood savored the "we've made it" sensation of progress. In time, the false limits of the past—Ritalin and its restrictions—yoked to the child would cease.

During Bobby's afternoon bow practice, the great brown bear calculated the trio of two-legged creatures with subtle indifference. Like a towering man at half a ton, upright in stance he commanded nine feet—the better way to study the human dwarfs.

"Bobby … do … very … still," whispered Bearhead. Snaillike, he drew out a solo stride toward the beast to form the apex in a three-person defense. He didn't have to tell Graywood to hold motionless.

The senior Raven brought palms together in the tantric ritual of splayed fingers before the face and raised both forearms parallel to cheekbones to enlarge his skull's appearance.

Ursa Major sniffed the air. His narrowed eyes darted back and forth on the triad to center on Bearhead. Two silent men and a boy faced nature's overlord.

Blood pounded to Graywood's pores, his mind raced what he'd risk to save his son should the monster charge. Only a bird pecking a far-off tree broke the quartet's mutual entrancement.

Grunting, the brown terminated his regal posture and dropped to all fours with a demeanor that indicated no imminent attack. With the right forepaw, he disdained the ground by plowing a lengthy ribbon of dirt as if searching for something. With rounded nostrils, he reviewed the bipedal beasts, relaxed his nose fur, and rambled to the ridge where wild berry bushes bulged heavy with fruit.

"I've dreamed of a majestic brown like him," spoke Bearhead. With reverence he watched the sovereign vanish on patrol of the realm. "He's a powerful king but won't attack today."

"How do you know that?" blurted Graywood, wide-eyed, clutching his son.

"He believes we're a pack of ugly-looking wolves belched from the big loon you've tied to the spruce tree. He's granted temporary rights to us to be here," said Bearhead to reassure. "I told him we'd move on before the full moon."

"What!"

"He's protected you every time you've come, Gary."

"Roe, get serious," challenged Graywood.

"Since the first time you've landed *Seneca* on the lake, he's looked out for you. Thought it strange you and the loon left a canoe and kayak the last time you came. Since you and the loon keep bringing more stuff, he thought it wise to make a showing."

"Roe, please …"

"Gary, that's what he said."

"All right," said Graywood, playing along. "Why does he think *Seneca*'s a big loon?"

"She's in the water by the shore."

"Why not an eagle or raven?"

"*Seneca*'s always sitting on water when not flying. He's never seen her any place else, like roosting in a tree. You haven't set her down in any trees lately, have you, Gary?"

Graywood ignored the jab and tried another tactic to trip Bearhead up. "Well, Roe, this time we didn't bring any more stuff."

"You brought Bobby and me."

"Huh?"

"Bobby and me. To a bear, anything not natural to his domain is stuff."

"Stuff?"

"Yeah, stuff. They've got another word for it in bear talk, but it's too hard to say … way too many guttural clicks to pronounce it right. Only my uncle could click-speak it."

"You can talk to bears?" Bobby marveled and let go of his dad's hand.

"It's not exactly talking. We speak a lot with our eyes ... and reach an understanding."

Awed, Bobby remained silent.

Graywood uttered a moan and gazed sideways at Bearhead letting him know he'd not suspend disbelief regarding inter-species ocular communication.

"He told me a couple more things," added Bearhead. "There're ample fish uplake and in the river. To them, we're welcome. But we're not allowed to go beyond the dirt streak he's made on the ground."

With the big brown in the area, Graywood appreciated Bearhead constructing a terrain limit so Bobby always adhered close to them. What better way to get his son to follow an instruction than when commanded by the bear king.

Curious, Bobby asked, "Why can't we go past it, Uncle Roe?"

"There's a mother bear with two yearling cubs feeding beyond the ridge. She's very protective and will kill us if we even look her way cross-eyed. It's really, really important, Bobby, we avoid her and her children. Our bear has warned us to stay right by the shore, and all should be fine. So don't dare go beyond the line he's clawed."

"I think it's time for a quiet," said Graywood, attempting to decompress his own surges of anxiety. Yet he'd been swayed by Bearhead's clairvoyance. How did his friend know of the resident sow and cubs? He'd never told Bearhead of them ... somehow that mystery had legs. Tonight once Bobby had fallen asleep, Graywood would get Bearhead to reveal how he knew.

And Graywood admired Bearhead's proffered ability to talk to a bear and remain unharmed. He imagined his mentor setting safety perimeters for Chitina's children long ago, warning them the brown bear was a great and horrible ancestor to the First Peoples—the embodiment of strength, courage, and cold belligerence—and how its bravery compared formidable and fearless to all other living things.

Graywood decided they'd fish the afternoon but depart the following morning. Tonight, Bobby would sleep in *Seneca.*

The airplane had cradled Bobby for hours, yet Graywood and Bearhead stoked the midnight campfire and conferred at length before they reclined in the nylon tent. The speckled Milky Way wrapped the August constellations within its thin scrim. Perched on the horizon, the crescent moonlight marred away none of the stellar formations marking the heavenly dome.

The two Ravens contemplated Bobby, Jennelle, April, May, Chitina, the university, the health-care dilemma, and the upcoming 2008 election. Only when the blaze burned down to chars did they fall into deeper exchanges.

"I look up, everything is one," said Bearhead.

"Amazing how infinite and eternal," agreed Graywood.

"But we have to split off pieces for a closer look," said Bearhead, with a sigh.

"Guess we do … to understand the parts better."

"Don't know if that gets us any closer to the truth."

"Guess so. Our splits are mostly arbitrary anyway."

"Look, a shooting star," exhorted Bearhead.

"Almost time for the Pleiades," said Graywood. "Maybe he's an advance scout. Want some more tea?"

"Nah. Don't want to piss too much in the dark."

"You worried about that brown coming back?"

"I believe he'll leave us alone," reassured Bearhead.

"I hope so." Graywood emptied two sugar packets into a metal cup and finger swirled the contents. "So, Roe, when I split off a piece of creation, I hope to learn something from it."

"Yeah, like it should grow your mind and spirit some. That's what I hope for me."

"Like splitting off a piece of myself and really looking at it," pondered Graywood.

"Yeah, but I have to be careful not to reduce myself down."

"Reduce down?" asked Graywood, confused.

"Yeah, make myself too simple."

"You're anything but simple, Roe."

"I don't know. Sometimes I think I'm only an amalgamation of Higgs bosons interspersed through eleven dimensions."

"What? For Christ's sake, you crazy? What've you been smoking?"

"Am I?"

"C'mon, where'd you pick up on Higgs bosons?" asked Graywood

"I think last month's *Scientific American*."

"Oh, haven't read it. What'd it say?"

"They're gonna fire up the Hadron Collider by Geneva," updated Bearhead, "and try to prove Higgs bosons exist."

"Remind me what the hell's a boson?"

"Supposed to be the fundamental component to the origin of particle mass," explained Bearhead.

"Come again?"

"A boson is the smallest piece of mass. It takes a gigantic bunch of 'em to make an electron and way more for a proton or a neutron."

"Ah, for a second I thought you said the origin of species."

"No, not Darwin, I said the origin of particle mass … as in physics."

"So you're saying Higgs bosons are in quarks and mesons and neutrinos?"

"Have to be if they're fundamental to physics."

"Can you imagine what Piper would say if told he was a huge blob of Higgs bosons?" kidded Graywood.

"No, what would he say?"

Graywood stood to think, reached for the last piece of wood, and tossed it on the fire.

Bearhead sipped the remnant of tea and repeated, "Tell me, Gary, what would Piper say?"

"There's a hell of a lot more to me than a bunch of Higgs bozos."

"Bozos," Bearhead chuckled, "that's funny."

"Then he'd spit on your boots and ask how many bozos were glued into a hunk of snot," popped Graywood, "and rant about all the tax money wasted on stupid theories like bozos."

The crackling coals hurled a shower of sparks into the celestial vault as the lunar rim tucked under clouds. *Seneca*'s moored silhouette vanished from the lake.

"So what you're saying, Roe, is theoretical physicists have reduced the universe down to Higgs bosons?"

"I guess that's what they're trying to prove," said Bearhead, fighting off the urge to smoke.

"Probably tougher to prove bosons than dark matter and dark energy," speculated Graywood.

"I wished physics had stopped at Newton," said Bearhead. "For our time and space, that's all we need."

"You bet, old man ... good old, everyday physics. Newt's brand is good enough to fly *Seneca.*

"Good enough for cellphones too?" teased Bearhead.

"Cellphones? Hell, only when I need to use one. What a plain nuisance."

"You sound like Piper."

"He's got a point 'bout how the world's full of useless contraptions with too many buttons to push. Makes it all too complicated."

"Most people practice their own brands of physics anyway; they just call it by another name, that's all," observed Bearhead.

"So what other names are used?"

"Oh, common names derived from science or religion, whatever makes the most philosophical sense at the time."

"Do you mean pieces of nature or some religious cult?"

"Those or bigger pieces or both mixed together."

"You're losing me," said Graywood.

"Don't want that. Let's say the hierarchy of physics points all science towards the Higgs boson. If the Higgs boson is the ultimate pinnacle of reduction in the universe, what's the ultimate in religion?"

"I suppose one of the faiths, but I know where you're going, Roe. You're going to say each faith is only one aspect of God, one of his faces ... that each faith is a single reduction of God."

"I wasn't following that line of thought, Gary, but it's pretty good. No, I was leading towards something like the hierarchy of any religion points you to God. It could be argued that both God and bosons are, fundamentally, our poor placeholders toward understanding all nature and the universe and whatever happens after we die."

"Ahh, that age-old question again. You ring it up whenever we gab under the sky. Are you okay, Roe? Is something the matter? Your breathing getting worse?"

"I'm fine, Gary. Just as slow as ever."

"If that bear had charged today, I'm not sure Bobby and I would've played dead. We'd have outrun you."

"I know."

"And tonight you'd be bear poop."

"Good poop, I hope."

"Yeah, the bear best, Roe. Thank God he didn't."

He was merciful," acknowledged Bearhead.

So what you're saying, God's the ultimate in religion for us?"

"Yeah, I'll go further and humanize it—Buddha, Jesus Christ, and Charles Darwin are three great examples."

"That's quite a trio. I suppose you picked Darwin for the secular religious example, right?" asked Graywood.

"Yeah. He represents the embodied pinnacle of the Higgs boson."

"Charles Darwin, a Higgs boson?"

"Yeah, but let's call him a tremendous group of bosons. Entertain this notion, Gary, that in secular religion you can condense biology and Darwin's natural selection down to chemistry and chemistry down to physics and, from there, presto, the ultimate supercluster of Higgs bosons."

"It's hard to imagine all those constellations up there as massive clusters of bosons. I'd favor the trio of humans you gave, but I gotta check on Bobby. Can you heap some embers over that last log?"

"Sure."

An agitated northern shoveler cautioned its companions with a "took-took" alert when Graywood trudged toward the aircraft. He whistled Tchaikovsky's *Violin Concerto in D* to ward off any larger animals he might cross.

Seneca secure. No restless bears … or moose. Bobby safe asleep.

Bearhead gathered some downed branches to prolong the flames … and their talk. Both men settled.

"Okay," resumed Bearhead, "we got to buzzing about nature and philosophy."

"You mean science and religion."

"Yeah, more or less. They're both philosophies to me. You're just making another social split to plow up the world differently."

"Yeah, I suppose you're right. Old Cashel Goodlette idolizes Carl Popper's reasoning 'bout science having its unique philosophy, which sets it apart from everything else.

"And there's the third split I'm partial to."

"Third?"

"Buddha's third way of compassion for all things."

"Please, Roe, put a hold on him and stick to science and western religion."

"Sure, Gary, and I promise not to mention the four noble truths."

"Not even once?"

"Not a word so long as there's a glowing ember."

The moon uncovered from the clouds, but the sickle of light erased none of the tiny sparkling orbs beyond.

"Lots of people look to nature for insight," stated Graywood. "From all that looking, they evolve philosophies of science."

"You can say the same for creating religious philosophies for why we're here at all. Science and religion compete with and complement each other. Maybe like chocolate and vanilla ice cream complementing and competing for our tongues."

"Two flavors of ice cream philosophy for the same universe ... uh, Roe, please don't go Baskin-Robbins on me."

"Nah, let's stick to two and say one's a reduction to bosons and the other's an induction to Christ, Buddha, and the other faces of God. So which do you prefer, Gary?"

"Trying to trick me, Roe? I know how you think. What if I trip you up and say I prefer both reduction and induction."

"I like both, too, but must admit I'm partial to Buddha and Christ over bosons."

"Suppose you're right, Roe. Reducing everything down to Higgs bosons seems futile. You'll wonder what makes up a boson next."

"For sure, that's been the pattern. Remember when atoms were composed of nothing smaller than electrons, protons, and neutrons? Then they smashed 'em up and got into quarks and meson soups and neutrinos. And string theory came along with branes, and eleven dimensions ... Who'd have thought it?" recounted Bearhead.

"And the collider in Switzerland shall one day confirm Higgs bosons exist, and we'll have to start asking what they're made of."

"Mini-bosons," Bearhead jested, "and it'll just keep going, smaller and smaller.

"Micro-mini-bosons!" trumped Graywood.

"You'll wonder what's the point of it all."

"I can hear Piper making mini-bozo jokes, like how many can dance on the head of a pin. Remember when he said that about neutrinos?"

"No, I don't. I wasn't there."

"Oh, right. You weren't. That happened round last year. Jen, Cash, and I were trying to explain subatomic particles to Piper before he flew Cash to a North Slope data collection site. I don't recall how it all started, but I remember Piper patiently listening and at the end asking us how they'd affect *Sky Woman* flying north and how many danced on the head of a pin."

"What'd you tell him?"

"Well, nothing. We felt kinda stupid."

"So to Piper, neutrinos and bosons are really science fiction," reiterated Bearhead.

"Actually fairy tales. They don't exist to him."

"Perhaps he'd say Jesus Christ is more real to him than a Higgs boson will ever be?"

"Well, he's a damn fine pilot and prays to the Almighty every time he flies. Says praying helps his dyslexia."

The combusting stack of branches abruptly condensed, and one rolled out of the circle of stones. Graywood flipped it back with a cottonwood stick.

"Gary, I want to tell you how fascinated I was a couple of years back when you lectured the WWAMI students about medical sensitivity and specificity."

"Really?"

"Yeah, and I borrowed the four-square grid you'd explained and adapted it to better understand and communicate belief systems."

"You mean you kind of made up a belief grid that displays true- and false-positives along with true- and false- negatives?" asked Graywood.

"Yeah."

"Well that's mighty curious." Graywood paused and thought, "Roe's latched on to the bivariate analysis grid epidemiologists employ whenever assessing for associations." Needing clarity, Graywood asked, "Can you give an example?"

"Well, try this out," offered Bearhead. "I match two cultural questions or viewpoints into the four squares. I call them intersecting dualities."

"You're gettin' ahead of me."

"Sorry. So, Gary, take two questions … uh, such as does Jesus Christ exist and do Higgs bosons exist. Assign the positive and negative designations that represent their existence or not and place them in your four-square grid."

"Let me get this straight. Jesus is a true-positive or a true-negative, or he can be a false-positive or a false-negative?"

"Right! But stick only to true-positive and true-negative for now and assign the same possibilities to the Higgs boson."

"And you place Jesus and the boson in the same four-square grid?" asked Graywood.

"Yes, the same grid that'll give you four subsets of peoples' beliefs for the conditions of existence or not as posed by the two questions."

"Let me work this out," said Graywood, making the comparisons in his head. "One grid square will represent people who believe both Jesus and the boson are genuine, the second will believe Jesus is for real but not the boson, a third square has no belief in Jesus but truly believes bosons exist, and the fourth thinks neither is legitimate."

"That's it, Gary. You and I accept that both exist, Piper believes in the second square, Darwin and his progeny to include our friend Cashel argue for the third, but I'm at a loss right now to name anyone representing the fourth."

"Okay, so you've got four subsets of belief."

"Yes. And the best part is all four are allowed actuality."

"Even the one having someone who doesn't believe in Jesus or bosons?"

"Yeah, even that."

"Whoever he is, what does he believe in?"

"Well, Gary, try another grid and see what's possible."

"Another grid?"

"Yeah, take the dualities of whether religion or natural selection best explains the mystery of our world."

"Okay. You'll have the first square representing people who believe that both religion and natural selection explain the mystery of—"

"Or that both explain a part of our universe," amplified Bearhead, "and when put together, they do a better job."

"Okay, sure. You need both to try to explain our existence."

"And the other three squares?"

"Well, you've got the one containing those who exclusively believe religion but not natural selection being sufficient to explain our cryptic origins; the third holds those who believe natural selection solely explains our being here, which makes religion a myth; and the last square garners the few who accept neither religion nor natural selection will deliver the really true insights about the universe."

"It's kinda fun to imagine all sorts of grids like this."

"I have to admit I've never matched up Jesus and a boson," said Graywood.

"Substitute Charles Darwin for bosons. Rethink him as natural selection in the flesh, just as Jesus Christ is God incarnate.

"Oh, I see. Use Jesus and Darwin in the grid as respective personifications of God and the boson."

"So where's your belief set point in this grid?" asked Bearhead.

"Tonight under the Milky Way, I'm definitely in the square that's positive for both Jesus and Darwin."

"Or the similar grid square that matches up God and the boson as both positive."

"Yeah, sure, that too."

"You prefer to be a lumper rather than a splitter," declared Bearhead.

"Yeah, I tend to lump more the older I get. But I still split the world apart when needed."

"Do you ever think you'll change perspectives and migrate into one of the other three squares?"

"Never."

The golden-orange flames had reduced to rivulets. Graywood stretched and said, "I'm tired, Roe. I'll check Bobby and head off for sleep." He enjoyed getting into Roe's head … and might borrow Bearhead's intersecting duality model and compare the Campsite method of treating Bobby's ADHD against Doctor Timm's extended-release Ritalin. Eyes focused to Polaris, Graywood stepped out of the fire's light and gasped, "Look, a shooting star!"

But Bearhead studied Graywood's profile—a shadow merged to the black forest wall. Gary's frame had flattened into two dimensions. Bearhead doubted his friend's "never" and yearned to ratchet duality grids up a notch and reason with Graywood the resultant plus-and-minus comparisons between western philosophies, such as Plato and Immanuel Kant or Descartes and Occam's razor. More so, he wished to contemplate how a major change in one's personal spirit might propel the soul into any one of the territories marked off within the four-square realms.

But none of that happened tonight. Still, for Bearhead, it had been a day of great wonder with Graywood, Bobby, and the bear. He banked the ashes and slept gentle into the good night.

CHAPTER TEN

ADVENT

A broken axle on one of the two Volkswagens delayed the team's return leg.

Brazilian and CDC public health personnel had compiled outcome data from rural clinics situated 120 to 170 kilometers northeast of Brasilia. In Doctor Daniels's seventh visit to the country in three years, the search for answers remained elusive to the how-and-why questions regarding the worldwide HIV vaccine failure.

Jennelle and a co-worker elected to overnight at the village near the sidelined clunker while the rest squeezed into the serviceable vehicle and headed to the capital. A repair crew would retrieve the stranded volunteers the following morning.

Accommodations approached Spartan. Coin-flipping her partner for the choice between two rooms above the canteen fronting the plaza, she won the bed with box springs. Oppressive heat negated the need for blankets. Both chambers lacked window screens.

The unisex bathroom at the pinched hall's far end offered a pipe hole to toilet squat. Tepid, rust-tinged water dripped from a decrepit faucet to a cracked basin and spotted the wooden floor. An empty soap dispenser, lying helpless on stained floorboards, had broken off the wall over the sink. The local version of an Australian bucket shower, missing curtains, hung in the corner. Parked aside the crap hole, a quarter-filled lime pail with yellow-stenciled Portuguese instructed the user to dispense ONLY ONE 30 c.c. scoop of powder down the orifice to tamper malodor when finished.

Throughout the stagnant night, Jennelle welcomed tobacco and marijuana fumes braiding up from the downstairs pub to mask the stench. When asked to supper, she declined her colleague's offer out of fear of food poisoning and cautioned him to do the same. Bearing the nocturnal ordeal, she rationed bottled water timed to their pending rescue.

Hoards of mosquitoes attacked without mercy at sunrise and roused Jennelle from spotty sleep, too often interrupted by the bellicose drunks and sultry air. As applied the prior evening, she rubbed on DEET repellant yet shunned the poncho for skin cover to avoid overheating.

Three days later in Brasilia, fever, headache, and muscle pains struck. She suspected a bad case of flu. Her temperature abated the next afternoon, but the succeeding morning, she collapsed stepping from the shower. Rushed to intensive care, she had signs of shock with pinhead red spots scattered across her body. Worse, both nose and gums bled. She'd contracted dengue hemorrhagic fever from the mosquitoes. Jennelle almost died.

Letters, emails, and postcards to Graywood and Bobby ceased.

Romances never endure when challenged too long by distance and …

The August adventure to Campsite became an annual rite for Graywood and Bobby. Thrice, Bearhead accompanied.

Bobby stood in the ky-canoe's hatch the third summer, pulled Bearhead's bowstring, and shot an arrow seventy feet from shore toward the target tree. Missing the bull's-eye by a yard, the point penetrated a gnarled knot deep. When Bearhead extracted the shaft, it splintered off the metal barb.

"Now, alderwood, you're marked by a tough little spike," mumbled Bearhead. "If Overlord saw, I pray he forgives us leaving behind more stuff."

Unforeseen Chitina tribal issues forced Bearhead to decline the fourth Campsite sojourn. Piper, however, rearranged his hauling schedules and trekked there with Graywood and Bobby. In tandem, *Seneca* led the Beaver after the Lake Hood takeoffs—Piper had conceded to fly as Graywood's wingman.

The flight coursed south from Anchorage over the breast of blue sea abutting the west coast of Cook Inlet to Augustine Island—a 4,025-foot volcano vectored ten miles southeast from Tignagvik Point on Kamishak Bay. Its cauldron had erupted in 2006 to form a fresh dome.

Beyond the crater, the route veered to Bruin Bay. Guarding the coast and access to the Seven Sisters stood Big Hill, topping four thousand feet.

Skirting the tidal flat, the aircraft followed the river that flowed from Lake Venturi to the sea. Two miles short from the basin, they banked north and zipped the *V*-gap cleaving the two Sisters ahead of the unnamed triangular tarn. Shooting the chasm to glide onto placid waters gave a visual treat to any pilot introduced to the enclave. Graywood imagined Piper's enchantment when he pierced the tight valley and set the Beaver on the aquatic, glass-smooth surface.

A modest river drained the Sisters' backsides through the northern strand. Graywood anchored *Seneca* aside the channel's mouth. Piper followed. The parked floatplanes surrounded by virgin mountains rested in stark contrast to Lake Hood's flying-machine congestion engulfed by modern, overbearing Anchorage.

Piper stayed two days to capture the ever-changing countenances on the Sisters. Dawn, afternoon, and dusk, he sketched their dazzling faces and backed up the impressions with digitals to sharpen the natural lines. Come freeze-up, he'd brighten the drawn transitions with colored solar hues.

"How'd you find this place?" Piper asked the evening they arrived.

"More by accident than design," replied Graywood. "I was working my southwest clinic assistance loop but took a different route on the back leg between Naknek and Seldovia."

"A bit out of your way. Bad weather forced the switch?"

"Nah," answered Graywood in a reflective, softer tone. He ambled to the easel.

Piper had edged bold shades to a graceful portrait of the prominent Sister, denuded by the fading twilight. He noticed Graywood comparing the natural wonder to the artwork and pronounced, "That Sister's gotta be mother watching over the lake. Don't you see it belongs to her?"

Caught off guard, Graywood uttered, "You're talking like Roe."

"Guess ol' Monroe would've said something good like that," confirmed Piper. "Cash would've too. He thinks all mountains are mothers." Piper dropped back eight feet to eye the rendition. "If no air turbulence day after tomorrow, I'll snap a few shots from six thousand feet. From there, she'll look the big tit she is."

Graywood grinned. Piper sounded back to normal.

"So why the change on your route back?" queried Piper, touching up the picture.

To render in-person assistance visits three times a year between thaw and freeze-up, Graywood navigated a southwest, five-day clinic loop from Anchorage to King Salmon and Naknek and then circled back via Seldovia and Seward. He reviewed out-patient procedures and provided updates and advice. Most of all, he assessed staff morale.

But three years ago after the Naknek stopover, an inclination had compelled him to soar northward over Iliamna Lake. Upon reaching Kakhonak Bay, he banked eastward and flipped on his mental terrain compass for Augustine Volcano. As *Seneca* approached Cook Inlet, a curious force from the Seven Sisters reached out and beckoned him to look at the lake they protected. The tranquil water sparkled as a crown jewel, and he touched down on the glazed surface.

To tell the discovery to Piper that way oozed too much sentiment. So Graywood said, "I got a yearning to take a different route to Seldovia. Had plenty of gas and some extra time."

"It's prime country, Gary. Don't think it's been sketched before. Damn straight glad I'm first."

By Graywood's invitation, Piper's code of conduct required obtaining permission, direct or indirect, for commercial uses of the area, be it camping, hunting, or drawing. "What should we call this piece," asked Piper, "when I'm done paintin' it?" Letting Graywood title the work meant getting consent.

There were more unnamed lakes in Alaska than all the lakes in Minnesota and almost as many nameless mountains. Graywood scanned the panorama that had posed for Piper's creation yet decided against an inscription. He might ask Bobby for a name, but they already called the place Campsite. That unadorned term for their fond escape touched best. Besides, to title something fancy implied ownership, and no one should have rights to all this. Graywood felt blessed just to skim in and stay awhile.

"Call it what it is," declared Graywood. "View from Campsite."

"That'll work," grunted Piper. "Skeeters ain't too bad here." He put the pencil's stub to his lips and hand-rolled the day's efforts into waterproof map cases.

"Yeah, that's the case most of the times we've come," confirmed Graywood. "The new air force bug repellant works better than DEET. That helps too."

"DEET juice does a damn fine job. What's the new stuff called?"

"You'll like the name," said Graywood. Elaborating each syllable in the primary chemical compound and repeating it quickly as he did for any long first-time word for Bobby, he said, "a-cyl-PIPER-i-dine, acylpiperidine."

Piper smiled enough to show teeth, and the pencil dropped from his mouth. "Damn straight name, but a bit too much. I'd shorten it to Piper-juice." He reached down to retrieve his tool. "Suppose it'll be fine to draw some more tomorrow?" Piper half-asked, half-telegraphed for any camp agenda Graywood might have that included him.

"Do as much as you want," granted Graywood. "After breakfast, Bobby and I'll lake fish." He extracted beers from the ice chest and offered one for their nightcap. "You see that expanded ridge along the upper part of the river?"

"Yep," said Piper, taking a can and popping its top.

"It splits the valley up where there's a big brown sow who claims it every year for her cubs. We don't provoke her. So never go there."

"She ever come down to the tents?"

"Nope. We make heaps of noise and stink up the place. She knows we're here and stays away. She'll shepherd upstream or give us the wide berth. Closest she's come with cubs was three hundred yards over there by that stone crop stabbing into the water."

"Think I can get a bear family portrait?"

"Christ, Piper, do what you want. Just remember Bobby and I'll be out in the canoe and can't help when you piss momma off and your butt gets bit."

"Gotcha, Gary. I'll keep put."

The imposed human order of the day gave way to creeping moonlight and the pilots' evening ritual. If Bearhead had been here, they'd have stoked the fire and philosophized awhile. With Piper, it played opposite. Rationalizations yielded scant merit on a short summer night. He preferred solitude underneath the stars or a self-possessed friend.

And Graywood welcomed either way as well.

Piper traced eleven picture backgrounds without a bear encounter and tagged each to four photos of contrasting brightness for the wintertime studio assembly with paints. Rich ripples outsourced dark shades of coming nightfall and controlled the landscape's mood to create the black-silver mesh on which Piper hung the bold palettes of color.

Natural light hailed as the artist's supreme friend, and light reinforced its primal importance whenever Piper sought out the better way to land the Beaver or *Sky Woman* in all types of weather on half-thawed tundra or makeshift, potholed runways. If he misjudged the brilliance in a descent onto cracked ice fields or gravel river bars, both plane and pilot might be damaged, or worse. Piper marveled at how light beautified the harsher terrain and how it kept him alive.

Often in the studio when he compared a sketch to its photographs, he'd discover the horizon's details had been roughed out in reverse. But backwards never happened with views of the ground from above. For that he thanked the God-given radiances and the ability to judge them from on high. Old pilots and good artists respected the light. Younger amateurs who didn't, didn't last.

Piper and the Beaver departed Campsite to resume their back-country hauling schedule. At Katmai National Park, they retrieved a smart-assed party of government surveyors. Suffering their obnoxious bravado, Piper vowed to keep Graywood's refuge secret and never show or sell its artwork. He respected his partner's hidden sanctuary as he did the light.

Jennelle phoned Graywood to explain five months of avoided communication. She recounted the bout with dengue and how her CDC colleague, a pure godsend, had nursed her recovery. After catching up on Bobby, Jennelle stated her co-worker had proposed marriage. Graywood agreed to cease contact so she, in fairness, could consider accepting the offer.

A year lapsed before Jennelle declined.

She wished to restart the letters and emails to Graywood and Bobby but honestly could not without a face-to-face encounter to reassess their emotions … if ever that occurred.

Graywood reckoned she'd married. Would she ever tell him?

For three years from the 2008 election, failure persisted in the nation's leadership. Stark, factional divisions embedded within polarized politics drummed out discontent from both the Democratic and Republican parties. Despite Democratic majorities in both houses of the 111th Congress and the passage of a stimulus package, long-term conservatives outnumbered the liberals. The fundamental tension that pitted zealots wishing a never-ending governmental stimulus against those adamant to rein in federal spending permeated throughout Washington.

Egotism for retaining one's district or senate seat prevailed over nation building. Votes cast had eyes on how they'd play back home. Power and mind-game mentoring mixed well with special interest groups resourced by larders of cash. Incumbents who represented districts that swung back and forth Republican and Democrat held the most influence because their fears limited their courage and greased the gridlock.

Voters beyond the Beltway wanted government to work but worried how it over-promised and under-delivered. They prayed for legislators to solve problems, yet each political party degraded the other and therefore discredited Uncle Sam altogether. Anxious Americans yearned for change while the nation's wealth stagnated and retracted. Everyone feared scarcity the most—its empty, withdrawn hands shrinking their lives.

Belief in government had declined for years, and it nosedived in 2005 after the subpar responses by local, state, and federal officials to Hurricane Katrina. Trust bottomed with the 2007-2008 financial crisis. The spirited words meant to bandage the public's shredded faith at the 2009 presidential inauguration—change, responsibility, hope, and leadership—had barely pierced the chilled air before contrary, truncated truths stalked the capital and fanned the country's flaming rage.

Ideological warfare in Washington mattered more than the citizens' day-to-day concerns from Delaware to Des Moines to Deadwood. Insincere, out-of-control factional politics defied reason and devastated the country. "Washington is broken" and "Does anybody hold anyone accountable for anything?" were kinder declamations emitted beyond the Beltway in tandem with congressional approval ratings rarely topping the teens.

Many concluded Washington perverse and useless as droves of lobbyists and kleptocrats—acting like surrogate, subterranean politicians—pulled the levers that affected large swaths of the administration. These power-brokers believed the common people and their elected proxies were too callow, too uneducated, too sympathetic, or too stupid to fully comprehend preservation of the fiefdoms stitched into the fabric of Beltway factionalism. Their fiendish cultivation and pursuit of divisive clout strengthened political rivalries to cause even more missteps and scores to be settled by blunt payback. Out of these managed plots of domination, the controlling class of lobbyists maintained their petty political agendas. By campaigns of fear and innuendo, they negated impulses toward the unity needed to solve the great issues that threatened the nation's welfare.

But the electorate pushed back. The seven-hundred-billion-dollar rescue package for Wall Street, major banks, and businesses cobbled in Congress during the final months of the Bush administration had radically restructured the conceptual roles of government and business and had shifted the interface between Big Brother and his citizens—laissez faire had fallen out of favor. The media echoed street sentiments such as:

> If you can find funds to rescue banks, then you can come up with effective employment schemes and employment subsidies.
>
> If government can take on the role of lender of last resort, then it has to be employer of last resort, and the doctor and nurse of last resort, too.

Community firebrands coupled the credit market debacles to an earlier decision by the United States Supreme Court—viewed as an unjust ruling in favor of New London, Connecticut—that allowed a municipality to condemn one's home in order to give private property to a real-estate developer. Other festering issues—such as the excessive cost of health care, fear of climate change, the Alternative Minimum Tax, the Iranian nuclear threat, and the country's haphazard responses to the social meltdowns in Pakistan and Afghanistan—reinforced the public's confirmation of a fickle, unresponsive Beltway. Yet foremost in national distrust was the middle-class anger over no solution to the cancerous creep of financial insecurity. The howling rage yoked to the equity turmoil fueled a grassroots movement to bypass the political partisan game-playing.

Minnesota's legislature was first to call for a nationwide Constitutional Convention—as specified under Article Five of the United States Constitution—to save the country. The Gopher State's proposal centered on six critical issues: property rights, health-care reform, a social security rescue plan, an inflation-indexed permanent fix to the alternative minimum tax, term limits, and the national debt. Its principal motive sought to degrade the power of the self-proclaimed Beltway elites by reinvigorating rank-and-file government of the people, by the people, and for the people.

Across Internet chat rooms, blogs, twitters, and electronic mail, citizens advocated and advanced the national convention tidal wave. Out of the non-profane quarter of cyberspace, one read:

> This is the twenty-first century, and we've got to lead the way for change now.
>
> No more partisan game-playing, pandering, and breaking of election-year promises.
>
> Bad people and screwball priorities created this mess in Washington.
>
> We will hold government accountable by convening a Constitutional Convention in accordance with Article Five of our great Constitution of these United States.

Not to be eclipsed, multiple newspaper editorials promulgated subscribers and local civic organizations to sign on to the national convention crusade. They printed:

> People want dramatic change from the current way politics works, the money, the dark lobbying, the whole obscure thing.
>
> We've lost democracy and must re-establish it from the ground up.
>
> We can make the middle class stronger from the bottom up, not the top down.
>
> If there is going to be class warfare, let it be against the political class, whatever their stripes.

Fresh community organizations, such as Chapters for the Convention, were spawned with large memberships that represented diverse occupations and religious beliefs.

By the 2010 bi-election, the national convention movement had mutated from theory into substance: twenty-six states, by referendum or legislation, had voted to officially place the federal government on notice that their chosen representatives would assemble for a national constitutional convention. Article Five of the United States Constitution stipulated legislatures of two-thirds of the several states were required to approve a call for a convention to propose new amendments. With twenty-six states on board, supporters marshaled their swelling resources to bag eight more ahead of the 2012 national election. A crescendo of hope swept each corner of the country—the stagnating logjam of critical, unfinished federal business would break at last.

The convention's political agenda centered on resolution of the Minnesota Super-Six, plus other diverse issues annexed to the movement. Like the initial twenty-seven amendments to the Constitution, any subsequent modification voted out of a national convention had to be ratified by the legislatures of three-fourths of the several states or by state-wide conventions in three-fourths thereof to become embodied in the document.

The potential to beat the silly lobbyists and their elected lackeys spilled over into the lengthening list of controversies to be resolved. The original six that Minnesota proposed had ballooned to thirty-one. Other matters advocated for convention deliberation crossed the entire political spectrum to include a resurrected equal rights amendment tied to women and gay rights, abolishment of the Electoral College, farm-subsidy reforms, wider broadcast airwave access, a comprehensive immigration policy, a ten-year loss of individual suffrage whenever personal bankruptcy was declared, the ending of capital punishment, the return of abortion control to the states, tort reform, codified limitations on the judicial branch's ability to ad hoc legislate, and a comprehensive energy policy linked to good paying jobs with the promotion of alternative energy sources in support of the nation's wars against dependence on foreign oil and climate change.

However, a lens emerged and refocused the blurred interfaces between the national government and its citizens. Every country has had defects in its political system. The means to endure those defects without resorting to a massive overhaul as advocated under an untested Constitutional Convention—or even worse by a state's secession from the union or overt civil war—had become apparent to congressional leaders and the president: with past coast-to-coast movements, the two major parties had co-opted the grassroots or the progressive third party platforms. To abort the convention's avalanche, the congressional and executive branches joined forces, led from their behinds, and followed a similar script.

Pain avoidance and gaining pleasure through the control of power were the fundamental motives that underpinned congressional and presidential vacillations or decisions. Summarized, national government favored stalemate over action; hence the nation's greatness eroded to brass mediocrity. But the threat from the nationwide convention forced a colossal shift below the Capitol dome and along Pennsylvania Avenue into a golden era of pragmatism and palpable compromise. Staunch positions were trimmed to fit the political gales blowing out of the recharged electorate. The nuanced view aimed toward the center became vogue and persisted throughout the 112th congressional session. The polarized reflex to cast whatever problem that plagued the country into all-or-nothing terms got abandoned, and at long last, rare wisdom abounded the Beltway.

Congressional leaders created a super-committee to draft a grand compromise to address Minnesota's initial six issues ahead of the additional twenty-five on the belief that achieving those first half-dozen would derail, if not evaporate, the convention's groundswell. Yet in private chambers, it was agreed only five of the original six would be debated and signed into law prior to the 2012 election. The sixth, congressional term limits, required extensive committee reviews. And to insure all deliberate speed faithfully exercised, a joint task force of judicial, executive, and legislative leaders was sanctioned to study term limitations to the greatest depth necessary to get it done right. Only from there could the legislative leaders prepare the recommendations for the subcommittee hearings, as many deemed required …

A month before winging to Campsite with Bobby and Piper, Graywood had submitted retirement papers to the Public Health Service. The part-time teaching salary from the University of Alaska coupled with the PHS annuity would provide sufficient financial security. If needing more, he'd contract and oversee any state epidemiology program.

Graywood planned to enjoy the free time with Bobby and pursue his penchant for historical medicine. He toyed with writing an anthology on cultural interpretations of diseases throughout the centuries. Bearhead had offered to collaborate.

The PHS office phone buzzed on the final workday in July while he packed files and reference books. He craved it to be Jen updating her life. Instead, the United States Department of Justice spoke.

The majority of voters had cast ballots for believable change in the 2008 national election, and change had come one way or another. Subsequent the severe recession and Washington's impetus to usurp the constitutional convention movement, two issues from the proposed thirty-one debated nationwide had become laws within the 2011 Grand Compromise framework which affected Doctor Graywood's immediate future: the Alpha-Omega Federal Health Care Act that mandated governmental financial participation within everyone's medical insurance and the death penalty for capital crimes replaced by lifetime banishment to a prison outside the United States.

The Justice Department contacted Graywood regarding the latter.

A multi-nation bidding process held at the executive level under congressional oversight, and followed by State Department negotiations with the Russians, had selected Kamchatka—a 750-mile-long Siberian peninsula between the Sea of Okhotsk and the Bering Sea—for American prisoner deportation. Via a groundbreaking treaty, the new facility operated under the auspices of the Justice Department's Federal Bureau of Prisons in liaison with the Siberian government.

The prison needed an interim medical director. Unknown to Graywood, his superiors had judged him the best-positioned expert to assess and plan the immediate medical care for the future staff, guards, and prisoners at the subarctic penal institution. They'd forwarded the recommendation to the United States surgeon general, the attorney general, and the White House. Once Graywood completed the vetting process, he would develop and implement the maiden business plan for prison health support that also complied with the congressional mandate for facility self-sustainment.

To support this mission to exile, Elmendorf Airbase had been tasked to coordinate and execute all logistical requirements between the lower forty-eight states, the Departments of State and Justice, and Kamchatka.

From pride and sense of duty, Graywood accepted the challenge. Leading a cutting-edge staff, he'd work from offices located at the airbase medical center. He'd hand off the position to the permanent medical director, once selected, within a year or less.

Graywood reviewed the points argued for and against the death penalty and found they varied no less than the number of members in Congress. Mainstream and cable news talking-heads tried to condense the broad range of opinions printed in the Congressional Record. Hosts of media bigwigs assisted and hindered the public's moral comprehension.

If one railed against the death penalty, then the alternative, life in prison, needed to be severe enough to deter committing murder. Living conditions at the incarceration locale had to be frill-less yet sufficiently humane to satisfy society's sense for justice. Nationwide polls reflected the strong sentiments that killers expatriated in lieu of death should not be coddled, must work for their upkeep, and should forego access to the press and conjugal visits. Majorities in twenty-six states still approved putting to death any sane adult convicted of murder, yet they yielded to the 2011 Grand Compromise as the preeminent law.

With any agreement attempting to capture the center, almost all factions voiced dismay at the guidelines negotiated for maintenance of ostracized prisoners: whittled down, the rules stipulated the banished were to receive fair treatment and support to sustain a lifespan equivalent to the denizens in a third world country. Again, most considered this level too beneficent, compared to what the felons had rendered unto their deceased victims. And by allowing murderers to escape death row, American society had granted the condemned a measure of control over their lives that immeasurably exceeded what they had lethally meted out.

Regarding their health care in Kamchatka, the legislation that created "Prisontown" stipulated, in general terms, the exiles had access to adequate medical support, yet it excluded all extraordinary measures to extend their lives. If a prisoner succumbed to organ failure or terminal cancer, he or she received general aid and pain palliation—the equivalent of hospice care.

One prominent East Coast newspaper advocated banished prisoners receive health assistance to the level not to exceed what Doctors Without Borders provided refugees in Darfur or Somalia. Others championed medical care on a par within the United States. The toxic arguments running the blogosphere and newspapers magnified and played out in the federal courts.

With uncommon rapidity, the initial legal challenge bolted into the District of Columbia Appeals Court—the ACLU advocated equal health access and quality levels for banished prisoners as permitted for all Americans under the Alpha-Omega Health Care Act. Anything less was cruel and unusual punishment.

The federal lawyers argued against the ACLU and reminded appellate justices that the nation, for the first time, had reasonably compromised to eliminate all capital punishment, and the death penalty had previously been upheld as not cruel and unusual. If the ACLU insisted, the prisoners could be placed back on death row to meet their certain fates. The DC court ruled for the government, and the decision was appealed to the Supreme Court.

If not overturned, exiled murderers would die in Siberia. No heroic medical measures to save their lives would take place—no transplants, heart surgery, or emergency evacuations to the United States for life-extending, specialized care. There would be no sex-change operations, no treatments for erectile dysfunction, and no cosmetic surgeries. The convicts' rights to first-class American medicine had been abrogated by their capital crime convictions.

Thus the death-row inmate magnanimously lived and died by natural causes instead. He or she resided in a third world medical system, based on the triage concept—limited medical resources were expended to do the most good for the most people. Whenever a prisoner became boneyard ill, interventions that retarded the natural processes carrying one to the grave would remain unavailable.

Thus under the 2011 Grand Compromise was forged the sense of American justice and punishment deemed sufficient for the banished felons' murderous crimes. Thus became the alternative to capital punishment.

Graywood's initial efforts to recruit American physicians into Kamchatka under these criteria proved unsuccessful. Those who'd contemplated laboring overseas in a resource-limited medical environment had opted for the more beneficent, non-governmental organizations. To obtain Prisontown's medical staff, Graywood received approval to hire doctors from other countries. Because the requirement for hospital employees mandated English for the prime or second language, the first two came from India.

With 150,000 vacant nursing jobs in the United States, Graywood had to seek foreign nurses to fill Prisontown's positions. The chief nurse hailed from Quebec, Canada. He'd had prior military nursing experience with the Canadian Armed Forces in Afghanistan as part of NATO. Graywood signed thirteen Filipino staff nurses, six Russians, three Ukrainians, one who'd trained in Greece, and another from South Korea.

CHAPTER ELEVEN

Prison

Bobby's epilepsy during the month prior to his eleventh birthday initiated as short spells of vacant, undisturbed staring. Each frozen sense of awareness persisted for a few seconds, yet he could not appreciate the amount of elapsed time. By the birthday party, the malady had progressed to rare episodes of loss of consciousness. For three months thereafter, anti-seizure medicines controlled the incident severity and number.

Yet on Christmas Eve, Bobby revealed to his dad the appearance of a shaded figure standing behind Bobby moments ahead of an attack. The shrouded form approached by the boy's left ear and stood motionless. Bobby called him Shadowman after the second encounter. He couldn't tell Shadowman's intention. There seemed no malice. Bobby felt unsure if the visage possessed a left arm.

Graywood and Doctor Timm concluded the manifestation was an aura preceding an oncoming spell. Auras could be visual, auditory, tactile, emotional, or other complex experiences individualized to the afflicted person. Shadowman was Bobby's visual aura.

Within a year, Bobby also smelled burnt rubber with Shadowman's arrival. The increasing complexity of symptoms agonized Graywood. Auras showing two components—visual and olfactory—warned the scourge might be spreading within Bobby's brain. Was it expanding out of one focus or from two connected locations simultaneously sparked? A repeat EEG confirmed the earlier epilepiform activity but also indicated two abnormal areas.

Graywood rebooted his knowledge on brain anatomy with its folds, called gyri, separated by grooves and valleys, called sulci. These varied from person to person in number, size, thickness, depth, and position. Like a fingerprint, the gyri and sulci together formed a unique configuration for each individual. Comparisons between the serial CT and Magnetic Resonance Images over subsequent months revealed flattening of Bobby's gyri—a net loss of brain mass.

Bobby's physical movements had become outwardly clumsy as well. Once he'd skated smooth, flowing lines, but now the ability to track leg timing for a natural pace on ground or ice had emerged sluggish. The transmitted feedback loops of peripheral touch and positional senses to his brain displayed subpar integration and foreshadowed ataxia—disjointed extremity motion indicating potential damage to the cerebellum, the hindbrain that sat back and below the cerebral hemispheres.

CT and MRI derived the structural information about Bobby's disease progression, and EEGs showed more than one abnormal trigger. Doctor Timm suspected two locations: one forward in Bobby's cortex by the olfactory nerve and one cradled on the cerebellum.

To better understand the scope of the epileptic activity, Doctor Timm ordered a three-dimensional MRI reconstruction of Bobby's brain. It merged MRI radio waves with single-photon emission computed topography, or SPECT. As the MRI revealed anatomy, the SPECT traced blood flow and brain activity patterns via a radiotracer compound promptly injected after a paroxysm. Because the brain cells involved in a seizure episode were busier than the non-involved neurons, the radiotracer would concentrate there. The SPECT in the three-dimensional MRI should light up the part, or parts, of Bobby's brain with increased metabolic functioning and localize the abnormal tissues prone to discharge attacks.

Graywood prayed the test revealed a single abnormality. If so, it might be possible for a neurosurgeon to excise the damaged locus and end Bobby's epilepsy. Yet cutting away affected brain tissue also risked a new impairment.

Unexpected, the SPECT displayed a bizarre, Swiss-cheese appearance indicating non-uniform blood flows that equated to no localized lesions. The smudged and dimpled 3-D MRI, combined with Bobby's developing ataxia, propelled Doctor Timm to consult neurologists in Seattle. They recommended a magnetoencephalographic study—MEG—at the University of Washington. MEG superimposed on the MRI images ought to nail down one and all locations of Bobby's abnormality.

On the commercial flight to Seattle, Graywood rehearsed over and over Bobby's medical history: negative for brain injury, near drowning, infection, or exposure to known environmental toxins. Bobby never had anemia or hypothyroidism. Significant past medications were simply extended-released Ritalin for ADHD and stopped more than a year ago. He had never become a meth-addled tween or used other illegal drugs. Graywood's prime question for the Seattle specialists: was Bobby infected with something not known?

Graywood studied the MEG brochure printed from the university's website:

> MEG is a biological application of the nineteenth century Maxwell-Faraday discovery where an electrical current has an associated magnetic field. In the same fashion, the minute electrical discharges along the brain's neural cells create a magnetic field within the skull. MEG research often maps specific regions of the brain active for certain functions, such as speech and language.
>
> Sensitive detectors supercooled internally beyond 300 degrees below zero Fahrenheit are placed next to the head to measure the miniscule changes produced on the surface of the cranium associated with the electrical signaling activity within the brain. MEG can measure the existence of magnetic fields one hundred million times smaller than the Earth's.

Seattle specialists proffered that MEG combined with MRI could detect the pattern of signals emitted from an area or areas responsible for the abnormal electrical discharges in Bobby's cortex. Once the location or locations were precisely identified, Bobby could be assessed for definitive epilepsy treatment—possibly a combination of advanced medications with or without surgery.

Over two exhaustive days, the University of Washington performed three distinct MEG studies yet could not pin down the focus or foci of Bobby's seizures.

Conflicted and devastated, Graywood started over.

He categorized the basic pathology to all chronic neurological diseases into a pattern he could understand: something harmful accumulated in the nerve cells; something critical within them was lost; or both. Bottom line, either the brain cells were scarred, damaged, or polluted, or too many went dead too soon.

Bobby's age at twelve years made Alzheimer's and Parkinson's disease not applicable.

In contrast, closer to him was Tay-Sachs disease, a genetic disorder that predictably killed its victims by age five. A child developed the illness only if both parents carried the rare mutation: a gene flaw that prevented production of an enzyme called hexosaminidase A. Without hex A, a fatty substance accumulated to abnormal amounts inside the body's cells, especially the nerve cells of the cerebrum, and caused them to swell. Once bloated, the polluted nerve cells functioned poorly, could not repair routine damage, and eventually died.

Out of desperation Graywood pursued each long shot to find any occult cause for Bobby's illness. He shipped his own cell sample to a genetic laboratory for the Tay-Sachs mutation test—it was negative. The result ruled out the inherited death warrant, even if Bobby's mother possessed the trait. Bittersweet, Graywood felt the compromised fool for ordering it but also gratitude for not having to track down Maren had he tested positive. He chastised himself for entertaining such a wild speculation about Bobby having an unknown variant of Tay-Sachs that allowed its victims to live beyond five or six years. Bobby was twelve. No one of record with Tay-Sachs had ever survived so long. By clinical history alone, he should have skipped it, but the fear for the boy's life had obstructed his professionalism.

Graywood continued his hunt.

Multiple sclerosis manifested as localized regions of inflammation anywhere throughout the brain's deep white matter. Why these pockets originated remained a mystery, and where they evolved varied from patient to patient. Most when diagnosed were between twenty-five and fifty-five years old. Many experts suspected MS as an autoimmune disease where the body attacked itself.

Bobby was too young for MS unless he had an unknown childhood variant. Was it possible? Adult rheumatoid arthritis had a juvenile variant, so why not MS?

Graywood discarded these questions and ceased ruminating on the absurd existence of an early MS variant. He wished not to repeat the Tay-Sachs fiasco.

Next, he probed mad cow disease and its cousin, Creutzfeldt-Jakob disease, or CJD. Both pathologies were caused by misshapen proteins, called prions, that eroded brain tissues. At autopsy, victims of either disease appeared similar. In CJD, a spontaneous mutation caused neural cells to manufacture the disordered human prion instead of the normal form, and the irregular entity gummed up the neurons to cause them to die. The incidence of this mutation in humans remained extremely rare.

Sheep and cattle had deadly prion counterparts that rotted out their brains—identified as scrapie in sheep and mad cow disease in bovines. These hardy prions resisted environmental degradation and crossed species barriers to decay human brains whenever contaminated mutton or beef neural tissues were consumed. Since all cuts of meat had nerves within them, in theory, anyone eating the meat of a diseased animal could ingest the brain-destructive prions and suffer a horrible death.

A human-to-human cultural variation of this sequence had occurred in New Guinea at the twentieth century's onset when a novel funerary practice of eating the brains of the deceased—most often done by women and girls—came into vogue. By 1920, the first incidence of brain-wasting disease occurred, and it spread until the brain-devouring feasts were banned in the 1950s by Australian health authorities. From this local custom and its resulting disease, called kuru, many villages became devoid of young adult females.

Graywood weighed the prion's efficiency at depleting human neural matter as equal to molecules of aerosolized Freon—emitted by the millions in hairsprays—punching holes in the ozone layers over the North and South Poles.

Excluding O'Malley's school lunch program, Bobby had eaten the same meat choices as his father ... plus a few reindeer hotdogs. That pretty much ruled out mad cow, unless an unknown prion existed in domesticated caribou.

At length, Graywood considered whether Bobby might have developed CJD by spontaneous mutation. He reviewed the clinical literature for tests to be done. None existed, other than submitting an autopsy sample.

Graywood overreached a second time for an etiology—this time a polio variant.

A person could become paralyzed following an exposure to one of the three varieties of poliomyelitis after ingesting contaminated water or food. And the oral polio vaccine itself might cause the disease as an untoward complication.

Like kuru, the polio virus survived beyond the human digestive tract but invaded the motor neurons in the spinal cord instead of the brain. Worldwide, cases persisted in remote areas of Nigeria, Afghanistan, Pakistan, and India.

Graywood had administered the injectable polio immunization to his infant son instead of the oral product to nullify the miniscule risk to contract the disease. To mitigate the boy's tantrums over shots when he grew older, Graywood enlisted Cub to take a booster prior to Bobby's. Without a grimace, brave Cub played the part well and double-dared Bobby to do the same. It worked. Thereafter, whenever Bobby required inoculation, Graywood reviewed Cub's medical record for needing a similar dose, and if so, injected them together.

Graywood concluded Cub's stellar health and comparable vaccine record to Bobby's negated any chance polio had caused the illness. To have regarded the possibility seemed outright foolishness as well.

The father's ever-looping mind probed unusual manifestations for other disorders, such as Lou Gehrig's disease, Guillian-Barré syndrome, and Duchenne muscular dystrophy. Online sites and pathology textbooks brimmed with examples for neurodegenerative maladies where subsets of cells had become compromised or killed. He imagined rare or unheard-of presentations for whatever disease he'd read as a potential cause for Bobby's condition. If his boy had been fated a tragic neurological sickness, Graywood bargained with God that it be akin to polio rather than kuru.

When Bobby tripped in the kitchen reaching to lift Brandy Belle, Graywood had a revelation: except for mad cow disease and scrapie, he'd not reviewed the veterinarian literature for other animal degenerative illnesses, especially those that may present in house pets. Perhaps Bobby had a zoonosis—an animal disease—that had jumped across species.

For days he searched the web … and found the lethal condition dysautonomia. It wrenched his heart. Fatal within weeks, dysautonomia attacked the nervous systems in dogs, cats, and horses. Cause unknown and without a cure, only palliative care gave the creatures comfort until the end.

In 1986, it appeared in a Kansas City housecat and remained localized to the Midwest and Rocky Mountain states. In 1988, it also affected dogs in southern Missouri and swept to the canines in Colorado and Wyoming. Every year thereafter, hundreds of animals died from the affliction, and it showed no sign of going away. The disease tended to occur in late winter and early spring, yet by summer its frequency diminished. It preferred younger dogs and those that roamed wide territories.

Graywood also uncovered reports of an epidemic among cats in northern Europe beginning in 1982. The contagion had faded out at decade's end after hundreds of cats and a small number of dogs had perished.

Horses in Scotland had suffered dysautonomia's plague one hundred years earlier. Local residents had dubbed it "grass sickness" from the belief the animals became ill upon grazing in certain pastures. A rare human form had appeared too, but nothing else on past epidemiology was known.

Dysautonomia's origin had two competing theories: an autoimmune disease, like multiple sclerosis, in which the animal's immune system attacked its own nerves; or an undiscovered bacterium that produced a toxin to poison the victim's nerve cells. Because the disease had remained limited to the Midwest in the United States, the toxin or the autoimmune reaction might have been triggered from one or more intrinsic agents within the local environment.

Autopsies of canines with dysautonomia revealed dead or dying neurons or their absence in the animals' autonomic nervous systems. This portion of the nervous system controlled many vital functions, such as regulating the heartbeat, stimulating bladder and intestinal contractions, allowing eye glands to produce tears, and making the pupils expand or contract with light changes. From the brain and spinal column to the intestinal wall, everything had been afflicted.

Dreading that Bobby's positive tilt-table test had demonstrated a sign of this disease, Graywood marshaled his wits: could the child have the human form like the handful of Scottish victims had a century ago?

At work the following day, Graywood uncovered no past or current Alaskan reports of dysautonomia in cats, dogs, or horses.

It still didn't feel right. Bobby displayed one of the physical characteristics—a compromised ability to maintain blood pressure whenever he quick-changed positions from lying down to standing. If he rose too fast, he'd become lightheaded to the point of almost passing out.

The disease had come and gone in northern Europe once. Might an unrecognized variant have come to Alaska?

Graywood wept.

The human brain was so plastic and complicated with abilities to adjust and recover from assaults on its integrity. Over and over, Graywood reasoned through Bobby's unfathomable condition. Yet no diagnosis appeared to fit. Perhaps in time he'd discover the cause behind his child's worsening condition … or maybe …

God, help me please …

To only find a definitive conclusion, a label, or one simple concrete thing welled up as Graywood's sacred wish. Not knowing drained. He doubted his endurance. Whatever malady lurked within his son, he prayed it would cease and reverse. Then he'd have precious Bobby back.

"How's Bobby moving around the house? Is he playing outside?" asked Doctor Timm at the exam's conclusion. She observed a fresh fasciculation in the child's left deltoid muscle, plus a hyper-reactive elbow reflex when compared to the right. She also detected a subtle change inside the right eye.

"He's slower than last year," Graywood replied. "I think it's the anti-convulsants."

"That could be. But the left-arm signs are puzzling. What do you make of them?"

"I don't know," Graywood grimaced. "I'm worried it's not good."

"Well, let's set Bobby up for another EEG and MRI. Compare them to past ones."

"I fly out to Kamchatka next week for a site evaluation at Prisontown's hospital."

"How about I schedule both in three weeks and see Bobby back in a month," said Doctor Timm.

"That'll work," confirmed Graywood.

"You're still doing the prison job?"

"They couldn't find a permanent medical director so asked me to stay on," Graywood recounted in mixed tones.

"Must be, ah … exciting?"

"It's a pain. Devising health care to meet bare-bones budgets is pure headache. Leaving Bobby isn't a picnic either."

"How'll you manage it?"

"The Justice Department lets me take a leave of absence whenever I need it for Bobby's sake, and I've got a network of great friends who'll look after him too," replied Graywood, reassuring Doctor Timm as well as himself. "What I do for him isn't much different from what gets cobbled together in Kamchatka, just a whole lot bigger there." Graywood left out how Washington wanted someone to blame and sack if anything went big-time wrong with the prison's health situation.

"I admire you, Gary, for what you do," said Doctor Timm, touching his arm.

"Want to see my new sled dog?" yelled Cub as Graywood dropped Bobby at Rachel's house before boarding Elmendorf's prisoner-modified Boeing 767 for Kamchatka.

Graywood's downcast eyes observed the methodic child ply out of the Subaru and tail Cub to the dog run. He recalled a medical professor's summation on clinical neurology as a long history and long hallway—it took a lengthy timespan to make the correct assessment on what's wrong with a patient's nervous system. The brain's not a simplistic pump, like the heart, or a mere recycling and waste-disposal plant like the kidney.

Tagging after Cub, Bobby's gait appeared jagged but not ataxic. A couple of years earlier, he'd have challenged a race. Then the world was his to explore and own. Now it slipped away as if belonging to a slow old man. Graywood's eyes moistened when the boy fought to construct a normal stride.

"I heard you drive up," said Rachel, standing on the front porch. "How's Bobby?" In Graywood's tired face, she saw how spent he'd become keeping his world together. If he allowed, she'd nurture him and his son without reservation.

Graywood pulled a handkerchief to clear his nose. "I think a tad better," he lied.

They entered the bungalow and crossed to the kitchen.

She assembled bread and spreads on the counter to make sandwiches for her boys. "I got my CPR updated last week, Gary." She pulled a butter knife from the drawer. "Any changes to the emergency contact numbers?" she asked with raised, highlighted eyebrows.

Exemplary Rachel … Graywood wanted to hold and tell her so, but he resisted the urge and answered, "No changes." He opened the bread's wrapping, thumbed out four slices, and thought Piper the worst damn fool ever to have left her.

"I'm working from home next week so I'll watch Bobby real close and get him to special ed."

"Raych, you're the kindest person I know." Graywood wrapped both arms about her shoulders and squeezed. "Thank you," he whispered.

Had he embraced for other reasons? Panged, he released. Had he crossed to where he wasn't ready?

Rachel sensed confusion. "That was nice." She turned to the sandwiches. "Hug me whenever you want. Bobby does it all the time."

Graywood never forgot the compliment mixed with permission and assurance he'd done no wrong.

Yet she added an unexpected slant. "I was thinking of Piper when you arrived."

Graywood didn't interrupt.

"I don't love him like I used to, but I still love him. It's hard to put in words. Gary, you still love Maren?" She'd pierced Graywood's heart.

Breath tripped out of his lungs. "I stopped loving her five years ago," trailed his voice toward inaudible.

"Have you heard from her since?"

"No," he said, mouth drying and bitter. "Not even a Christmas card."

"Does she know Bobby's condition?

"I've sent her emails and a helluva lot more to her father in Maryland. Zero back."

"You try calling her?"

"Goddamn," he muttered, "when we divorced, she said never call under any circumstances. And she meant it."

Rachel shrugged, sliced the sandwich in half, and smoothed her pink apron before fixing the second. "I don't mean to criticize Maren, but Piper loves Cub and is a good father and was so after he married Sheila and is now with Mary."

Graywood's spine slouched from wearing parental failure. With disheartened eyes, he declared, "I believe Maren never loved Bobby, and sure as hell, she lost her love for me. Raych, that's something I'll never understand."

She laid a hand to his. "I won't understand too. You're a wonderful man, and Bobby's the sweetest child." Each gazed at the other saying nothing, eyes searching to wherever the exchange might lead.

A yelping husky broke loose from the dog run and blitzed past the kitchen window. Cub yelled like a banshee in pursuit.

Trance broken, hands pulled back.

"Raych, I warned Piper about Sheila. I told him she's a gold-digger."

Her short laugh had an edge. "You got that right," she said, making a face. "And I'll tell you something else." She stabbed the knife in the peanut butter and flung out a huge wad. "Piper despises what he calls the tyranny in Juneau, but he's really hooked on all their shortcomings whenever down there." She spread the wheat slice not missing a corner. "He won't admit it, but when he led those rallies to move the capital to Willow, Sheila had him sized up first, not the other way around."

"Piper went there a lot for that," said Graywood.

"Sheila saw him in the Beaver and *Sky Woman*." A faint smile creased Rachel's lips when she grasped the raspberry preserves. "She was convinced he was rich since he owned two planes, and so she left the Juneau fisherman for her next prey but found he wasn't worth much at all." Rachel erratically layered on the red jam. Her face soured. "Gary, I could never go back to Piper once he'd bedded her in my house."

Territorial for the art studio and home she'd made with Piper and Cub, she'd never return. It wasn't the only reason. "I'm over his betrayals," she sighed. "I just want to hold on to memories when he was my Piper." She placed the sandwiches on paper plates garnished by sweet potato chips and carrot sticks.

Graywood wondered if Maren had ever felt this way for him, or if Jennelle still wished to keep memories when they had been a couple. He refocused to Rachel after she called the boys to lunch.

"I'm getting Cub an authentic reindeer harness they use in Kamchatka. Can I bring you something, Raych?"

"No, I'm fine. You just come home safe."

Cub darted through the back door. Bobby trailed. They cornered their meals. Graywood embraced his son and refrained from kissing his forehead in front of Cub. Manlike, he shook Cub's hand and instructed him to watch after his mother and Bobby.

Rachel walked Graywood to the front door. They hugged. He stayed silent when they broke. She softly assured him, "We'll be here when you come home."

On the road to Elmendorf, he mulled over what had stopped him from falling in love with her. She's pulled toward him. Like a surrogate mother, Rachel picked up Bobby from special ed, took him in tow, and looked after him most times whenever Graywood was away. She was the main woman now in their lives.

Piloting *Seneca* on a string of clinic visits, he'd often imagined being married and returning to Raych's warm greeting … Bobby with a mother and older brother.

Would she live in the Snowline Drive house with its Maren memories or stay in the cottage she'd maintained since her divorce? How much would she accept filling in for Maren? How much should he acknowledge the same in himself for Piper? What baggage would both discard to move on and try for a bit of sustained happiness? Was it fair for her, for him, for everyone? Marriages made out of necessity were common throughout the world. But shouldn't marriage made from love be the idea?

The 767 waited.

Graywood could not commit to Rachel if he desired her for what she'd do for Bobby yet not for what she was and what they might become over the years together. Foremost, she had been Piper's wife, and for a time, they and Cub had been a blissful family. Graywood never forgot their perpetual face-beaming swoons at the first gallery opening of Piper's landscapes.

And the friendship with Piper would spew turmoil if Graywood married her. Piper acted the rogue, but for sure, he'd feel betrayed by his partner. Yet Graywood would shout him down to hell and back if the chemistry existed for Rachel. But his adoration brewed incomplete—never on a par with what he'd held for Maren or Jennelle.

As with most things in Graywood's life, conflicting motivations combined to create a comforting stalemate. He boarded the jet and reconciled to leave all as is.

When the 767 zoomed over Mount Susitna, he had an enlightening thought: "You don't marry to replace a parent for your children. They'll grow up and move on. Despite what romance experts say, you marry ultimately to grow old together."

Graywood couldn't imagine doing that with Rachel. With Maren, he had wanted so. If fate ever brought Jennelle back, he would hope for it.

CHAPTER TWELVE

WWAMI Land December 2013

"Good morning everyone," said Graywood, stepping aside the lectern to hunt for the laser marker.

"Good morning, Doctor Graywood," replied several of the twelve students clicking laptops and devices in unison.

Naked willows scraped the outside windows from turbulence blowing off Knik Arm. "Weather's a challenge," thought Graywood. "Heavy snow to come evening. Hope Piper is home painting and not bush hauling in the Beaver." He found the pointer, and asked, "Where are you all going for the holidays next week?"

The trio of Parker, Margot, and Samantha confirmed plans to meet respective families in Juneau, Sitka, and Wrangell. Carl, Aubrey, Kip, and Correy—the "Fairbanks Four"—had organized a two-car convoy to Alaska's interior metropolis. Caitlin and Jennifer anticipated skiing at Alyeska. Masi's parents had booked a hop from Nome to join him in Anchorage for Christmas. Melissa and Joshua remained smug on what 2014 might bring besides broken New Year's resolutions.

"Let's begin." Graywood passed out CD copies on the PowerPoint lecture. "Today we'll cover our new health-care system, how it blends in with other health programs, and several of its strengths and weaknesses."

He returned to the podium. "The practice of medicine is as much about its history as its attempts to forge fresh frontiers. When I sat in your seats in the 1980s, I never received a summary on our health-care system as it then existed. So much has changed."

He clicked to the initial slide, EPIDEMIOLOGY AND ALPHA-OMEGA, and highlighted the first word. "Epidemiology is the big picture for diseases and health in a population, and today we'll discuss our population's interaction with its health-care system in terms of access, quality, and cost and how those parameters relate to our new universal Alpha-Omega Health Act."

The second slide displayed an equilateral triangle supporting an inflated dollar sign atop the apex with the words QUALITY and ACCESS, each anchored on a corner at the triangle's base.

"Question number one." Graywood peered beyond Aubrey and asked Correy, "Does universal care mean universal access?"

With paced words, Correy answered, "Probably not 100-percent access … but better access at least."

"That's a good hedge," Graywood replied. "Universal health care does not, I repeat not, mean universal access or universal quality."

Graywood expected the confused looks on their faces. "It means a basic level of care delivered, or rationed out, to a universal standard throughout the population so that when you access the care in Alaska, it is equivalent to care given in Florida or any other state. In theory, different standards of basic care are not allowed to exist. The non-basic care is rationed by the need to control its cost, and that's done by placing limits on access and limits on new health technology."

Graywood didn't intend to substitute "new health technology" for "quality," although the wording rang comparable. For him, cutting-edge approaches and advancements, whenever compared by clinically derived evidence over time to the older treatments, often proved no better or even harmful. But he deferred such elaboration. Instead, he declared, "In all countries, there are tradeoffs in providing medical care. A reasonable way to understand those tradeoffs is with this triangle of cost, quality, and access."

The following slide depicted two oil barrel stacks—one column piled four drums full with the word SUPPLY printed topside; the other showed six empty kegs under DEMAND. He laser-danced between the two highlighted words saying, "Medical care is rationed in every health system designed, whether a decade ago by private plans in the United States or today under a country's universal plan, such as Canada's, Great Britain's, and now our own Alpha-Omega. Rationing happens because the demands for health access and quality always, I repeat always, exceed the funding committed to pay for it. There's not enough money in any country to ever meet its population's perceived demands for the highest quality, anytime-access, ever-ready medical care."

Graywood paused until laptop chatter slowed.

"Who can give me examples of limits on either access or quality?"

Joshua piped up, "Very few doctors and nurses in rural Alaska, so those who live out there have a long way to go to get treatments."

Jenny added, "And waiting times for surgical procedures. There're very long for hip replacements in Canada."

"Two fair examples," Graywood confirmed. "Jenny's demonstrates an overall constraint on resources. The cohort of Canadians needing their worn, rusty hips replaced exceeds the number of available orthopedic surgeons, or perhaps the total number of decayed hips exceeds the supply of operating rooms, recovery-room bed availability, or some mix of all three. Any deficit in the availability of surgeons, ORs, or recovery beds will back the system up and force a waiting list. It's like wanting to see a rock concert that's already sold out."

Graywood swallowed to refresh his mouth and said, "Joshua's example highlights the maldistribution problem of medical assets across the country. There are too many doctors in plush urban and suburban areas and not enough working in the inner cities or rural areas of the United States. Why's that?"

Graywood scanned the students and picked the one close to falling asleep. "Melissa, I bet you were studying late last night." Shocked clarity surfaced on her face. Graywood forced a cough and rephrased, "So, Melissa, why are there so many doctors in places like Beverly Hills, California?"

Rolling her lower lip, she ventured, "Because that's where the money is." Giggles filled the room.

"She's partially right," Graywood said. "If given a choice, people in any occupation, including doctors, migrate to better economic areas to live with more choices and avoid the sparser ones."

Graywood sensed tepid acceptance by the students and amplified, "This inherent maldistribution by doctors choosing to avoid inner cities and rural areas was one of the realities that sunk Hillary Clinton's health-care reform effort back in 1993." Several heads cocked forward seeking elaboration.

"At that time, Hillary advocated three flavors of health-care delivery for the country." Ticking them off on fingers, Graywood said, "A standard fee-for-service system, a preferred provider network model, and a health maintenance organization." Graywood jumped to the slide HILLARY'S FLAWED 1993 MODEL.

"The PPO and the HMO were supposed to save enrolled patients money by competing for health-care market share. However, Hillary had made a huge mistake. There weren't enough competing hospitals, doctors, and nurses in the rural areas to make any PPO or HMO viable, especially the HMO option. You'll only find HMOs in metropolitan areas where there're perceived excesses in health-care capacities that are essential for creating market competition."

To illustrate, Graywood said, "You don't see big-name rock concerts staged in Homer, Alaska, as often, if ever, as in Los Angeles."

Graywood advanced to a photograph of Doctor C. Everett Koop. "Congressional representatives from rural states backed away from Hillary's plan because it wouldn't work for their constituents. In fact, her shortsighted program wouldn't have worked for over half the country." Graywood pointed on Doctor Koop's white beard and emphasized, "Even the surgeon general at the time verified that truth."

"Doctor Graywood, you said I'm partially right," Melissa said. "What did I miss?"

Appreciating her question, Graywood enlarged, "Most people want quality in their lives, and that includes doctors and doctors-to-be. It's hard to get educated people to live and work way out in the sticks. It's tough to find volunteers to accept hardships in the boonies. To correct the doctor maldistribution in our capitalistic society, we'll need incentives like additional payments for services, early forgiveness of tuition debts, or some other set of rewards and benefits."

Then with a veiled challenge to the class, Graywood added, "But of course, there are some who'll find practicing country medicine very appealing." Jumbled, non-vocal responses trumped back.

"Now before I go to the Alpha-Omega program, let's condense the two areas we've discussed so far." Laptop-key tempo increased.

"First, health care has been and shall always be rationed in every system designed because our demand for quality and access will always exceed supply. Anyone who promises health care won't be rationed is either lying or ignorant. There's simply not enough money to totally meet our massed desire to live longer, disease-free lives, regardless of our chosen lifestyles. We all die. We may slow down death's pace a bit, may prevent some mortal causes. That's the best we can do, but we all will die. As Professor Bearhead often tells you, our culture massages our ethics and politics to determine into which groups we'll ration additional resources and which unfortunates will receive only devoted prayers, if that.

"Second, health-care resources are not evenly distributed throughout the United States. There're geographical barriers to access, and there're social resource maldistributions. There're too many places with not enough clinics, doctors, nurses, and hospitals for the local people to acquire even basic health care, as well as too many places with way too much."

Doctor Koop's picture got replaced with ALPHA-OMEGA HEALTH CARE ACT.

Graywood asked, "What's Alpha-Omega?"

No volunteers.

"Carl, you look awake. You tell us."

Carl squinted and said, "It's our national health program that covers prevention tests and pays for the really big expenses."

"That's a good start, Carl," complimented Graywood. "Alpha-Omega provides two components of care for all US citizens. It covers the cost of preventive services recommended by the USPSTF, and it provides a catastrophic disease coverage plan."

"Doctor Graywood, USPSTF stands for US Preventive Services Task Force, right?" asked Kip, peeping over the laptop ready to key if confirmed.

"Yep, it does."

Graywood popped on the slide with the word ALPHA aligned with PREVENTIVE CARE, and OMEGA linked to CATASTOPHIC HEALTH INSURANCE. “It’s a clever name,” he said, with a twinkle. “The Alpha represents the prevention portion, and Omega pretty much tags into place whenever a patient seeks treatment for a costly major illness.”

Graywood picked a student who hadn’t yet participated. “Margot, answer for us … does the Alpha cover preventive services recommended by all medical specialty and non-medical advocacy groups?”

“Nothing ever covers everything, so I’ll say no.”

“You’re so right, Margot. It covers only those preventive screening tests, procedures, and counseling found through clinical practice to have actually made a positive difference in a population’s mortality and morbidity.”

Graywood projected two slides in succession, each listing ten examples. “We’ll cover these effective Alpha preventions in later lectures.”

“Now look at this trio of groupings,” said Graywood. Advancing deliberately, he displayed three lists of fifteen offset bullets. “These forty-five recommendations didn’t make the cut. There are many people in medicine and pseudo-medicine who advance their own priorities about prevention which seem initially to have a rationale for helping patients. But after rigorous clinical trials, they show no evidence of improving peoples’ overall health.”

Graywood back-clicked to the OMEGA/CATASTROPHIC HEALTH INSURANCE line. “So, Carl, you said Omega paid for big health-care expenses. What exactly did you mean?”

“Ah … it pays for treatments when they cost more than a gazillion dollars. I can’t remember the amount.”

“You’re right, Carl, but the threshold is nine thousand per disease per year. Does it pay for all diseases?”

“Not all of them. As Margot said, nothing covers everything.” The class tittered, and even Graywood grinned.

Graywood took an example out of the vast catalog of medical procedures. “Does it cover cosmetic surgery, Carl?”

Hesitating, he answered, “No.”

“Well it does cover reconstructive cosmetic surgery after a total mastectomy but doesn’t cover Botox, facelifts, tummy tucks, and things like that.”

Graywood shifted gears. "There's a financial cap at the other end on the Omega payout for a catastrophic disease too—it will stop paying once a treatment exceeds two hundred fifty thousand dollars. Why's that?"

No takers.

"Anyone care to offer a speculation?"

Still nothing.

"Okay, let me give a little background. Recall that for part of the Great Compromise in 2011, Congress and the White House hammered out Alpha-Omega in response to their overwhelming fear the Constitutional Convention movement might diminish their political power in Washington. The enormous expense of health care—compounded by fifty million uninsured individuals and the systemic need to make it more affordable across the board without ruining the tax base to pay for it—had to be addressed. After much rancor, Alpha-Omega became the plan selected out of eight competing proposals, and the subcommittee that worked on it hit on the idea of providing proven preventive services to all Americans and coverage for 80 percent of the cost of catastrophic diseases. From crunching the numbers over and over, they believed this reimbursement level significantly would decrease the cost of all the other health insurance programs, both private and public, and make it affordable for businesses to provide health insurance as an employee benefit as well for the self-employed to purchase individual policies.

"Said another way, Alpha-Omega was meant to only augment, not replace, private insurance and all the other governmental directed and mandated health insurance programs, such as Medicare, Medicaid, SCHIP, and workers' compensation. With total annual health care approaching three trillion dollars, Congress wanted all those other insurance programs to continue with their reliable funding streams, and they didn't want people to stop purchasing, for example, the bodily injury coverage on their car insurance and then shift costs for auto-injury treatment and recovery to Omega. So Congress devised the two thresholds. Omega pays once the diagnosis and treatment of a condition exceeds nine thousand bucks per calendar year and stops paying after two hundred fifty thousand dollars.

"All individuals will still need insurance to cover that first nine grand of an acute or chronic illness before Omega kicks in as the primary payer, and they'll need coverage once the treatment exceeds two hundred fifty thousand dollars per calendar year when Omega drops out.

"This satisfied the health insurance lobby. And business groups, led by the auto industry, jumped in as they focused on the nine thousand cost-share they'd be at risk for each employee. They already were paying the equivalent of that or much more per worker per year, and their past experience had demonstrated very few employees would cost beyond the larger quarter-million cap. And so class, why's that?"

Together two students voiced, "The healthy worker effect."

"Very good!" encouraged Graywood. "You were listening in last week's class."

"So," asked Margot, "how was it decided to set the upper cap at two hundred fifty thousand dollars?"

"As I touched on before, Congress didn't want people to drop their medical liability from their auto insurance. If you read any policy, there's a limit on liability for bodily injury per person per accident. And I didn't mention it earlier, but there's also a stated limit for medical payments for which a comprehensive insurance policy for a homeowner or a business is liable if someone's accidentally injured on the premises. Bottom line, most car insurance policies require at least $100,000 for bodily injury liability, and nearly all will recommend more.

"Congress borrowed the cap idea from the accident insurance industry and compromised on two hundred fifty thousand dollars as the best coverage limit while searching for sufficient tax money to pay at the same time for both Alpha and Omega. Combined with Medicare and Medicaid coverages and all the other programs, like SCHIP and workers' comp, Alpha-Omega with its threshold and its cap appeared to be the best fit."

Half the class reflected dazed expressions from too many terms thrown out too fast.

"Some of you look confused about the integration of Alpha-Omega with Medicare and Medicaid," concluded Graywood. "I'll give an example ... Say a fifty-year-old man, let's call him Bill, is employed at Alaska Airlines and is diagnosed with hypertension by his primary care provider during a preventive screening. Who pays for Bill's prevention screen, Alpha-Omega or the health-care policy he has from Alaska Airlines?"

"Alpha-Omega should," replied Margot.

"Correct. The Alpha part pays for all approved preventive screens. And screening for hypertension at age fifty is one of them. No doubt Bill got evaluated for other appropriate things at the same time. Now who first pays for his treatment of hypertension?"

"Bill's health insurance from Alaska Airlines, right, Doctor Graywood?" volunteered Jenny.

"Yes, and for how long?"

"For the first nine thousand dollars."

"That's right, Jenny, the first nine grand in the calendar year. Now if Bill has uncomplicated essential hypertension, that amount is more than enough to cover his care for a year using the average number of visits and tests needed to follow and treat it. So Omega is not tapped at all for any payout."

"Who pays for the drugs to treat Bill's high blood pressure?" asked Jenny.

"If Bill signed up for a policy sponsored by his employer that included pharmaceutical coverage, then it pays. If not, then Bill pays out of pocket." Graywood continued, "Who pays for his hypertension care if by chance it exceeds nine thousand in a year?"

"Omega pays," answered Melissa.

"And for how long?"

"Until Bill hits the two-hundred-fifty-thousand-dollar cap," she replied. "Does Alpha-Omega pay for drugs after the first nine thousand, Doctor Graywood?"

"Nope. Alpha-Omega doesn't pay for pharmaceuticals. The money for drugs comes from other various insurance components that the individual selected or was qualified for."

Graywood skipped past six slides to one entitled PHARMACY. "Alpha-Omega pays for diagnostic, surgical, medical, and mental health treatments and the necessary follow-up visits and tests, but it excludes drug costs. Why do you suppose drugs got excluded?"

No answer.

The AARP subtitle was printed near the bottom of the PHARMACY slide. Melissa placed hand to her chin, and volunteered, "Did it have something to do with the AARP?"

"Yes, indeed it did," verified Graywood. "AARP was very happy with its Medicare Part D once the donut hole got closed. They did not wish to lose that benefit. Too many in Congress feared the AARP voting block, and AARP was against incorporating any part of Medicare into Alpha-Omega. That's why Alpha-Omega pertains only to citizens less than sixty-five years."

"So you can't get drugs paid by Alpha-Omega?" asked Melissa.

"Remember, Alpha-Omega wraps around all the other programs, such as employer-sponsored health insurance, Medicaid, Alaska's Basic Health Plan, SCHIP, workers' comp, and auto insurance liability coverages. Those other programs can pay for medications—some completely, some with co-pays. But on that, I'll have much more to say later."

Graywood paused as he gazed out the window at the falling snow. The students needed a speaking break, anyway, to enter into their external e-brains what he'd explained.

"Here's an easy question," said Graywood, after a twelve-second time out. "Does Medicare pay for Bill's hypertension once he turns sixty-five?"

Many confirmations came back.

"That's right. Once Bill hits sixty-five, Medicare takes over as the primary payer. And he'll get his meds paid for if he has Medicare Part D.

"If Bill exceeds the two-hundred-fifty-thousand-dollar cap in a calendar year before reaching sixty-five, who pays?" asked Joshua.

"Then Alaska Airlines becomes the primary payer again, if he's still employed there. If Bill has changed jobs, then his new employer's insurance pays whenever he exceeds the yearly cap until he turns sixty-five; then Medicare takes over."

"What if the new employer doesn't provide health insurance?" asked Jenny.

"Very good question! Alpha-Omega in Alaska requires all businesses with forty or more employees to offer a commercial health insurance policy or pay into the state's basic health-care plan. The other states vary on the threshold number but pretty much do the same. Two states, California and Maryland, for example, have set it at twenty employees. Most other states are pegged between thirty and fifty. If Bill's new employer doesn't provide health insurance, then Bill buys an individual policy, or he's pooled into Alaska's basic plan. Although Bill may want to, he cannot go bare."

The permutations of health-care coverage had glassed over many students' faces. Graywood restarted. "Let's recap the money sources for treating Bill's hypertension per calendar year. Over time, payment is shared by four insurers: Alaska Airlines for the first nine grand, Alpha-Omega from nine thousand to two hundred fifty thousand dollars, Alaskan Airlines or Bill's new employer after the treatment costs exceed two hundred fifty thousand dollars, and Medicare when he turns age sixty-five."

Fingers whirled on peripherals until Graywood asked, "But what if Bill loses his job because of poor work performance and drowns his depression in a perpetual alcoholic binge? Now who pays?" He looked straight at Samantha.

"I don't know," she mumbled.

"Okay, let's review Bill's increased number of diseases. He has hypertension, depression, and alcohol dependency. He has worked long enough to qualify for Medicare if he lives to age sixty-five, but let's make him sixty years for this part of the example. Bill has no employer-based health insurance because he got fired for poor work performance. Before he got canned, his hypertension treatment had exceeded the nine thousand dollar threshold, so it's covered by Alpha-Omega until it's over two hundred fifty thousand dollars. Bill has three diseases: hypertension, depression, and alcoholism. By each condition, what financial source or sources pay for his health care?"

Caitlin volunteered, "Alpha-Omega continues to pay the hypertension treatment because he's past the threshold, but he has no employer health insurance for the other two. So would it be Alaska's Medicaid for them?"

"Very good, Caitlin. Medicaid pays the first nine thousand for treating Bill's detox and another nine grand for managing depression. But if Bill happens to be married and his wife, let's call her Hillary, has a job with health insurance benefits that cover both of them, then her employer's health policy pays the initial nine thousand of Bill's detox, and the nine thousand for his depression treatments. Thereafter, Alpha-Omega is the primary payer. Are you starting to get the concept behind the catastrophic insurance component in the Omega piece?"

Most of the class voiced or nodded okay.

"There's one more wrinkle in all this you need to know. Alpha-Omega is the primary payer after nine thousand up to two hundred fifty thousand dollars for each disease Bill suffers per calendar year. But Congress decided to employ another parameter to limit the cost by spreading out the payment risk. By that I mean Alpha-Omega pays 80 percent of the costs between nine thousand and two hundred fifty thousand dollars, and that means the employer-sponsored insurance or the state's basic health-care plan or Alaska Medicaid, whichever applies, pays for the other 20 percent. So why do you think Congress did that?"

"Because they're cheap."

Laughter erupted.

Graywood wasn't sure who'd spoken, yet continued, "Many agree with you, whoever said it. But let's keep it simple." Class order returned.

"Congress set the eighty-twenty coverage split in order to spread the financial risk and responsibility for payments," said Graywood. "They believed this division level would influence positive behaviors from each insured patient, each provider, and each payer not to go hog-wild with medical care. Again it's that triangle of cost, quality, and access with which we started out our talk today."

Graywood flashed up the triangle slide with the QUALITY and ACCESS at the base and the dollar sign atop the apex. He followed with another slide: SHOW ME THE MONEY.

"Where does the money come from to pay for Alpha-Omega?" Graywood's eyes signaled out Samantha.

"Everyone knows, Doctor Graywood," she said, like ice. "The VAT and the tax on being fat."

Chortling swelled until Graywood popped to the next slide, VALUE ADDED TAX, and said, "Yep, you're right, Sam. During the 2011 Compromise negotiations, Congress borrowed an idea from the European Union and decreed a value added tax levied on all US goods and services in order to pay for the bulk of Alpha-Omega costs. The Congressional Budget Office number-crunchers calculated a 2.4 percent VAT would work so long as all the other streams of money—Medicare, Medicaid, and SCHIP revenues and appropriations—continued and Alpha-Omega did not replace the private health insurance plans provided by employers or take over any part of the state's basic health-care plan, workers' comp, or individual auto and home accident insurance policies."

Graywood advanced to the next slide: WHO SHOWS ME THE MONEY?

"So the VAT is levied at the wholesale and retail levels every time a product is bought or a service is performed. We pay VAT whenever we buy something or upgrade whatever.

"In contrast, Medicare is funded from a payroll tax levied on workers and employers, and the remaining shortfall is covered by congressional appropriations. Employers pony up for the workers' comp. Auto and property owners pay for motor vehicle and home liability insurance policies, and Medicaid and SCHIP are resourced through a combination of shared federal and state general funds, augmented with taxes on social sin commodities, such as cigarettes and alcohol."

Graywood advanced to the next slide: TAX EXEMPTION LOSS.

"Now let's spend some time on the fat tax as Sam calls it. It's not a direct tax like the VAT."

"Yes it is," interrupted Sam.

"No, actually, it's the partial or complete loss of the standard tax exemption on your Form 1040 if you, the taxpayer, are overweight or obese when you file your annual federal taxes," declared Graywood. "But before we go any further, we have to define overweight and obese. As dictated by the government for tax purposes, what parameters dictate when one is overweight or obese?"

"It's based on BMI," said Masi, "but at different thresholds than what's used in medicine."

"That's right. To lose one's tax exemption, the government chose body mass index calculations, yet set them to higher levels. In the hallowed halls of Congress, you're defined as overweight if your BMI reaches twenty-nine, and you're pegged obese once you hit thirty-three. These numbers are three points higher than our medical cutoffs of twenty-six for overweight and thirty for obesity. Why do you suppose more lenient ones got written into law?"

"Fat congressmen with too much girth to meet medical standards," hooted Sam to sniggering from the rest in the room. "They inflated them to make the cut."

"There's really quite a bit of truth to all that," said Graywood. "It's called the Frank-Franken rule and named after the congressman and senator who proposed it."

Graywood moved on to the slide comparing the different weight standards. "The CDC lobbied hard for the medical definitions, but the politicians wanted even higher BMI cut-offs, in spite of all the critical evidence showing BMI measurements of thirty or more increased the risk of premature death from heart disease, diabetes, and kidney ailments, as well for multiple cancers, including breast, pancreas, and colon. Eventually, they compromised to the current legal grades, but it got very entertaining to read the blogs and newspapers waxing on and on about bipartisan paunches of portly men voting belt-and-suspender in ample solidarity."

To hilarious roars from the students, Graywood raised both hands in mock surrender to the political will in Washington. He repeatedly cleared his throat to reestablish class control and added, "By the way, the congressional BMIs are so generous they overlap abdominal girth tape measurements, which most authorities believe assess health risks better for unhealthy amounts of body fat."

Some students appeared confused, so Graywood reloaded. "Abdominal girth measurement is the preferred predictor for unhealthful body fat, rather than BMI levels. All men who exceed the congressionally defined BMI obesity level of thirty-three will certainly exceed the unhealthful medical girth measurement of forty inches, and all women likewise with a BMI thirty-three or more will have unhealthy girths for their sex greater than their threshold for thirty-five inches. It's all these girthy people—men whose waists expand beyond forty inches and women over thirty-five—who are most likely to suffer the highest risks for all the illnesses that derive from obesity."

The slide LIFESTYLE CHANGE took over.

"A lot of social change came from the 2011 Grand Compromise. Capital punishment was replaced by overseas banishment. Social Security taxes and benefits were restructured, and there were many other changes too. But most critics on government and culture will tell you that the creation of Alpha-Omega did the most to rewrite the social contract because the embedded weight standard joined necessity to purpose ... our bloated ways as a nation could no longer persist, and the legacy costs of obesity—like the legacy costs that forced two Detroit automakers into bankruptcy in 2009—had to end. Our elected leaders exhorted Americans to give it their all to lose excess weight for the common good. The solutions for our country's health crisis emphasized lifestyle change over more and more medicine. That's why the weight standard got added to Alpha-Omega and into the tax code. And for the common good, our government vigorously applied the stick of partial or complete loss of one's standard tax exemption if you're overly fat. So class, how's this stick applied?"

"You lose half or all your exemption if you're overweight or obese," disclosed Sam, with a sharp edge.

"Correct," confirmed Graywood. "It is part of the behavior change the White House, Congress, and the CDC wanted to implement to stem our country's obesity epidemic. If your BMI is between twenty-nine and thirty-three, you're legally defined as overweight and lose half your tax exemption. All gets forfeited whenever BMI measures thirty-three or greater because you're legally defined as obese.

"Let's look at an example. Say our good friend Bill has a BMI of thirty-four, which, by the way, makes him more than a third fat. Come April, he'll file federal income taxes for the 2013 tax year. Because Bill is legally obese, the standard income exemption he had prior to Alpha-Omega is now voided, and he's now taxed on the once exempted income at whatever rate fits his current bracket. That extra tax revenue goes straight into Alpha-Omega's ledger to help pay, for example, for an overweight diabetic's additional costs for health care when compared to a taxpayer who has normal weight and blood sugar.

"Let's say the standard single exemption rises to ten thousand dollars in a few years. If all ten grand is taxed at the 20-percent bracket, that's an additional two thousand our corpulent Bill surrenders to the IRS, and it's credited to Alpha-Omega.

"But if our man Bill is only legally overweight, sporting a BMI between twenty-nine and thirty-three, then half, or five thousand, of the standard deduction is taxed at 20 percent for a one-thousand-dollar contribution to Alpha-Omega. And that will continue every year until he reduces to the normal, non-taxable, legal weight now defined for our citizens.

"So how does our government know if Bill is obese or overweight?" asked Graywood, flashing up the slide: BEHAVIOR REINFORCEMENTS.

Jenny answered, "Bill has to get BMI authentication at an approved height-and-weight center."

"Where are those?"

"They're all over," she replied. "The university's student health clinic provides weight certificates, and doctors' offices can get approval to e-print verification forms."

"I've heard malls and shopping centers and Nordstrom have applied to become certified locations in California and Washington State," added Carl.

"Before you know it," huffed Sam, "it'll happen at vehicle emission stations too. Certify your weight while your car's exhaust is checked."

"Why not churches or beauty parlors and barbershops?" returned Carl, louder.

"Or post offices, like they do passports?" retorted Sam.

"All right, that's a little farfetched," intervened Graywood. "But you're right. Not everyone will go to a doctor's office to get weighed, or people will put it off until the last minute and can't get an appointment. But let's assume our friend Bill goes to an approved height-and-weight center to get his BMI validated. When and how often does he go?"

"Every two years in his even-numbered birth year," answered Carl.

"I'm disappointed in you, Carl. That's way too simple," joked Graywood. "We're talking about a governmental mandate that involves paying additional taxes. The procedure must be more complicated than that because the IRS is involved."

After class-wide laughter abated, Graywood proceeded. "So here's how it works. Bill can get a valid BMI for tax purposes up to three months before to three months after his even-numbered birthday whenever he turns, for example, sixty, sixty-two, sixty-four, and so on. If Bill's birthday is 17 July, he should get validated between 17 April and 17 October. What happens if he's weighed too late?"

"Something very bad," said Sam in a tense wobble.

"Samantha, you're absolutely right again," said Graywood. "All of us know that when you're late filing taxes, the IRS fines you. You're similarly penalized whenever you miss your weighing window—you're assessed a whopping noncompliance fee of two thousand dollars on your Form 1040. But let's say our honest Bill is not tardy and gets his weight and height certified right on his birthday, and his BMI is calculated at twenty-nine point four, making him overweight."

In hopeful tones, Jenny asked, "Can Bill lose some pounds over the remaining three months in his window and get measured again?"

"Yes, he can go every day to a certified weight center until he makes the BMI cutoff of twenty-eight point nine or until time runs out at midnight, October 17. More likely, Bill will go to his doctor for counseling on shedding some pounds and will return to the weight center ten weeks or so later and have a twenty-eight BMI. He happily pumps a fist in the air and covets the updated verification form, which he receives in duplicate from the weight center to use for each of the next two tax-filing years."

Before Graywood clicked to the following slide, he asked, "Does anybody know what that verification form is called?"

"The 1040WT," fumed acerbic Sam.

Graywood flashed it on the screen and said, "Bill's a happy camper now. Come April, he'll attach a 1040WT to the rest of his tax forms and use the duplicate the following year. In the meantime, he can chow down on donuts and burgers with abandon. For the federal weight requirement, he's good for two years, no penalty, full tax exemption guaranteed, slam dunk.

"Now let's look at the other side of the time window. Why would people want certifications earlier in their weighing windows prior to their birthdays?"

"They've got a normal BMI but want to pig-out later," kidded Kip.

"A possibility," returned Graywood. "Or they plan to be out of the country later and can't get to an official weight location on or after their birthday.

"I also want to caution you about all the gaming-the-system potential that exists to get a normal weight certification during that six-month window period. So expect it to happen whenever you're seeing overweight patients."

NEGATIVE FEEDBACK replaced the 1040WT slide.

Slanting to a related topic, Graywood said, "The income tax cuts made under Bush 43 took many taxpayers off the rolls and made it easier for Congress to pass the 2.4 percent VAT for Alpha-Omega. In contrast, the weight requirement made it harder to push the legislation. What have you heard about losing part or all your tax exemption if your 1040WT validates you're overweight or obese?"

The room ignited:

"It caused gigantic scream-fests on talk radio and blogs, just like the VAT."

"It's an invasion on individual rights. Weight is a personal choice and responsibility. We need better school nutritional programs, and communities need to encourage walking."

"The government's an interfering nanny."

"Worse, it's a bully!"

"People should be free to make wrong choices about their weight."

"All the talk about health-care reform and controlling health-care costs is absurd if the obesity epidemic continues. Massive numbers of obese make any reform unaffordable!"

"It's a regressive tax, which hurts the poor more."

"Money talks, and taking away money also talks."

"Hold yourself accountable for your own weight."

"Tax a thing, and you'll get less of it, so tax body fat like cigarettes and booze."

"Some places pay you to lose weight."

"Yeah, Italy pays fifty Euros if you lose nine pounds in a month and two hundred more if you've kept it off for a year."

"And most companies charge higher health insurance rates if you're overweight or smoke."

"They'll charge even more for both overweight and smoking."

"Smoking and drunk driving are health hazards and are priced higher by taxes and fines than non-smoking and sobriety. It should be the same for obesity."

Like a school crosswalk guard holding up a hand, Graywood intervened, "Okay … okay. Let's flip the coin to its other side. What do you recall are the government's comebacks to these criticisms?

"I read where officials claim obesity costs one hundred eighty billion dollars per year," offered Correy.

"Yeah, I saw that article too," added Aubrey. "It costs twenty health-care dollars for every pound someone is overweight."

"Yeah, that's what it's all about," yelled Kip, "the medical carbon footprint."

The class erupted again:

"Alpha-Omega slashed away the movement for state protections to overweight workers."

"But there're forty-eight million lost workdays each year due to obesity."

"Lifetime employment with one company is no longer the norm. Today's worker takes responsibility for her career, her retirement, her health, and especially her weight."

"And sixty billion dollars lost every year to employers."

"Even Al Gore minces support for reducing his carbon butt-print! He backs Alpha-Omega whole hog and says we must reduce for the greater good."

"All right, everyone," interjected Graywood to regain order. "You've brought up just about everything. Now allow me to summarize what you've said. It sounds as if a lot of political psychology exists out there to get our citizens to live healthier lives and reduce health-care expenses. Government and private businesses want to change our unhealthy behaviors because no collective life changes will break the bank. But we resent the policymakers for forcing us to change. Society can help or mandate most people to make good decisions through a combination of carrots and sticks. This isn't new. Society encourages you to own a house and allows you to write off mortgage interest. The government allows church and charity deductions on tax forms—more nice carrots.

"On the other hand, government taxes cigarettes and alcohol. Government fines you for speeding or not wearing a seatbelt. It takes away your driver's license if you drink and drive. Any problem with officials enforcing those examples of sticks?"

Dead air. Graywood accepted the silence as unified agreement and said, "With the VAT and the over-fat tax, government now pays for many health-care components for all its citizens."

Graywood spun more analogous examples. "We pay gasoline taxes to maintain and improve our roads. The gas tax is regressive. If you drive a car, you pay it whether you're poor or not."

"If you want cable or satellite TV, you pay the going rates for the bundles of channels, fewer bundles if you're poor. There's no special rate given the poor for TV, only less choice.

"A drunk pays taxes levied on Old Crow, whether he's poor or not.

"To access medical care, there's no free lunch as well. The feds decided that VAT and fat taxes would fund Alpha-Omega and made the most sense for our country. Look at what it does. It provides prevention services to everyone. It mandates all to have health insurance. It financially shores up other government and private health-insurance plans. It lessens cost shifting between government and privately funded programs. And when an illegal alien buys something in the US, he's charged the VAT and is, at least, partially paying in advance for future care in an emergency room he might someday need. Do you think taxing fat deposits might motivate many obese citizens to lose some weight and impede others from gaining extra pounds … and therefore reduce health-care costs for us all?"

"There's a lot of demand for gastric surgery," observed Kip. "I'm thinking about becoming a general surgeon."

"Kip, have you seen the new 'Consume One Hundred Calories Less Each Day' public service announcements?" queried Aubrey. "If those catch on, you won't be needed in surgery."

"And if kids slept more," said Caitlin, "it would lessen their obesity too."

"Your weight's a concrete fact," fired back Kip. "You can rationalize to the moon how it's what it is, but obesity is simply more calories consumed than what the body needs for tissue generation, maintenance, and activity level."

"What you've all said pertains to the here and now," interrupted Graywood. "But let's take a different viewpoint and look at some medical economic history and then transplant it into today's situation to better understand what's now going on."

Graywood forward pressed images to a man in a uniform.

"Over half the adults smoked in 1964 when the US surgeon general, Doctor Luther Terry, first warned that habit was hazardous to health. Since then, all levels in government have discouraged tobacco use, and today less than a fifth of adults smoke. Lung cancer rates in men have dramatically fallen, and they've stabilized in women.

"Now let's go back two years to 2011. The rising cost of health insurance continues to accelerate, and it's more and more imperative for government to meddle into the private lives of overweight people as it did smokers back in 1964. Two-thirds of the adults are overweight or obese, and our current surgeon general proclaims excess body fat is bad and obesity is extremely detrimental to health. Diabetes rates in adults and children are skyrocketing. There are over twenty-five million Americans diagnosed with diabetes and most from excess weight. In essence, being overweight in 2011 is to diabetes what smoking in 1964 was to lung cancer.

"Our government believed that taxing a behavior or losing an exemption would change the human conduct in question. Look at what happened to smoking when cigarette taxes increased—it dropped like a rock.

"Similarly in downtown London, British officials found taxing the use of private cars at peak driving times changed motorists' behaviors and reduced traffic congestion on business days. Major cities all over the world now follow London's lead.

"Bottom line, some people will change their behaviors, and some won't, regardless of the carrots and sticks applied. Those who don't change, pay more. Those who do, pay less. That's what social and personal responsibilities are all about. If you want something to go away, tax it.

"A few more things regarding revenue generated from VAT and losing the tax exemptions: Medicare receives a portion of the VAT each fiscal year that's estimated to have been paid by its beneficiaries the year prior. This VAT transfer shores up Medicare's ability to operate through its designated payroll taxes and less from the supplemental appropriations by Congress. The annual VAT money shifted into Medicare also delays the urgency to increase payroll taxes to cover future projected Medicare deficits."

Graywood moved away from the lectern to the center of the screen. With head and torso blocking Doctor Terry's back-lit picture, he said, "You can just imagine during the Grand Compromise debates how those legislators slapped each other's back when they'd figured this out.

"And of course if you're over sixty-five years and overweight or obese, you lose part or all of your standard deduction, just like anybody else—and all that money goes back to Medicare's budget too. Bottom line, weigh too much and you pay more for health care. So our elected leaders believe paying taxes by the pound is the fairest way to do social business.

"One more point," said Graywood. "The VAT is not assessed on care approved by the Department of Health and Human Services, but it is collected on any provided care that's not approved. What is and isn't taxed is detailed within the supplemental annual billing guidances confined by geographical locales that HHS publishes. Each year, some services get added, others excluded. So do any of you know how a medical screen, test, or treatment is approved for Alpha-Omega payment?"

"Whatever works that makes a real difference," said Joshua.

"Yes. Now I want to show you a typical—" Graywood stopped.

Jen … Graywood's brain froze … and so did his heart.

With Bearhead, she'd entered the room and sat in back.

The three closest in front, Masi, Aubrey, and Caitlin, caught Graywood's attempt to thaw.

They kissed and kissed … sincere, delicious kisses. Long kisses freely given, short kisses, and kisses to burst for relief.

"Jen, I've waited for you."

Bearhead and the students witnessed the pressed faces—the perfect shudder—and their bodies thrilled too.

"Jen, come with me."

At Kobuk's Town Square Espresso, they kissed and spilled hot tea against the popping fireplace where he proposed to marry.

Her delicate, vermilion lips cooed, "Not now, Gary," stopping him short.

They tango embraced and tongued before the full-length mirror bolted to the Sheraton's twelfth-floor corner room. Her golden-brown tresses fell loose over shoulders after he'd swept away the cambric chemise, trimmed in cream lace.

Bliss-raging ardor cantered to impetuous gallop … exquisite when sucked in and out. Tandem kisses rose on vigorous heaves and thrusts in search for treasure.

Melting bliss confused the blood mixing down every channel within … simply kissed away.

Dying bliss wove through joyous pinnacles too great to express in thought, word, or deed. Over parted mouths, two souls hovered, creating love anew … and dared so assuredly thereafter.

Rubbing Jen's neck, Graywood wondered out loud, "Why'd you come back?"

"For you." She inched closer and stroked his cheek. "Tell me about Bobby."

"Bobby? No! This isn't true."

Touching this child's name vanquished illusion.

Muted, Doctor Graywood dropped the pointer. Confused, he swallowed between resonant breaths, head cocked pensively to the ceiling. Derailed, he coughed thickened spit and resumed the health-care discussion with the rafters.

"Uh, ah … Alpha-Omega isn't trying to be our parent in regards to extra pounds," he plodded. "It merely categorizes obesity risks and assesses them the way financial markets price the risks in stocks, bonds, and other commodities. Regarding the business of medical care, you could say that in our dire economic times society views overweight people as sub-prime."

Eyes dropped to the students, Graywood plowed on. "Smokers have been viewed as sub-prime for five decades, and their increased lifestyle risk has been priced in and paid out as higher health insurance premiums. Likewise, since 2011, the obesity risk has joined tobacco."

The lecture had a quarter hour left. Perplexed, Graywood stared at Jennelle, and stumbled, "Students, ah, often I've gone into Professor Bearhead's time." He zeroed on Bearhead and teleported intention. "We'll stop here today so he can get some time back."

Bearhead nodded up and down once. Gary and Jen had *beaucoup* to catch up on.

"Take a break," said Graywood. "Doctor Bearhead will talk in ten minutes."

Student cliques shuffled out. Bearhead exited too.

She came to him.

He couldn't move—like six years ago when she'd faded beyond airport security.

"It's been too long, Gary. I'm sorry for that."

The miasma from past-love awkwardness filled within the four walls. Appealing as before, she appeared even more—no ring on any finger.

He knew he couldn't say a thing right except, "Coffee?"

"I'd like that."

She ordered tea at the Starbucks aside the Consortium Library.

Jennelle had adored Gary passionately, but an alien had blocked him within to elude her love. That nameless, wretched unknown had persisted in their personal correspondences—always the guarded extra inch of caution inserted to prevent revealing all the heart.

Her starry-eyed feelings faded with years on the road circling the planet. She wanted to forget him, and it worked for some time.

Yet he was here before her. Despite the cratered romance, she remained drawn to this complicated man.

"Rita called me last week," he opened. "She told me you were coming back to your old office."

"Not quite. I'm in Cash's. He needed more space and took over Glenn Olds Hall."

"You'll manage the new hepatitis C vaccine program, right?"

"Yes, Gary, the Alaskan arm in the worldwide field trial. I'll implement it here and see how it truly works."

Graywood brightened and said, "That's wonderful. I've really missed you."

To erase leftover confusion after six years, Jennelle refocused their minds without delay and set the ground rules. "This time, Gary, can we be purely colleagues and friends?"

Jolted, he answered, "Well, ah, of course." Rebuffed, he longed to say, "I ache for you." Whatever way she'd let him have her, he'd take.

Jennelle smiled to his spoken confirmation.

He loved her. Always would. Lungs exchanged air with less effort, and blood resumed normal courses into his skull and legs.

Less tense too, she asked, "How's Bobby?"

Graywood shifted away—never done in the past whenever the boy was brought up. Brow stiffened, and his eyes rotated as unhinged bearings. She leaned forward to hear the faint words, "He's very sick, Jen."

Astonished, she bit her inside cheek. The hundreds of stories that had danced upon his powerful face had become one ominous nightmare—Bobby's fragile illness. Monroe hadn't mentioned the condition, only general stuff about Chitina and Gary's new job at the Kamchatka prison.

"It's an unknown seizure disorder," Graywood rasped, palms pressed upon his lowered forehead. Overwhelmed breaths ejected, "No one … can … figure it … out."

The hepatitis C summary would wait. She pulled Graywood's limp body to her breasts.

They teared up together.

"Hi, I'm Cub. You must be Doctor Daniels." He swung open the double door in grand fashion to Graywood's home. "May I help you with your coat?"

"Thank you, Cub." She had not expected him—six feet plus, muscular, confident, destined for a lady charmer like his dad—and he sensed it. She had accepted Graywood's Saturday dinner invitation to see Bobby and review the CDC's field trial.

"Mister Graywood hires me to look after Bobby every other weekend. He's told me all about you."

"Was it Mister Graywood or Bobby who told you all about me?"

"Well … ah, both kinda did."

"Oh …."

She handed Cub fur gloves and parka before changing snow-covered boots to the flats she carried.

"Where's Mister Graywood now?"

"The kitchen. I'll show the way."

"No need, Cub; I've a good memory."

"If you need me, I'm watching Bobby in the great room."

Christmas decorations bedazzled the entrance filled with wreath aromas. Hallway lights were strung up the banister. A giant red and green bowed ribbon hung from the chandelier.

From the kitchen's entry, she viewed Graywood folding a roast beef slice into the food processor. "Hi, Gary," she said.

"Oh, you're here." They exchanged a brief hug. "I'm pureeing for Bobby. Once I've mashed the spuds and cut the rest of the meat, we'll eat."

"It smells good."

"Have you seen Bobby yet?"

"No."

"Cub was supposed to take you."

"I told him I knew the way to the kitchen. Can I help you with anything?"

"Sure. Please fill the tall glass on the counter with 2-percent milk. It's for Bobby before we eat." Graywood pulverized the potatoes.

Jennelle paused, grabbing the carton from the refrigerator … two shelves crammed with every soft drink … and hidden in the back lived her sourdough starter. After she'd poured, Graywood added one dropperfull of an emerald fluid.

"It's one of Bobby's seizure meds," he explained.

"Gary, is it all right if I know about it?"

"Oh sure. It's Regard." He stirred the glass to uniform pea-green. "Just so you know, I make sourdough pancakes every Sunday morning Cub's here," he said as if he'd read her mind by the fridge. He mixed in three more droppers of a clear fluid. "It's twelve K units of vitamin D."

"Why that?"

"There're articles touting it prevents multiple sclerosis. Who knows, it might help whatever Bobby's got."

Graywood detected her glance of pity. He set the glass down and pivoted away. Grasping the carving knife, he slashed the roast with hardened gusto.

For the first time, Jennelle perceived his pernicious fear.

He stopped hacking and said, "Jen, I'm desperate." His eyes stared upward as charred stones. "I don't love the God who's done this to my child and me." Like night's veil descending on heaven and earth, his slackened body contracted before her.

She hadn't yet seen Bobby, but Graywood's misery broke her heart in three. She'd help him and the child live through this. Steadfast, she'd support them in whatever was necessary to survive.

"I'm sorry, Jen. Sometimes I lose it."

She went to him. "It's okay, Gary. I understand. It's okay."

"I'll be fine the rest of the evening, I promise."

"It's okay, really."

With shoulders pulled back and filling his chest, Graywood handed her the medicated glass. "Go ahead and have Bobby drink every drop. I'll have dinner prepared by then."

"Sure, Gary."

"But don't go right up to him. Make him walk to you. It'll help him physically."

Bobby and Cub were seated at the play station. Cub toned down his game to a tie score while they dueled in an action contest set at level two. Bedecked for Christmas, a Noble fir illuminated the great room's windows with miniature stars reflected from its interwoven strands of bulbs. Stuffed underneath were twenty-odd presents. The yellow cedar statuette given by Bearhead to Bobby at the potlatch six years previous commanded one side of the fireplace with four toddler-sized socks divided around its base. Three red stockings trimmed in white hung from the mantel.

Holding Bobby's beverage tight, Jennelle drilled deep to find courage and chided herself for not bringing a gift.

"Hi, Bobby. It's me again."

"Yah … ah … dinner … ah … Dad an' Jen an' Cubber … Satoorday … sled ride … dinner … yah … Cubber fall off sled … we eat four cookie!" Bobby pumped the right arm to let Cub know he wanted to stand.

"Four cookies," corrected Cub. "We ate four cookies." He braced Bobby as they struggled toward Jennelle.

Cub's aid and support reminded her how April had assisted May in Bearhead's lodge before the potlatch. After five awkward steps, the gangly, crippled, golden-haired boy clasped Jennelle as hard as possible … far weaker than their first embrace at the lady moose.

"I've got sled dogs," explained Cub. "This time of year, we get ready to race, so Bobby rides as my extra weight."

"Yeah … ah … in month … Cubber an' hiss dad … Janu'ry … sled … yah … funs for Cubber!"

"Fun for Cubber, Bobby."

"Fun for Cubber," he repeated, wide mouth grinning.

Devastated by Bobby's hollowed appearance, Jennelle gathered every gram of strength to maintain composure.

"Here, Bobby, time to drink this," she said, cheerful as a holiday carol.

The right hand pinched the glass. He slurped away.

Jennelle sized up the mauve-colored sweater draping Bobby's torso to the mismatched muscle loss between the left and right upper extremities. "I wished I'd seen you two gliding across the snow today," she said. "Did anyone take a picture?"

"I don't think so," answered Cub.

"Oh, that's too bad," said Jennelle, disappointed. She remembered the photographs in the den Graywood had shown with pride the first time she'd dined at Snowline Drive.

Bobby burped and handed her the emptied glass. "Yah ... ah ... gooder from you. Aah ... best ... today gooder!"

"Today good, Bobby," she coached.

"Today good," he giggled and hugged her again.

"So you're helping Bobby with speech therapy," said Graywood from the great room's entry.

Jennelle's face revealed a how-could-I-not look.

"The therapist says he's got impairments with control and processing grammar. His ability to comprehend meaning is good."

"Is the grammar getting better?" she asked, crossing to Graywood.

"Not any worse with Cub's drilling," he answered, masking a sigh.

"They said they went for a sled ride today. Did you get a picture?"

"No." Casting narrowed eyes down, Graywood adjusted ornaments on the tree that were not out of place.

Jennelle mentally kicked herself for making him sullen again. Once he'd been the obsessive photobook hobbyist. She didn't know he hadn't taken one of Bobby since the seizures had begun.

"Mister Graywood, should I help Bobby to dinner?"

Perking up, Graywood brought back the brighter side. "Yeah, go ahead, Cub. It's ready." Graywood motioned Jennelle toward the dining room.

She resolved to avoid misunderstandings, however slight. "Cub's sure great with Bobby."

"Yeah, the best at Bobby-sitting," said Graywood, flicking off the play station.

Foregoing the field trial review after dinner, Jennelle appealed for details on Bobby's medication regimen.

Graywood opened a log book kept in the great room: each seizure, earliest to most recent, was recorded and indexed to anti-convulsant dosages and adverse effects. Two-drug and three-drug combination failures were catalogued on the final five pages.

"We try to stay away from four-drug mixes because of compounding side effects," he said.

"How often does Bobby have an attack?"

"Well, a new regimen knocks them down to one every ten days or so, but they lapse back to two or three times per week," he replied.

Graywood's bewildered eyes diverted to the corpulent Christmas tree. His raw voice, frayed and fatigued by seething rage, said, "Jen, we're running out of therapeutics. I'm afraid I've got to accept two or more seizures each week … but then I'll lose all of him."

"I don't understand, Gary."

"Every convulsion has some neuron loss. Bobby's brain has to reboot, reprogram neural networks, and start over."

"I'm so sorry, Gary," she said, touching his hand.

"Jen, I'm even considering an experimental anti-epileptic."

Recalling his apoplectic aversion for any cutting-edge medication until twenty years of clinical experience had uncovered all its side effects, she half-probed, half-asked, "That's quite a change for you, isn't it?"

"I've got no choice," he said, shifting facial semblances between a biblical Job's resignation and Jonah's dread. "For my child, I'm forced to risk an unknown and hope for no lethal consequences."

"Please tell me, Gary, about the drug. I might be able to help."

They entered the den and accessed the National Institutes of Health website. Jennelle surveyed the room—same furniture and wall pictures as six years ago except a computer upgrade plus three extra albums in the walnut cabinet dated 2008 to 2010.

"The unnamed drug's a magnesium channel blocker," he declared. "NIH sponsors the research."

"Do you know the RO-one project officer's name?"

Graywood scrolled attachments and found the headshot for Doctor Nicholas Severstal.

"Gary, I know him. He's one of their best," effused Jennelle. "NIH stole him from FDA."

"He's heading the search for volunteers with very difficult seizures for the clinical trial," said Graywood, glued to the screen. "He's looking for patients with hard-to-control epilepsy."

"Like Bobby," Jennelle concluded. She ran a hand across the 2010 photo album, patted it, and perused the shopworn one lacking a year stenciled to its spine.

"Yeah," said Graywood. "Through the Human Genome Project, they've discovered magnesium channels. If more magnesium goes into a neural cell and gets blocked from coming out, it lessens the neuron's excitability and makes it less able to trigger a seizure. It's like sodium channel blockers bringing down blood pressure in diseased kidneys and calcium channel blockers dampening the heart." He spoke methodically, as if to convince himself for the umpteenth time on merits exceeding risks.

"Gary, if this eliminates Bobby's seizures, then with a load of physical therapy you might get him back closer to his original self … at least like what had helped May Coldsnow, maybe even more." Jennelle replaced the unmarked album to its prominent spot on the shelf.

"I've read every drug trial," said Graywood in biting short tones, pupils adhered to NIH's website. "It's experimental. I'd feel better about Bobby taking it if I knew the cause for his condition and if blocking magnesium was a plausible cure."

"Gary, magnesium channel blockers are as revolutionary as Cashel Goodlette's climate change theory."

Graywood chuckled the first time that evening.

And Jennelle witnessed the former Gary she remembered.

"When Cash's theory got published," Graywood said lightheartedly, "it sure caused a racket in scientific circles and all the media. Jen, do you know how he got the grant money?"

"I actually asked him that when I saw him in the parking lot behind Grace Hall," she said, with a faint smile. "He smirked he got a seafloor research grant in 2011 that came out of leftover 2009 stimulus money."

"Whoa, they sure weren't kidding when they said it'd take years to spend the federal stimulus on whatever—"

"Gary, wait," interrupted Jennelle, "here's the good part. Cash said he broke down and purposely rewrote research proposals to say he was studying potential man-caused global warming. He laughed how that had done the trick to get Washington to send the money pronto."

"Well he sure buffaloed those bureaucrats. Now he's the darling of the fossil fuel industry and the bane to all those one-track environmentalists."

"But he'd be the first to say his theory wasn't rigorously tested to Popper's standard," defended Jennelle.

"Jen, Roe and I've talked a lot about Cash. Roe's been following what's going on in geology journals. He believes Cash is the third way in science … like a Buddha."

"Regardless, Gary, we really don't know the causes behind climate change. What if Cash is wrong?"

"Well, it's not carbon dioxide footprints according to him."

"Yes, I know that."

"We need to forget about charging after carbon dioxide," said Graywood, in an attempt to move away from Bobby's mystery and cling to any certainty or even Cash's theory. "Changing CO2 levels won't change climate outcomes or mitigate its effects. The world needs to reinforce levees and dikes instead, not waste money controlling CO2 levels—"

"Gary," inserted Jennelle, in edged tones, "you and I are good at researching the causes and errors in thinking." Then she lifted Gary's right hand off the keyboard and pleaded, "For Bobby's sake, maybe this time you should stop going after the cause for his seizures, unlike what Cash does in climate change."

"You lost me, Jen."

"Stop looking for the disease that you'll never find. Search for better ways to treat Bobby's condition. Epilepsy is like climate change. Both are symptoms. We don't know the cause, so treat the symptoms the best you can."

Defeated, Graywood pulled away and stared at the floor.

"Climate change is like a fever in parts of the world, like a seizure in others," nudged Jennelle. "Fevers and seizures are symptoms for things we may never understand, but NIH has a promising drug to control it."

Stunned, Graywood rubbed his forehead.

"Of course the insistence in many circles to go after CO_2 is wrong," said Jennelle, shaking her head. "But Bobby's seizure treatment utilizing that magnesium blocker could be crucial."

Silent, Graywood refused to commit.

"Mitigate the effects of Bobby's disease by eliminating the seizures. Gary, you said every episode loses neurons. It may become too late before you're ever satisfied about causes and side effects."

"It's experimental, Jen. I'll think on it."

Jen remained respectful, honest, and good to Graywood.

He wanted to be with her. Maybe God had brought her to tell him to try the exploratory med. Maybe she'd come for other reasons too … perhaps for him … like Mary Tarf bringing the light back into Piper's life.

Don't press …

The ruinous conflict within Graywood's heart and head made Christmas Day a battleground where a parent fights for one's sick child. Burnt-rubber Shadowman had knocked Bobby out twice—first by the tree opening presents and then at dinner when he lit the centerpiece candle.

Graywood agonized six days over the increased seizure occurrences. The aggressive tempo forced a decision between the experimental drug and surgical intervention on Bobby's brain.

An operation could mitigate severe epilepsy by severing the deep white matter connection—the corpus callosum—between the cortical two sides. Split-brain persons functioned remarkably well, but they processed information in a disjointed manner when compared to those having the left and right cerebral hemispheres linked and communicating both ways. In contrast to people with integrated brains, each part of a divided-brain individual could learn something the other half would not recognize. If Graywood chose surgery for Bobby, he'd lose the son he loved and second-guess adoring the modified boy.

Graywood's prejudice against experimental medications impeded as much or more. His father had died after enrolling in a heart drug trial at an acclaimed Seattle hospital. The test medicine was withdrawn from the market by FDA only months subsequent the funeral because it caused more harm than good. Thereafter began the smoldering grief and chain-smoking in his mother. Sorrowful memories resurfaced of the suffering and resentment against lung cancer not averted by the innovative chemotherapies championed as her last best hope for survival.

Graywood evaluated a drug's risk by how it matched to survival: the benefit was low if survival risk without the medication was high; or the reverse, a high benefit if the survival risk without it was low. This inverse correlation made no logic if reasoned in Bearhead's four-square method: risk and benefit did not have to be at opposite ends of the seesaw—a novel medicine could be both high risk and high benefit, or low risk and low benefit.

Each fresh morning approaching the New Year, Graywood policed the Christmas tree's desiccated needles and repositioned Bearhead's quaint Brandy Belle carving on the fireplace—an inch leftward one day, a hand-width back the following. To the wax-tipped angel crowning the Nobel fir, he appealed, "Jesus, what should I do?"

Leafing through the Kauai photo album on New Year's Eve, he recalled Bobby's words when they'd left Kilauea Point lighthouse: "Dad, you always take so long to do things."

Graywood stopped vacillating.

Jennelle helped register Bobby in the NIH trial.

"Epilepsy is a disease for which we don't know the cause, but we've got treatments, and that's so much better than diseases where we know the cause but don't have any treatments," reasoned Graywood when exiting the Glacier Brewhouse with Bearhead to their parked vehicles.

Bearhead kept silent. The crystal evening bit cold hard, and tonight he willed not to smoke.

"What's causing Bobby's seizures doesn't really matter so much," Graywood chortled, unlocking the Subaru. "They're controlled now."

The experimental medication had worked—no seizures for five weeks. Graywood welcomed the hope that pressed like a coveted greatcoat in Arctic gales. "Thanks to science, I'm getting my son back," he chattered. "We don't know what's causing the seizures, but we can treat them. One day science will explain that too."

Unlike the global warming debates, there existed no corruption within the meticulous pieces of fundamental neuroscience advanced by the NIH. And with extensive physical and occupational therapy, Graywood believed he'd have Bobby at or near the levels he'd paraded on Kauai and Campsite. From his wallet, he showed Bearhead a two-by-three digital taken the week previous—the confident boy balanced on Cub's sled runners without holding the handgrips. With Cub's assistance, Graywood would take Bobby back to the smooth, carefree lake cradled in the Seven Sisters … watch the boy ky-canoe and fish and shoot arrows hitting or missing the target on the alder tree.

Bidding goodnight, Bearhead caught a shooting star not dimmed by the city's nightlights. He pondered how to live with risk, accept uncertainty … Time might give cheerful endings or maybe not. Either way, one had to adjust. Life was possible, but never easy. Whatever happened, one had to try to grow one's spirit.

To the faint stars, he spoke, "I'm glad for you, Gary and Bobby. You both can now follow your bliss."

Through Bearhead's mind-eye, happiness tended to split in arbitrary quantities. From their qualities, one's spirit could grow or be made smaller. So how should one choose?

Bearhead yearned to get comfortable with joyful endings. Yet too old to fully believe that way, he still believed in having good days. This was one.

By June, the world made sense to Graywood. Bobby had remained seizure-free for four months. Jen had inched back into their lives.

Science had led the way.

Graywood thanked the gracious God.

CHAPTER THIRTEEN

FORWARD

Dogs rolled in the bright, blinding snow, laced in the rich smells from other sled teams. In fine frenzy, they reveled in the cold out-of-doors at the starting line by Meiers Lake Lodge.

Severe weather tumbled out of the Gulf of Alaska to blast frigid hardships. Yet Cub's huskies and crossbreeds strained in harness, eager for action on the out point. Piper hand-signaled he'd been cleared to fly ahead to the mandatory rest stop and wait with Cub's resupplies.

Cub spent a moment to thank old Sable. Canine lymphoma had wasted the pack's matron and First Sergeant to a hoary trunk on compacted stilts. She'd died at home two winters past behind the backyard pissing stone. Yet her sense for order somehow stretched through Cub's lead dog, the intrepid Balthus, the prime from her sole litter.

Cub had revered Sable's pure intelligence and staunch loyalty. He'd never called her bitch.

The Copper Basin 300—held each January prior to the Iditarod—stood the best qualifying dogsled competition among serious mushers. Slotted forty-third in the initial out times against 116 competitors, Balthus and Cub pressed forward and overtook seven ardent teams.

But the long intense miles at minus thirty degrees deluded Cub's wits and created interludes with demonic self-doubts he might not finish. Facing them down, he reached every checkpoint the first day and assessed the team's stamina for injury, despite clever canine attempts to cover up weaknesses: separated and left behind loomed the worst for a trained animal whenever others remained linked and were commanded away.

At the supply stations, Piper scrutinized Cub too. Like a seasoned doctor who assessed patients, he applied the unobtrusive manner honed from decades instructing student pilots toward solo flights.

Piper sparkled as the most capable aviator to sky-hop harsh conditions along a trap line of break sites. Backing up Cub with encouragement and provisions in a major race like the Copper Basin or the upcoming Iditarod reconfirmed Piper's arctic airborne skills and buried the age-old rivalry between bush pilots and dogsledders on who owned true back-country supremacy. Gruff yet cautious toward unpredictable atmospheric conditions, Piper most wanted Cub to complete the contest and, with luck, place in the top twenty.

Cub craved his father's respect as well. But when crossing vast snowfields and guiding around drifted obstacles, Cub failed to fight off the relentless fatigue, so ached and heavy and chased by mental meanderings. Uppermost, he grappled with the tragedies Bobby endured … *How brave. He's suffered so much loss—limping steps, weakened arm, broken speech, and that sneaky Shadowman …*

Cub felt fortunate with the challenges in the ordeals he'd picked—tests having ends. Sifting over perpetually frozen, whitened tracts, he weighed the horrible fate that had hobbled Bobby so. Why had destiny brought his young friend so much harm?

Cub had chosen the pitiless exhaustion and squeezing cold off the flagged, wind-whipped trails pierced by ice spit. Yet in Anchorage, Bobby had no choice but to trust the experimental drug he swallowed six times a day for seizure control—its magic had to work.

Come third nightfall, a revelation seemed to glaze from the magenta-hazed dusk. Howling winds that had plastered gritted frost into one's face since daybreak shifted to Cub's back. An uncanny zest tingled his skin. Like the training runs near home, Bobby's crippled profile appeared blanketed and propped audaciously in the sled's bay urging Balthus to win. For eight entranced miles, the sublime mirage animated an unbound eagerness in Cub's frigid trial … and formed his most coveted memory.

Forever brother-like, Cub embraced becoming Bobby's physical proxy. Two fortified minds in unified spiritual fire persevered against the savages of uncertainty.

The team raced not only for themselves but for Bobby too. Cub never let down his dogs, his dad, or best friend. Strengthened, they streaked over the ivory-colored reaches to the final pennant.

Cub had chosen this rite of passage. He'd come of age.

Summer rain glistened on the pavement and then faded to dull silver under the pale dawn sun. Anchorage had added a dozen square miles to its grey urbanity in the six years Jennelle had been based at Atlanta. City fathers promoted Alaska as the Pacific hemisphere's center and Anchorage its hub. Worldwide among cargo shippers, it ranked third in metric tons, ahead of Tokyo and Shanghai.

The Centers for Disease Control and Prevention had relocated Jennelle the previous December to its Grace Hall offices at Alaska Pacific University. Elated to leave behind the unrelenting Arctic winter, she succumbed to the days smudged ever so slightly in evening's tepid darkness, which forced blackout blinds pulled down on every window. Surrounded by brightness, she coerced herself to cease work and sleep. As had happened years earlier, her rhythms adapted to the perpetual midnight glow.

Alone, she drove to the Lake Hood landing strip to catch the double-hop to Glennallen and Chitina and finalize procedures in those villages for the new hepatitis type C vaccine trial. She took Cashel Goodlette's recommendation and hired Piper for swift shuttles into bush country—no equipment barriers, baggage delays, or security bottlenecks to impede time. She enjoyed Piper's banter as well. Curt and perceptive, Piper in many ways was a kindred spirit to Cash.

Jen wondered if there existed any roadblocks between Piper and his partner, Graywood—probably not. They still owned equal shares in *Sky Woman.*

But two obstacles impeded her and Gary from hooking up as they'd done ages ago. Bobby's bizarre seizure disorder had forced Graywood's total commitment to the child. That understandable masonry would crumble as Bobby improved on the investigational medication she'd argued for last Christmas. But the second wall stood impenetrable: Gary's hang up on his ex-wife. He wasn't diamond material yet. Weaving through the warren of airport hangars, Jennelle measured Maren's imprint on Gary, an unalterable seal of ownership …

There's that one special person whom you'll probably never get over, although your friends and family say, "You'll get over it …"

Graywood remained clutched by what adult amours were supposed to be—first true love, dazzled by supernova sheen. For a significant number of people, first love, even decades later, remained as fresh as yesterday. Many would reunite with their first love if they could. Stuck, Gary was one of them.

Jennelle deduced she'd become an idealized Maren replacement. Graywood defined self by relationships, emotional dents and all, and foremost those with Maren and Bobby. That's how she reasoned when she parked behind *Sky Woman*'s shed.

"My little bird's ready," Piper said. "Got equipment to load?"

"None this time. Just me, a laptop, and my smartphone."

Buckled in, they taxied toward the airstrip.

"Oooh, look Jen," gasped Piper, pointing out an open bay tucked in a row of maintenance shelters.

She craned her neck.

"They're getting a vintage Stinson ready for a run," he sighed, thin lips pursed wishing to kiss its taut wingtips. Two men hovered at the forward landing gear of a silver-colored Stinson SR Reliant. Another inspected the black-trimmed tail. "God, such a sweet piece to fly. Makes me just sizzle to see her so spiffed."

"Why so?" asked Jennelle, leaning back and unzipping the carry-on.

"Ahh, for one thing, she's my age," Piper answered through a drawl grin. He nudged *Sky Woman*'s throttle back to slow entry to the runway and wait for clearance. "If we wanted, she and I'd start collectin' Social Security, but I'll hold off till sixty-six. But damn straight, I bet she'll fly forever."

He switched to control tower talk and got the go for takeoff.

Jennelle slipped a preliminary data disk into the laptop. Hepatitis type C had imprisoned victims for years without parole—a biological confinement tantamount to diabetes, paralytic polio, or HIV infection. Caused by a virus analogous to its type A and type B cousins, hepatitis C had worldwide distribution. Greater than four million Americans carried the chronic infectious form, and each year, over twelve thousand died from its related liver cancer or cirrhosis. Those complications often lurked as silent maladies, and victims remained unaware how debilitated they'd become until their livers had failed.

A long-standing mystery, hep C was identified in the 1980s, yet scientists were unable to develop an adequate screening procedure for the elusive virion until 1992. Thereafter, donated blood and organs were tested for it. The virus had spread by transfusions, accidental puncture exposures to health-care workers, or dirty needles utilized in drug addictions and tattoos. Sexual transmission also had been documented as a risk but remained far less efficient.

Not everyone affected progressed to advanced liver disease. The disease acted in dissimilar manners within varied groups. Many victims carried the infection throughout their lives without major problems. For others, it harbored a death warrant.

Once researchers created a method to replicate the virus in human liver cells, instead of from standard culture media, then viable immunization development moved ahead. Cellular biologists reconstructed the intricate automations that type C self-triggered in order to mutate and remain covert within its host—the virion, in cunning reiterations, donned disguises, like a fleeing criminal, to avoid detection and destruction by the host's immune system. Scientists targeted the products critical for the masking mechanisms to make it vulnerable to immune attack.

In stark contrast to the crapshoot mentality speculated for the biological workings behind the HIV inoculation trial, which had failed in 2007, the basic science that underpinned the novel hepatitis C vaccine elucidated all the meticulous components deemed critical to induce disease protection and to what degree. Borrowing earlier knowledge on human immune activation when exposed to hepatitis A and B immunizations, a viable hepatitis C inoculation was readied for effectiveness trials on diverse volunteer groups across the globe.

Not wishing to lead a hepatitis C study arm slated for Chicago, San Francisco, or Houston, nor overseas at Capetown, Naples, or Bangkok, Jennelle volunteered to direct the Alaskan program. Akin to Jane

Eyre retuning to Thornfield Manor, most of Jennelle's motivation had stemmed from discovering whether Graywood had changed and if embers still glowed between them.

Although not afflicted with Edward Fairfax Rochester's blindness at the end of Bronte's novel, Graywood had indeed about-faced: enigmatic eyes searched for bitter secrets instead of truths. A decade in years older than Jennelle, he appeared like her father with mental vitalities contracted to running on fumes instead of bolder substance.

As *Sky Woman* arched the Chugach Mountains, Jennelle's mind spoke on Graywood's apparent state: "When I think hard on you, Gary Graywood, I admit sometimes I dwell on my one-time fiancé back in Georgia. That's over, but he didn't compare anywhere to your constant clinging for Maren. I really don't wish to know about her, but you still keep your ex too much deep inside. It's natural to have a few leftover emotions, some keepsakes of past lovers. But for all your suffering with Bobby, is there space inside you for anyone else—enough room for me when so much Maren swirls your heart?"

Piper opened the intercom and motioned Jennelle to don the co-pilot's headset. "Cub told me he signed up for your shot study last week."

"Yes, he did," she confirmed. "Being eighteen, he's ideal to follow long-term and see how protective the immunization becomes."

"How long's that gonna be?"

"Depends on funding for the project," she replied. "I hope five years at least. Ten's better; twenty is best."

"Shoot! You track people that long?" Piper said, mouth puckered as if he'd swallowed a lemon.

"Yes. It's easy with electronic medical records everyone's got."

"Hells bells, I don't know," Piper groaned, head shaking sideways. He banked *Sky Woman* toward a landmark bend in the Matanuska River beyond Palmer. "Jen, I like and trust you. But the government's got way too much power. I ain't happy 'bout people probin' my family's private records."

"I share your concern."

Piper remained silent. They maneuvered past a moraine and tracked Glenn Highway for an easy ground guide to Glennallen. "Jen, what'll you look for anyway in Cub's records?"

"General health history, if any allergies, what vaccines he's taken," she said matter-of-factly. "That's about it. Nothing more."

"So when'd you shoot him?"

"A few days ago."

"Hmm. So he's protected against whatever you're studying."

"He might be," she replied. Piper's raised eyebrow hinted distrust. To clarify, she said, "Every volunteer gets the new hep C vaccine or the old hep B one. I don't know which one Cub's gotten."

"Why not? Ain't you s'posed to be in charge?"

"To limit bias in the results," she explained, "everyone's blinded as to who gets what. It's called a double-blind cohort study."

"Well … How do you know it'll work?"

"A few people down in Atlanta know the code for whom got what," she said. "At a future point, like five years or so, they'll reveal it and compare results."

An abrupt air pocket buffeted *Sky Woman* into sharp descent. Clenching teeth, Jennelle clamped the laptop. The altimeter spun down nine hundred feet.

"Didn't feel that bastard comin'!" Piper screeched. "Damn, not at all." He steadied the aircraft and increased airspeed to regain elevation. Offhand, he added, "You know Gary keeps my boy current on all his shots."

"I'm sure Gary keeps good track of everything as Cub's doctor," she said.

"Nah, he ain't his doc. Cub goes to Doc Timm, same as Bobby," Piper corrected.

"So why's Gary involved?"

"Oh, in the past, he'd ask if it was okay to stick Cub with a booster of whatever when he needed to shoot Bobby. The boys got shot together." Piper winked at Jennelle and added, "Before Bobby got real sick, every time he'd be stuck, he'd bear scream to Barrow. Cub teased he'd take any shot like a man and wouldn't cry and then dared Bobby he couldn't."

"So Bobby accepted the dare?"

"Ahh yep. Gary's pretty clever 'cause it sure helped a load when stickin' the little guy. Bobby never liked losin' a dare to Cub."

That was the Gary she'd known before Bobby's illness.

"How long's the Glennallen layover before we hop to Chitina?" asked Piper.

"I have to check the clinic, look at their implementation plan for my protocols, and see if they need equipment for the field trial."

"So how long?"

"Couple hours."

Piper calculated flight times in his head and announced, "We can get early supper in Chitina with the Coldsnow sisters."

"I wouldn't want to impose."

"Nah … they'd be insulted if we didn't spend time with them."

"You're certain we'd be welcomed?"

"Jen, back in *Sky Woman*'s tail are four full supply boxes Roe wanted me to drop off to them." He winked again. "Believe me, they'll be happy to see us."

Bearhead had urged Jennelle to include Chitina and its surrounding villages in her Alaskan field study. He'd googled hepatitis C for history and impact—a scourge on all populations but more so to Native Americans and other minorities.

Bearhead had recounted to Jennelle how his first wife, Ume, had died from liver cancer caused by hepatitis C in the blood transfusions needed for her hysterectomy in 1984. And he described the meningitis suffered by his daughter, Sophia. Her death would possibly have been prevented had she lived a decade later when state-of-the-art childhood vaccines existed.

"How's your wife been?" asked Jennelle, curious about Piper's state of matrimony.

"Oh, Mary's wonderful," he said, cracking a full smile. "She retails my paintings at damn good prices. Took a bunch down under to Sydney last year and sold the lot for top dollar."

"How long you've been married now?"

"Six years next month."

"That's great, Piper."

"Damn straight! Longest ever been married to one woman."

"You're so lucky you found her," she murmured.

The primary order of business at the Glennallen clinic dealt with vaccine storage at the proper temperature—the refrigerator units required reliable checklist procedures and a backup power source. Keeping the cold chain intact stood the most critical component for any inoculation trial. A product lost efficacy whenever maintained outside its optimal temperature range. When Jennelle had investigated the suspected causes for the international HIV immunization failure, the first parameters assessed were warehouse and monitoring records: only two locations had failed—one in Jamaica and another in Brazil. All the African sites had maintained the correct conditions.

The Glennallen clinic's cold storage capacity and tracking procedures met Jennelle's standards. Almost error free, the documentation and injection log passed scrutiny, except for an unusual discrepancy: forgotten in the main refrigerator behind the routine inoculations hid an unopened vial still wrapped in cellophane. Manufactured by Cannes Pharmaceutical Internationale, the European casing label had instructions printed in French and English. It prevented chickenpox.

What a curiosity! How did it get to Alaska of all places?

Jennelle recalled CPI from the prior HIV investigation when in South Africa. The biotech firm had developed a novel method to produce inoculums, but sometime in 2008, the South African Ministry of Health had cancelled its CPI contract due to insufficient funding from the World Health Organization. A British-Swiss holding conglomerate swallowed up the company after the global financial meltdown. The foreign product she now held brought back the exciting hunt for the bedrock answers to the HIV vaccine misfortune.

Moisture had diluted away the first part on the printed expiration date to reveal two smudges with a decimal in between followed by the number 070815. The log book had no record of the bottle ever being opened, but notations only covered the past five years. When questioned, the clinic's head nurse assumed the contents remained potent until 07 August 2015 and, therefore, had not discarded it.

Under her breath, Jennelle kidded how the French believed their immunizations aged like a Roquefort cheese or Bordeaux wine. Then she explained to the nurse how the French employed a dot instead of a comma to separate thousands. The correct expiration date must have been 2.0070815, or 2007 August 15.

Perplexed why this product had made its way to remote Alaska, Jennelle decided against tossing it. Her biomedical skepticism toward current scientific dogmas had magnified after all the never-ending, international bird flu scares plus the unprofessionalism that had birthed the worldwide 2007-2008 HIV vaccine debacle. If she ever carved out some spare time, she'd track the vial's lot number through the FDA and trace where other CPI shipments might have gone in the United States.

She borrowed a portable ice chest and transported the tiny glass puzzle back to CDC's cold storage locker in Grace Hall.

Graywood did not meet Jennelle and Piper at Lake Hood as planned. A text message vibrated her cellphone: "At Providence. Bobby + seizures. Double shit!!"

CHAPTER FOURTEEN

Knik Arm's Far Reach—2016

Tapestries in dreams, shattered glass, goodbyes …

"He's a huge sleeping dragon who blows in the mist,
and he lives far beyond the great mountain in a secret cave
on the wild side of the island."

"I can't hear you …
"I can't make you out … Your eyes should be as big as eggs
when we go searching for him. Hold my hand!"

"God, there's mud over my eyes. Help it off! Is that your hand?
"Now, I see them. My eyes! Get hold of my hand."

"He's a huge sleeping dragon who blows in the mist,
and he lives far beyond the great mountain in a secret cave
on the wild side of the island."

"I can't hear you …"

"I dreamed of you last night. Must I, then maybe again … not. Your fingertips, ten fleshy temperature pads, clean, keratin-rimmed, electric!"

"Gripped.
"I swallow possessed, sighed the full breath over dimensions filling voids between the gas stars. The sigh we each know once."

"We pursued adventure or a birthday?
"I can't remember …"

"A mirror … an octagon reflector. There! I stared it.
Tense skulled eyes winced back, penetrating, horrid hot,
ever searching the blank black blur. My eyes. God, MY EYES … only."
"Was something more there? Were they yours?"

"Try to remember the dream. An apparition like Hamlet's father?"
"No, none at all."
"A dragon? Yes, a dragon! Maybe you're telling me you're okay there."

BRRRING … BRRRING … BRRRING!
Wake-up clock. Damn! Oh goddam!
"Phhth!"
Dreaming about dreaming again. God, how long looped I on that tarn?

BRRRING … BRRRING … BRRRING!
Okay, okay! Shut off, damn it!
Done.
Move legs.
Can't.
Try feet.
Don't want to.
"Ugh!"
Dig your fourth fingernail into thumb and exhale, inhale,
repeat and again. Face rub sheeeet … breathe slowly into nose.

Graywood pulled off blankets, floated a gut snort, and then mouth-sucked air.

Exhale.

He yawned.

Exhale.

Slit eyes open? Well … maybe …

Damn! Legs won't move. Useless. Where's the damn will?

Get up. Oh, Jesus Christ, get up!

Think yourself up. Will it. You damn well better!

You know he can't. Only now in dreams can he get up if you'll remember them.

Morning broke to a young raven's caw-caw. He rose to it. Refusing re-possession of the bed, he dragged open window curtains. No sun to flood on the sojourn to toilet.

"There you are," he spat out, passing the eight-sided mirror. "You and your buddies invade my dreams." Old and silver with faded edges, it telescoped absurd labyrinths of mirrors diminishing within mirrors beyond forever in the dream about dreaming. Yet he remembered no more on his son than fingertips.

He brushed lather to stubble. Blade across beard, metal dragged skin like a bird's claw.

Arm nailed to chest, he froze after one stroke.

Graywood's torso shuddered.

"Why'd you have to die?"

Salt burned his eyes.

No ferocity in the sun.

Damn You, God, where are You?

Endless grey clouds. A pubescent storm had ripped the birch leaves and stuck them to morning's window.

My child's funeral … today …

"How's that, God? Is this what life's about?"

The kitchen coffeemaker beeped completion to the 7:10 a.m. routine brewing. Gharrett Graywood had received the programmable contraption as a gift when he'd retired from the Public Health Service.

Legs burdened as barrels, he descended the staircase and dragged toward the double sink. No stomach for caffeine. Not yet.

Brandy Belle nibbled dry cat food by the back door to the garage, her metal tag tinging the porcelain bowl with each tongue-spear of food. He listened to the cadence. Feeding her twice a day was Bobby's chore.

Do something.

Toxic grief glued lower limbs like deadweight logs, shellacked and motionless. Nothing but brain ache and guts cha-chunged across a gnawed, crass chasm lacking a dram of fortitude.

Heartless … courage had vanished beyond oblivion … vanquished with his child. The worst day in his life, more wretched than when Maren had abandoned Snowline Drive fifteen years ago.

A cone of sunlight intruded through the great room's center windows. Graywood limped to its glow. Fresh glinting snow crested the Alaskan range to mark the cold night. Pearl-topped coastal waves chopped high and beckoned him. Mountains to sea—Knik Arm to Cook Inlet, Susitna to Talkeetna—he scanned June's panorama.

A pedantic awareness crawled along both arms. He lifted binoculars from the walnut end table and scanned the incoming tide thankful he'd done something.

But the water shurled frothy sprays. Limbs lowered, Graywood grasped an emerald-glass dragon figurine from the sideboard. Framed by denial that comes easy in the early mist to hold death's demons at bay, he embraced an escape to Kauai.

"Puff's a huge sleeping dragon who blows in the mist, and he lives far beyond the great mountain in a secret cave on the wild side of the island."

"Why's he's sleeping now, Dad?"

"To build up his magical powers. And it's time now to go and fix some supper."

"How big is Puff?"

They started for the Hanalei Inn with Graywood spinning out more thick threads of the tale.

Alone on the lanai after Bobby had settled to bed, he thought of Maren and what might have been …

Stop!

Kauai happened nine years ago at spring break.

Father wanted to take son to a warm spot. More so, he wanted a time out from Bobby's school. At winter's parent-teacher conference, Graywood had been told Bobby demonstrated signs of attention deficit hyperactivity disorder.

Do whatever's best for the boy. The evidence for treating ADHD favored medication helping while in school, yet he waited until Bobby started second grade …

End these unwelcomed shades.

"Dragons live forever but not so little boys." Not little Bobby whose blue eyes once outshone the Kaua'ian sun … Prophetic lyrics sung by Peter, Paul and Mary. Yet boys were destined to grow up and become men. Not die.

The crystal statue fell from Graywood's grip and struck the window sill. One wing cracked, the other in three pieces.

A massive, arsenic-grey band erased the golden rays. More scuds seethed out of the gigantic storm parked in the Gulf of Alaska. Graywood punched on the weather channel.

"Intermittent showers with afternoon sunbreaks."

Bobby never minded rain, but Graywood wished for one solid spell of light, timed to carrying the casket to the gravesite.

Stodgy steps lugged back to the kitchen. Empty-handed, he slumped beside the lacquered oak table: the central meeting place for catch-me-up dinners followed by more catch-me-up homework; the oft flour-dusted surface flagged as the official sponsor for monthly cookie-eating contests; and its brown-grained, rectangular boardwalk brimmed by eager breakfasts of scratch-made, sourdough pancakes or mixed-up cereals sprinkled with wild blueberries they'd stolen as a team from the bears at Hatcher Pass.

Eyes closed, Graywood regressed in time, lungs as hollow as his will.

"What're you eating?"

"Sugar lumps with honey," volunteered Bobby. He groped inside a Frosted Krispies box, liberated from the floor cupboard.

The bare boyish truth made Graywood mute. Preparing hot oatmeal topped with sliced banana had to wait another day. Head shaking side-to-side, he carried to the table two ample bowls, spoons, and milk.

"They're good with cinnamon too!" crowed Bobby. He relished combining breakfast foods into concoctions Graywood punned "sonny bunches of oats."

Rain battered the roof and ripped Graywood back to the terrible present. Not hungry, he trudged to the den.

Two o'clock funeral … plenty of time … too much time … No, not enough …

He clicked Maren's lone email.

"Gary, this is so sudden. What a loss for you. I'm sorry. Will try to come. M"

Just like her. The mistress of short replies. Not a paragraph in response to pages he'd sent. Graywood mulled on Maren and interment obligations and realized all the time he'd known his ex-wife she'd never expressed "I'm sorry." She was probably the only woman in America who saved all her I'm- sorrys only for funerals. At least by that she was authentic.

"Oh, sweet Jesus Christ, Maren," Graywood yelled at the screen, "Bobby's a loss for us both! He's your son. Acknowledge him and come."

He jerked a photo album off the bookcase's middle shelf and tore each sheet of catalogued pictures to pieces.

There once had been a time when he was sure of her and most things. Then she deserted them.

"You can still go back to damn New York and pretend to be the eternal maiden denying ever having been a mother," Graywood half spoke, half cursed. "Just come to the church service."

From Maren, he hoped for a valuable step toward closure. For their Bobby, he needed her help. After fifteen years of avoidance, would she come or stay away?

Graywood remembered little about their nuptials—a sultry-hot, Maryland-elite Labor Day weekend extravaganza. It was not a 1999 New Age millennium close-out, marked by vows bubbled underwater in scuba gear or mouthed parachuting from seven thousand feet. Maren had toyed with the ceremony concluding on her sport club's high diving platform followed by stripping off their wedding attire to swimming suits for an instant plunge after the husband-and-wife pronouncement.

There was the nasty explosion with her mother over which gown to wear. Maren had hunted every Anchorage bridal boutique and online catalog once Graywood had recited his marriage proposal in tempo with the impressive Independence Day fireworks at Elmendorf Airbase. For three frustrating weeks, she'd discounted all formal garments in Anchorage as second rate and ordered a custom designed fashion from New York labeled "Snow Fairy." But the gown had grown mundane upon her return to Maryland a month before the ceremony. She had to revise it and all the other copious preparations—dictated in person to her mother and maid of honor.

Maren desired furrowed Belgian lace embellished on Chesapeake Bay taffeta. She shuttled to Baltimore, Philadelphia, and all the way to Richmond on the great quest. Over and over, every wedding detail was transformed. Her mother multi-tasked every tumultuous day with brilliance and held her pleasant demeanor while fighting the urge to strangle her daughter.

Without warning, Maren chose a trumpet gown with button back and sweep train to embrace her exquisite silhouette. She felt the beautiful, slim mermaid. It was she.

Her mother advocated "Snow Fairy."

They crescendoed into a two-day, pitched battle with all the mutual recriminations only a daughter and mother can manipulate. Maren won.

Exhausted from spite, they overdid making up and vowed not to tell Graywood about the gown change. They reasoned him so mesmerized in love he couldn't tell one from another. Men were like that.

Yet Maren had not anticipated the maid of honor spilling the secret blowup to the groom at the reception after too many flutes of Sekt. Graywood simply passed it off as a peculiar form of preparatory stress. Besides, weddings always were advertised as the happiest day in a woman's life. Seeming rather paradoxical, he surmised, the advent of so much joyfulness could indeed create ample discord between the bride and her mother.

When they departed on the honeymoon, Maren's mother cautioned: "Gary, Maren is delicately pretty and a carefully tended flower perpetually in slow bloom."

Uncertain whether his mother-in-law thought him stupid or intended him to be impressed by her elegance, Graywood inferred she'd meant him to be the perfect gentleman and take total care of her daughter. In short order, he discovered she'd warned about her daughter's out-of-bounds narcissism.

To bear Bobby for Graywood had become Maren's greatest sacrifice. And she'd steeled mind and body to never have another child.

"Will try to come. M"

Graywood read her email fighting its undertow.

Will she say goodbye?

What is she?

CHAPTER FIFTEEN

Pilot's Wife

Sited in the Hillside area of Anchorage on Snowline Drive, the Graywood home boasted jaw-dropping views of Cook Inlet. The mountain peaks within eye-shot took too long to count. The abode divided twenty-eight-hundred square feet among a great room, sun room, office den, formal dining room, kitchen, and three bedrooms. Large twin oak doors opened to a natural stone-floored foyer, illuminated by vaulted skylights and an Irish crystal chandelier Maren had imported. A granite fireplace opposite a wet bar anchored the lofty great room. Into it poured summertime's light, courtesy of etched French door glass, from a west-facing, tiled sunroom where one accessed the north and south exterior decks. The foyer's oak staircase ascended to the master suite with its gigantic walk-in closet and the smaller two bedrooms.

Huddles of spruce and birch bordered the sloping acre outside. The semicircle driveway, trimmed with thick perennial shrubs, connected garage to street.

O'Malley Elementary School sat a mile away, and Hanshew Junior High sprawled within two. Nearby Ruth Arcand Park maintained Little League diamonds. The Alaska Zoo, the Prospect Heights hiking trailhead, and the abutting Chugach State Park were short scoots down the road.

The location seemed perfect when Graywood and Maren signed the myriad purchasing documents: breathtaking views, not far to work or recreation, and plenty of space to raise two kids. Graywood would have done all things possible to make Maren and their future children happy.

He discovered Maren couldn't cook a lick after their New York City and Nantucket Bay honeymoon. She shunned culinary precision and hated time wasted cleaning up.

Graywood preferred meals at home and had cooked since medical school.

By default, he arranged the kitchen appliances, utensils, pots, and crockery to his usage pattern and coaxed Maren into splitting each week's dinner preparations. He managed Sunday, Tuesday, and Thursday nights while she concocted Monday, Wednesday, and Friday. Saturday evening they ate out. Breakfast and lunch remained solo endeavors tied to daily individual routines, although Graywood often created weekend morning platters of waffles, pancakes, or biscuits plus ham or sausage, garnished by sliced fruit, berries, juice, yogurt, and whipped cream with mugs of stout coffee. He even baked sweet cornbread from an old Southern recipe Maren's mother had sent.

He installed a kitchen window greenhouse and cultivated an herb garden to zing his creations. To Bearhead and friends, he gave fresh chives, parsley, oregano, basil, and marjoram.

In return, Bearhead offered cooking tricks gleaned from globe-hopping as a chef. Bearhead had summarized his itinerant cook-for-hire experience prior to pursuing university at Anchorage as the finest background for cultural anthropology. One core motto he often repeated was "One shall truly understand a people by what and how they eat." Graywood modified Bearhead's bromide: "A doctor must understand the patient by what and how much he or she truly eats."

Graywood hoped Bearhead's culinary skills might pass to Maren by osmosis. It appeared so until her initial battle with morning sickness on Valentine's Day. Thereafter, Graywood assumed full-time kitchen duties.

After Maren left, Graywood scoured efficient cooking techniques as he juggled career and raised Bobby. Bearhead shared many recipes that aided time management. One particular creation, Bearhead's Breakfast Souffle, was a savory bread pudding Graywood threw together in the evening to bake fresh once they'd started early school-day rituals.

He'd dice eight cups of one-inch bread cubes and pile them into a three-quart, buttered, casserole dish. After browning a pound of breakfast sausage links, he'd cut each into one-inch lengths and lay the parts evenly among the bread pieces. Twelve ounces of cheddar cheese were grated over the sausage and bread. A half-dozen eggs blended in a cup of 2-percent milk, three dashes of black pepper, and a teaspoon of chopped oregano leaves, dried from the herb garden, completed the assembly. He poured the mixture on the bread, cheese, and sausage and covered and refrigerated it overnight. Come morning before shaving, Graywood popped the container in the oven.

Bearhead's recipe called for salt, but Graywood eschewed it in harmony with his never-ending crusade to limit everyone's sodium intake. And Graywood never violated the cardinal rule learned from his mother—prepare breakfast to feed one's child before ever leaving home.

Swelling rain pummeled the forenoon of the funeral.

Graywood's rough-hewn physical appearance demarcated the fierce struggle to cling to reason. Never the glossy, gorgeous men's-magazine model, neither did he appear the opposite … yet today only worse.

He spurned leafing through the volumes of Bobby's chronicled photographs to select ten or twelve needed for the memory binder next to the condolence book. He drained his mind away from the home's hollowness; yet a part of him yearned to gather handfuls of remembrances that drifted within its rooms.

Plenty of time … not enough time … no, too much time …

He entered the sunroom to erase melancholy aches. Light-kindled shards pierced the turbulent clouds and revealed a red-and-white-striped Cessna 185 like the one he'd trained on with Piper. It chinked the western sky atop the coastal wildlife refuge and traversed the Fire Island wind turbines before its descent to Lake Hood's airport.

Graywood mouthed Piper's mantra: "Fly with skill and aggression. Swoop and roll updrafts, kite-waft downdrafts, never dart chopper-like. Always check the propeller once you've taxied to the hangar."

Piper managed adversity with outward aplomb, and Graywood envied his friend's stubborn strength. Partners since '98, they were straightforward, predictable men who each had a son.

Cub possessed Piper's verve yet possessed more practical sense and tact for others than his dad. Bobby … thankfully simple and terribly complicated … was gone.

The gentle Cessna joined the horizon. "It's God's will to land well," whispered Graywood.

He refused to accept God's will for Bobby. To delve on faith or the lack would numb Graywood senseless. Rather, he craved merciful blankness, or he'd doubt all connections to the Almighty. Better to flush the mind, climb the stairs, and pick the afternoon's suit to wear.

To failure's tempo, two feet shuffled the hallway. He lingered on the banister by the twin front doors … Each ascending step held a phantom of his boy. He welcomed some …

"Bobby, what a mess you've made!" exhorted Graywood.

The three-year-old munchkin had extracted eleven pairs of Maren's leftover shoes from the guest room's storage closet and lined them down the stairs two per step. Over his head, he fluttered the right tan slingback from its box and cradled the other on his lap.

"Well young man, what are you going to do with those?" Graywood asked, anticipating Bobby placing them on the last empty tread.

"Take 'em to my 'oom."

"Your room? Why?"

"I 'ear Mommy ooalking in 'em."

Dumbfounded, Graywood hesitated until Bobby climbed the staircase clutching one sole in each hand. Was it possible that an infant, not quite a year old, had imprinted the mother's cadence and recalled it later when a toddler? And why this pair? With dinner close to burning on the stove, Graywood had no time to ponder the mystery.

"Okay, Bobby, take Mommy's shoes to your room, and after we've eaten, we'll put the rest away where you found them."

Graywood, in time, suspected his son possessed a form of synaesthesia—on the boy's fourth birthday he proclaimed hearing frost freezing and, with closed eyes, recognized greens and reds by touch without a miss.

Synaesthesia existed as a trait not uncommon with artists. Bobby might be gifted with enlightened abilities, and Graywood anticipated with pride how the talent might mature once he'd started school.

It didn't. Bobby's kinetic energy and reluctance to master reading funneled him down into the world of attention deficit hyperactivity disorder. Once medicated, he responded less to every whim, and his brain shifted up to the long-term planner mode required of every American second grader. He thrived without any of the drug's known side effects, yet extended-release Ritalin pruned off synaesthesia's buds: he ceased hearing the frost or feeling green, red, silver, and gold. That unanticipated side effect wasn't deemed important to report to the Food and Drug Administration.

Graywood let in another phantom, not so filled with hope …

"Dad, was I adopted?" Bobby asked, having abandoned Lego assembly in the great room.

"So the seven-year-old boy actually listened today in church," thought Graywood. "Ritalin did some good after all." He stroked varnish on the half-dozen gouges in the banister, gashed by the wayward hockey stick. The Sunday-before-Thanksgiving sermon had talked of Jesus Christ adopting you when you feel alone.

"Why do you ask that, Bobby?"

"'Cause Cub has two moms and I don't have any."

The answer hooked Graywood deep but made sense—a week earlier Bobby had met Piper's fourth fiancée, Mary. All the past contact with Piper's second wife, Rachel, when he'd played with Cub must have sourced the question after he saw so many mothers with children in the pews this morning. What answer would he believe?

"No, you weren't adopted; you got adapted," rolled astonishingly off Graywood's tongue.

"Adapted?" Bobby's face filled with a what-do-you-mean grimace.

"I'll try to explain." Trapped by his own mouth, Graywood hunted for an acceptable response for Bobby as well as himself. "Ah, I meant to say your mother isn't here."

"Why's she not here?"

Graywood laid the stained brush in its aluminum tray and paused to come up with a better chestnut. "She had to go away. So you had to adapt to that." Searching for words, he sealed thumb-tight the resin bucket's lid. "I had to adapt too. So we both got adapted."

A close call, but Graywood couldn't relax. Another sharp barb snagged.

"Dad, why'd she go away?"

For years Graywood had rehearsed that response knowing someday the question would be asked. Yet his mind rubbed out when it counted most. He had to ad lib. "Your mother couldn't live here in Alaska like us for lots of reasons … so she had to go away."

"Why?"

Gaff number three, the gigantic one. Graywood pleaded inward, "Please, brain, don't fail me." He cleared throat phlegm and said, "Your mother wasn't born here like you. She was an outsider from a state called Maryland where it's a lot different from Alaska." With the brush handle, he tapped the lacquer can's top and added, "Our winters were too cold and too dark for her health. And our summers weren't hot enough." There, he'd answered with concrete facts instead of more triteness.

"Oh, okay." Bobby traipsed to the great room and resumed constructing Legos.

And Graywood rediscovered how simple and short facts, not vague feelings or creative wording, got farther with the seven-year-old.

Then he remembered what he'd wished to say. He wanted Bobby to know one of the biggest challenges to being a family was dealing with—adapting to—a member who behaved in ways that disappointed or distressed the others. The rest of the family could still choose to love her, even when they hated what she'd done. And he ached to have said, "Your mother still loves you even if she's far away." He couldn't after Maren's terse rebuff to join them on Kauai for spring break. It might confuse the boy. Graywood had been split-hearted too. That's why he couldn't recall it.

He trudged to the great room's entrance and watched his son erect a runway control tower. After a conflicted rumination on parents choosing to separate from children, he carried the varnish and brush to the den and commenced planning Jennelle's going-away party at the Glacier

Brewhouse. The CDC's main office in Atlanta had reassigned her to uncover answers to how the state-of-the-art HIV vaccine had failed.

But he put Jennelle on hold and opened the untitled photo album in the walnut cabinet. For the umpteenth time, he resurrected why Maren had refused Kauai.

An ambulance stretcher gashed the banister's railing the final time. Bobby's seizures had progressed to status epilepticus—abrupt toxic bouts of unconsciousness every few minutes with the spine arching with rigid feet and hands after arms and legs flailed. He never returned to Snowline Drive.

Graywood ascended the stairs to the guest bedroom. The tan leather shoes Bobby had heard his mommy walking in were lodged somewhere here or hidden in his room.

Maren had commandeered this unclaimed space as a makeover into a colossal walk-in closet for spillover apparel.

She hung meticulous gowns, blousons, caftans, wraps, sheaths, and cocktail dresses on movable metal tiers aside the walls and added two reinforced racks that trisected the room from window to doorknob. Graywood had the hinges reversed so the door swung unencumbered into the landing.

He remembered the room's footgear section the most and Maren's mission to own the utmost fashionable styles. She morphed the space into an enclosure crammed with four hundred berths divided by genre. These lucky pairs had survived the grand purging of their ranks before she married.

Maren refused wire racks or hampers and had Graywood construct extra shelves to the ceiling. Bins parked beneath the bottom slats enclosed territory for twelve sets of seasonal boots, sacrificed to nasty weather soiling. She kept half the shoes in original boxes, stacked by type, color, and heel height. The accompanying rod inserts and packing tissues preserved shape and protected from dust. She photographed each design and taped it to the carton's exposed end to aid recognition.

Maren convinced Graywood to confine his clothes to the third bedroom's closet. She reserved the master wardrobe to protect coveted Fendi, Marc Jacobs, Gucci, and Chanel. And Chanel outnumbered the others simply because, for Maren, Chanel worked forever.

"It's all about the look. Everyday people judge you by how you look," she explained. "Fashion is what's offered annually, and it's fickle year to year. Style is what you ignore first and select second in putting together what to wear each day. Outfits you select and assemble will be judged. You're judged all the time."

Thus she required the entire walk-in closet area. It seemed excessive to Graywood, yet he hoped her devotion to appearances was not a substitute for personal depth. He agreed to the third bedroom being his dressing area until needed for their first child.

Maren left behind the twenty-eight pairs of footwear she'd purchased in Anchorage. Graywood bulk-mailed the unclaimed mavericks to her father's Maryland address after Bobby had asked why his dad had a cubbyhole with women's shoes and boots. All were shipped away except the one tan pair. Whenever Maren wore them, she'd correct her husband on their charming color—taupe.

Graywood found the duo in the old genre pen: fourth rank, sixth slot. He'd take them to the memory table and tell Maren the quaint story about little three-year-old Bobby on the stairs.

And he'd place both next to their son, forever.

"Will try to come."

Graywood stood by the bedroom window, his right index finger oscillating along the heel of one of the taupe-colored slingbacks. Another cloudburst loomed over Tanaina Peak.

"Will try to come."

He shortened Maren's message to "Will try." He'd no idea what she meant. A gamut of disguised intent, commitment, and purpose encased those two tiny words. They could result in anything so meant nothing.

Then a spark flashed from an old conversation he'd had with his mother-in-law once Maren had fled: "My daughter has only one idea, Gary ... herself."

Futile?

Graywood tried to comprehend his ex-wife anew. Every person possessed threads woven from vanity. In Maren, too many had been spun into choking cloaks of narcissism. He recognized the colors and parts in the pattern but not all of it.

Born in 1971, Maren was an only child. Her father, a Maryland newspaper reporter, savored writing articles on United States history pertaining to the American Civil War. Her mother managed a mortgage brokerage and traced family genealogy in her spare time.

Maren's parents had excluded her from their work and interests. By default to please her grandmother, she practiced the cello. She recused from most childhood friendships, yet she'd never forsake the freedom discovered at Virginia Beach summer camps where she swam and windsurfed Chesapeake Bay's natural currents. She became a seasonal lifeguard at the neighborhood's pool and excelled to the degree she competed at ten-meter platform diving in the state's Olympic trials. Her goal—win a place on the 1988 national team.

Equally committed to the cello, she played it with secure musical artistry to obtain grandmother's acceptance. The instrument's timbre, vibrating to her focused strokes, brought out soothing assuredness and control. The strings responded without complaint, and the intimate music she crafted was her own authentic confirmation, not illusion. Resonant passages anchored her consciousness and aided the ability to decipher reality out of social mists. Maren believed she possessed first-rate musicianship but never pretended having her grandmother's professional caliber to perform in the Baltimore symphony.

Granna started Maren's discipline at age ten, taught the stern basic and intermediary techniques, and three years later, passed her to the orchestra's principal cellist. Maren's skills flourished, and at her pinnacle, she performed dutiful solo passages of Victor Herbert's Cello Concerto No. 2—an unusual work—for her parents, teacher, and a handful of studio guests. Thereafter, she set the instrument aside, hiding it in a closet. Four years passed until she stroked it again … alone.

By a fluke, Maren discovered her cello playing skill could augment the execution of her competitive dives. She'd double the descent difficulty score whenever she synchronized face, neck, arms, legs, and back arch to a four-measure excerpt from a Bach cello suite, played in her head. She integrated a unique instrumental phrase for each plunge and promised to thank the coaches, Granna, and most of all, her cello if ever she won an Olympic medal.

Maren garnered competition successes until nationals where she finished a heart-freezing ninth. She'd been judged and lost. She terminated the Olympic quest and resolved never to lose, never to forsake control again. She—and only she—would choose the judges in her life. To heal the contused ego, she chose fashion and placed it higher than people, especially men.

Maren had a Goldilocks approach toward males. She bedecked her figure as an appealing picture in search for a frame, and should she take an interest in a man, he had to be just right. A date, boyfriend, lover, and future husband were accessories to her personal wardrobe; the masculine physique a mere cut above a coat, handbag, hat, and gloves but not on par with jewelry, nail polish, and pumps. It was harder to find the perfect shoe than the perfect guy because men came to her willingly. All types approached. The way it should be.

Her *modus operandi* was "It's better to be looked over than overlooked, unless of course a Neanderthal gawks at you." Yet she still hunted for flawless high heels.

She readily recruited admirers, both male and female, into her fan club and tested their loyalty. Writing off defectors became her justice. Exquisitely aware of her power and privilege as a modern female, in time, she drifted toward boredom and attempted to flee.

Maren started out as a buyer for Federated Department Stores. As ambition and anxiety gripped her more and more, she switched venues into high-end merchandise that maximized accentuations for the apparel, accessories, and cosmetic displays sponsored by the elite brand names across the country. Ultimately, her savvy and impatience pushed her to market fashion-line shows on the gargantuan cruise ships sailing the 1999 Alaskan summer schedule.

And Alaska beckoned the essential escape she craved—an unbounded space to assess the static relationships between self, design, and commerce. She'd had her fill of plucky, pouty males who controlled the fashion industry and believed they alone owned the divine rights to shape the swaths of fabric and influence. Such men could never be near her center—too loaded with falsehood.

Maren pursued originality, a more genuine life, and ventured north to find life's real substance, instead of sham experiences that infested the eastern seaboard. Alaska's majestic landscapes appeared ready-made backdrops for her heroic discovery of newborn womanhood as the fresh millennium dawned. But as she mapped the future, another life flew in.

Maren met Gharrett Graywood at a Juneau Chamber of Commerce event, co-hosted with several cruise lines to kick off the traveling season. Food-borne illness outbreaks had stricken Caribbean and South Pacific leisure ships the previous year. Graywood's public health office had refined shipboard food service and hygiene inspections for vessels docked in Ketchikan, Skagway, Juneau, Seward, and Whittier. Alaska's tourist bureaus lauded Graywood's deft interpretations to the up-to-date regulations promulgated by the Centers for Disease Control and the programs necessary to monitor safety compliance without itinerary delays. They invited him to Juneau to acknowledge his leadership. Before returning to Anchorage, he planned to hop *Seneca* over to Turner Lake and cast for rainbow trout.

Maren wore a short black dress and valentine-red lipstick in carefree cahoots with flowing blond hair. She spotted him at the buffet twenty feet away. Slim with gentle eyes, he had the spot-on height of six feet, prominent chin, and mandatory non-obtrusive nose. The second time he looked up from the crab salad and smoked salmon pâté, she turned profile and refrained her smile knowing his face would open bright upon such a view. She'd judge his response by how long it took him to converge.

Smitten, Graywood's chest froze … hyacinth-blue eyes gathered her in … the ballroom's prime appealing visage. By instinct, his torso squared to her.

She glanced at the central chandelier to signal no engagement with the couple abreast. Waiting for him to come, she arched her back ever so slightly and half-pirouetted to present the opposite side.

He didn't advance.

Curiosity tripped through her internal limbic brain, tinged by irritation. *I'm doing what any woman with a pulse would do. Why's he not moving? It's kind of cute if he's doing this on purpose to show restraint. Or utterly stupidly insensitive if it's some type of crass, manly callousness. Maybe it's the retarded pace to life here from too many cold winds. Strange, or reverent, still he's awfully cute, but darn sweet darn, he's glued to the cream dip!*

She altered tactics and strolled to him, long legs stretching gracefully, feline-like. Had it been noon, hot jealous tears would have flowed off the sun's great orb peering down on her.

Achingly beautiful, not simply pretty, she ignited Graywood's torch to blinding white. Maren sensed the powerful, controlled temperament exuding from him, much like Timothy Dalton of James Bond fame, only impaired by a dishwater-blond mane begging for style advice. She assessed the fork of hair on the left with the pinch to the right and the in-between waving locks as tolerable for his face but not her frame. They could be altered.

"Gary, I like you," Maren said once the easy talk paraded beyond the second glass of Sauvignon blanc. Graywood had hinted of his passion for flying and then steered the conversation toward books, music, and films he adored. He'd mention not a single sport.

She appreciated he hadn't broached one of her pet-peeve questions that hounded the usual meeting scene preceding a date request. Even better, he'd asked nothing about her family.

"I like you too, Maren," he said, captured by her sapphire-blue eyes when not diverted as she angled coy, and he caught the faint circular borders for tinted contact lenses. What were the eyes' true color?

The remaining evening's banter skimmed among probing exchanges on their respective professions, other interests, and delicate sexy nuances. By ten o'clock, the mutual deeper comfort had settled in, and they sauntered to the ballroom's balcony to follow the sun disappear beyond Douglas Island and Nun Mountain.

He abandoned the plan to fish in the morning and took the leap. "Maren, would you like to go soar in my airplane tomorrow and see some glaciers from above?"

"I'd like that, Gary."

Takeoff time was negotiated—rendezvous at her hotel's front desk by half past eleven. To close the evening with this gorgeous woman, he concocted the elegant excuse of needing adequate sleep to meet FAA requirements since tomorrow he'd pilot for an extraordinary passenger.

Maren regarded the charm and tactful insistence on safety. She gauged the aviator while he bid goodnight to the hosts and exited the ballroom—intelligent, no problem changing the hair distraction, he didn't press, and he showed potential. No deal breakers so far.

She entered the lobby wearing a tailored, charcoal Armani blazer and Versace jeans. "Hi, Gary." Blond, svelte allure matched well to her lyric voice, rich as blended, twelve-year-old Scotch.

Projecting a gaze intense enough to blind an eagle, Graywood betrayed a swooned lover.

"Gary, your eyes glitter like gleam off a glass," she cooed and offered a cheek to receive his quick kiss. "I put on my no-fuss clothes. Hope you don't mind."

She carried a Hermes leather jacket. "Help me on with this?" she gently asked.

Worth a Klondike fortune to have a woman like Maren on his arm, Graywood winced not shining his boots. *Seneca*'s auxiliary heater was also broken. Thankfully a spare parka was stored aft should she feel chilled over the ice. She'd be the first lady flown by him in *Seneca.*

Maren scuffed the cherry-red nail polish climbing aboard *Seneca.* When settled in, Graywood began the passenger safety briefing. He demonstrated unlocking the doors on either side in an emergency and pointed to the Halon fire extinguisher stored beneath her khaki leather cushion. She fastened the seatbelt but let him adjust the Bose aviation headset to help him inhale her perfume and touch her soft hair. As he fitted the equipment snugly, the desire to be with her percolated his core.

Graywood had installed the cockpit headphones and audio control panel to dampen flight noise and improve ability to hear music or continuing medical education CDs when cruising to outlying clinics. Whenever Piper piloted *Seneca-Sky Woman*, he preferred gabbing with the passengers he was ferrying into the hinterlands. Piper had insisted they wire a redundant comm-switch, push-to-talk relay to doubly insure control tower and intra-cabin communications.

Graywood had filed the flight plan prior to meeting Maren at the hotel—a loop to the Canadian border and back that zoomed over Taku Glacier. Upon receiving takeoff clearance, he taxied the floatplane out from Juneau Harbor. Airborne, they ascended along Gastineau Channel to four thousand feet and banked toward Taku Inlet.

"Look off to your right and down," Graywood said. "That's a grand tidewater glacier fed by ice all the way from Canada."

Maren peered out but remained silent.

"The blue light shooting off its crevasses matches your eyes," he added, in a neutral tone as possible.

"Why's so blue?" She tested for sincerity, not tipping gratitude for the compliment just yet. She wondered how good he'd do fanning last evening's subtle romantic intentions.

"The reds and yellows in the visible light spectrum are absorbed, and the ice is so compressed its density almost equals water, so you get your iridescent blue … a truly magnificent blue." He didn't need to add, "blue like your eyes." She got that by the trailing timbre in his voice.

A complex answer, she concluded: two clever parts, which displayed a splendid head and heart. He showed respect for her intelligence as well as beauty. Indeed, he had promise.

Graywood would have spoken further but stopped short. He held great respect for glaciers—somehow they reached up and threatened airborne concentration. Piper warned how flowing ice lacked graded snow for approaching planes, compared to airport runways, during freeze-up. And ice masses uncovered rolling rocks all the time because middle sections moved faster than the sides; the tops, more than the bottoms. A single day might convert a safe surface into treacherous as the ice packs advanced or receded. To know the safest parts to approach and exit committed one to seek the pilots who risked it. The best ones tracked and remembered the mistakes others made.

Graywood had snapped off a Cessna's ski strut while learning to land on Spencer Glacier. Fortunately, Piper had mountaineer gear to climb off the *névé*. He always carried emergency equipment and rations whenever flying, even a spare propeller, but not an extra strut. Graywood never forgot the ribbing other aviators blew their way afterwards—the stud instructor and book-learned student stuck on an ice floe without a strut and forced into a long twilight hike. Unlike then with Piper, Graywood had no emergency equipment for Maren in the rear of *Seneca* other than rope and a sleeping bag … so today, extra caution needed.

Coursing over the Taku, Graywood ascended to 6,500 feet and vectored on Demorest Glacier and its brother Llewellyn. A mere four hundred feet over the jagged pinnacles, he swung to the back of Mount Ogilvie and sited the landmark to Mammary Peak.

"That's Mount Ogilvie," he said. "We've strayed a bit into Canada."

"Can you do that?"

"Well, we had to." Graywood desired a clear position high and far enough to showcase the upcoming magnificence of three peaks—Gale, Typhoon, and Blizzard—before they skirted Mammary. He needed a tad Canadian airspace to do that. The three mountains were called the Cloud Catchers. Graywood wanted them not to reach and become the plane catchers, as well.

"The Canadian Air Force won't mind if we don't linger too long," he said and winked. "If we're caught and forced down on one of their glaciers, I'll just have them look at you, and you back me up and say I got lost in something for a while, maybe a snow squall. They'll understand."

Maren smiled thin-lipped at the man's bravado and the implication to foreigners he'd gotten distracted by her. She queried, "You can land on a glacier?"

"Don't want to, but I've done it and walked away."

"How many times?" she tested.

"Once."

"So today would be the second time," she said, playing.

"Not today. In thirty seconds we're back in the USA."

"Oh darn sweet darn, I was so looking forward to seeing a Canadian jet," she teased.

He wished to invite her to Anchorage and lay eyes on American interceptors at Elmendorf Airbase but had to focus on the return along Avalanche Canyon or bisect the Berners Peaks.

Maren sensed air-streamed freedom when parallel to the white-dressed mountain faces and more so when the aircraft lifted above them without effort—a supercharged superiority never before experienced.

Midway over Gilkey Glacier, Graywood loaded music to accompany two pending flight maneuvers. He leveled the aircraft to reveal row upon row of snowcapped spines arranged to Aaron Copeland's "Fanfare for the Common Man." When Wagner's "Ride of the Valkyries" commenced, he plunged *Seneca* into an adjacent ravine's nadir like a skier racing an avalanche down the steepest alp … the dive from heaven, the ultimate gold-medal thrill, the Olympic ten-meter platform descent Maren never had experienced. She wanted more.

Graywood drank the adrenalin and blended in more emotion by swaggering *Seneca*'s triumphant wings. From bedazzled joy, Maren pressed a palm hard on his knee as they arched like Apollo across the approaching Juneau sky.

To extend their time together two additional days, they concocted plausible work-related tasks for excuses. She discovered his essence and compared him to classical composers: sensuous as Debussy and surging like early Schoenberg whenever uncoupled from the sweetness and strength of an older Brahms. He was the one she'd hang up her high heels for.

For Graywood, Maren held all amorous visions and beyond. Like copper ends plugged into a socket, love's mysterious madness electrified every synapse. He globalized her, unlike any woman before, as the beloved.

Flowing emails catapulted their sworn Juneau devotions into desperate rendezvous. She mailed perfume-scented cards, the first on his birthday, and continued sending every week they remained apart. Graywood positioned the treasured greetings, fragranced with jasmine, in the top desk drawer of his office desk to keep her presence at work.

Distance formed the primary obstacle to the vicarious trysts from Seattle to Seward. After two months, the time zone tango for Graywood had to cease. Senses heightened and perceptions lowered from raw adoration, he proposed marriage … She accepted.

By New Year's Eve, unexpectedly, they were pregnant.

"We'll sit over at the bar till the table's ready," directed Piper to the host. He ordered his martini and a lemon drop for his spouse, Rachel. Soft jazz settled from the sound system. An open-through fireplace separated the lounge from the dining area at the Glacier Brewhouse on the corner of Fifth and H. In the shale columned hearth, aromatic cedar and spruce combusted on the metallic, six-foot rack, shaped as moose antlers.

Maren and Graywood entered from the street to join the Gunlocks. He guided toward the warmth. "How you feeling tonight, dear?"

"Fabulous," replied Maren. She glowed upon spotting Rachel and Piper. "Honey, before meeting you, I bought shoes at Nordstrom. Hope you don't mind."

He looked at her feet. "D'Orsay?"

"No. That's a style."

"Jimmy Choo?"

"I wish, but not this time," she said, ready to strut and show them off. "But you're getting better. You like them?"

Graywood had given up regulating her footwear purchases. He simply insisted she discard an older set for every pristine pair bought but wasn't sure she kept her side of the bargain. Truthfully, he didn't care, although he tried to recognize the designers. She carried his baby and walked for two. That mattered most.

"They're nice, darling." His gentle hand pressed her abdomen. "Tell me all about our little one."

"Nothing unusual today." She sashayed toward Rachel and Piper like a runway model.

"You look marvelous, Maren," said Rachel, moving off the stool to hug.

"I treasure my newest pets." Maren's right foot pointed a strappy, taupe-colored Ferragamo with three-and-a-half-inch heel.

"They're quite a statement in your condition," said Rachel, holding back a lustful smile.

"But it's me. Other than no alcohol, I'm not giving a smidge to this pregnancy thing. I don't feel I should."

"That's my wife," admitted Graywood. "She delivered from Nordstroms another set of twins today. At home, we could open a complete women's shoe department at the rate she's going."

Maren refrained to correct her husband in public with "Nordstrom" as the store's proper name.

"Sounds like a whole lot of walkin's planned once the babe's born," Piper said and slurped his drink.

"A woman can never have enough shoes," retorted Maren. "You men will never understand until you walk a mile in our shoes." She looked to Rachel for agreement and got it in spades.

"Walk a mile in your shoes? Which ones?" kidded Graywood. "You must have close to a thousand."

"I'll have a diet Pepsi with lemon twist and three cherries," ordered Maren, ignoring the remarks. She parked beside Rachel.

"If I walked a mile in each pair of my wife's shoes, I'd traverse the Alcan Highway and halfway back," boasted Graywood. He winked to Piper and signaled the bartender for GB's handcrafted beer, an oatmeal stout.

"Worse for me," sympathized Piper, "walking a mile in my wife's shoes would take a lifetime."

"Why's that?"

"Too small. They'd hobble my feet real bad, like they'd do Chinese women." Piper drained the martini and motioned for a second.

"Please, dear, only one tonight," mothered Rachel.

"Most my wife's shoes pinch her feet too," muttered Piper, forcing himself not to hear her. "I can't understand that."

That sparked Graywood's curiosity. "Well, let's get some answers." He faced the women and asked, "Why does a woman buy shoes that pinch her feet?"

"They have to be cute," replied Rachel in common-knowledge tones.

"So you walk in cute shoes even though they pinch your feet?

"Well no, Gary, you wear them on special occasions where you're sitting."

"Because sitting in cute shoes pinching your feet is more important than walking or standing?"

"Of course."

"All the time?"

"No, you silly. Not all the time. You have to go to the powder room."

To the dimwitted males, Maren explained, "The hallmarks of good shoes are weight and balance, and they have to help attractiveness in the pelvic sway when you walk. If they pinch your feet, you do it. We suffer for beauty, honey, always." She licked Pepsi off a cherry, smacking her lips. "All you can ask for in a good set of shoes is comfort, looking fashionable, and making you feel sexy. They're like a good man, so they're very, very hard to find." Minus a smile, she stared sideways but not at Graywood and then away.

Graywood quaffed his brew but persisted, "So when do you ever throw them away?"

"Once they become old and ugly," volunteered Rachel. She paused to think about adding more.

"So once they're old, they're thrown away, right?" asked Graywood.

"Right, unless they're cute," said Rachel.

"Let me get this straight. Old, ugly shoes are thrown away, unless they're cute?"

"That's right. But I'd throw away those that don't fit my bunion or are out of style, even if I've never worn them."

"So does out of style mean they're ugly?"

"Well, if they're cute shoes they're not. Shoes that are cute are never out of style."

Frustrated, Graywood retreated to the stout and then asked, "Would you ever toss a cute shoe at Piper?"

"Never! I'd throw scratchy smelly ones if I had to …or give them away."

"Who'd want those?" thought Graywood.

"Gunlock party," announced the waitress.

Piper raised an unencumbered hand to order a third martini for the dining room.

Sliding off their perches, the wives led the way.

Graywood remarked cryptically to his friend, "I can't get the pairing of women and their shoes. If a man can't understand them doing that, how can he ever figure out the bigger mysteries, like nature or God?"

"I don't know about understandin' God," said Piper, "but I know you can't figure women.

"Why not?"

"'Cause God made us first. Women are improved models from Adam's rib." Piper teeth-grinned recalling the long line of makes God had made—and Piper had tested out. "With nature, you'll catch the drift for a few things, such as where moss grows on trees. And, Gary, for the record, some men can be mysterious too."

Graywood wasn't sure whom Piper meant.

Before they reached the table, Graywood overheard Maren say to Rachel: "I should have told those twits a woman stops buying pinched-toed shoes when she doesn't feel a desire to be attractive." She glared at her ripe belly while waiting for Graywood to act gallant and pull out the chair.

Piper tapped Graywood's arm and whispered, "It's better to keep 'em barefoot and pregnant. You're halfway there, Gary. Without them shoes gettin' in the way, you might understand her better."

"Piper, you're a mystery all right. You're all over the map," flipped back Graywood, helping his wife to sit.

Rachel was correct about Piper and seated herself—no more than one martini.

Lukewarm to cold about carrying Graywood's child created contradictions in Maren. She committed the cardinal sin of losing appetite control: First she ate only the broken pieces from a snack, but then she'd smashed the bag on the counter and orally mainline all fragments without regret—easy to devour, like from a feedbag. And serotonin-charged mellowness from sweet scoops of cherry ice cream topped the cravings off.

Maren never lacked attracting the opposite sex—men always seemed accessible and willing. But a showing pregnancy made them cautious to the baby-on-board status. Blond hair and fake blue eyes counted not even frozen crab cakes next to obvious bread baking in the oven. She felt like a passed-over brunette.

The gravid body maligned her self-image. The visible evidence fashioned extra tenacious doubts. Haunted by self-distrust, she could not face her blooming, ever-changing form. Worse, her obstetrician fought her will.

Graywood waited in the office diagonal from the exam room. Voices escalated halfway through Doctor Lansburgh's routine appointment, Maren's most.

"You have striae gravidarum, commonly called stretch marks," Lansburgh intoned. Pink-purple, atrophic lines marked Maren's abdomen, buttocks, and breasts. "Nine in every ten pregnant women get them."

"My mother had them, and they never vanished. This shouldn't happen to me." Maren's fingers splayed over her belly. "Can you make them go away?"

He applied a stethoscope to her heart and listened too long for the question to hang in the air. At last he looked up and reassured, "Your heart is fine," and patted her tummy. "After the baby's born, most streaks will shrink and fade completely or at least go pale in color."

She clenched fists and said in crescendo, "Doctor Lansburgh, I want them gone totally. How will this be done? You must treat them now!"

Taken aback, Lansburgh said, "Let me check your chart." He scanned lab tests and medication history buying time to formulate a satisfying answer. "Maren, scads of creams and emollients have been prepared to make stretch marks go away, but none has proven effective." He cleared his throat and amplified, "They won't add anything more to what Mother Nature does for you after the baby comes."

"I don't believe it," she shot back. "I've read magazines. There're plenty of treatments."

Lansburgh's jaw forced a tense grin at this formidable mother-to-be, and he said, "Well, we could apply Retin-A after the delivery and see how that works."

"How good is it?"

"There're some case studies that support use on stretch marks. Postpartum women in Europe who've declined to breastfeed have even taken it by mouth with some fair results, instead of only spreading it over the skin."

"What about both at the same time?" Maren said. Frustrated, her right hand rubbed her navel.

"I'm not aware it's safe to combine oral and topical Retin-A for stretch marks." Lansburgh returned to scribbling notes in Maren's chart and hoped she'd accept the caution.

Irritated, Maren slid from the exam table. "Are we finished?"

The physician attempted to favorably spin the exam's conclusion. "Maren, you're doing very well. Your baby is healthy, and size matches to dates on the button. I'll check my journals for what's recent on stretch-mark treatments, and we'll discuss at our next follow-up."

"When's that?" she huffed.

Not wishing to compromise trust further, Lansburgh shortened the standard four-week appointment frequency for her stage of pregnancy. On the billing tab clipped to the chart he wrote: "Progressing Skin Condition, Diagnosis Pending, Follow-up Required."

"I'd like to see how your stretch marks have changed in two weeks. Can you come then instead of in four?"

Maren wanted to return tomorrow yet yielded to compromise. "I shall see you then, Doctor Lansburgh," she declared. "And I'll check my sources too."

More cosmetic troubles blemished Maren. Melasma, the mask of pregnancy, smeared her forehead and cheeks with heavy pigmentation mismatched to the natural color on her chin, mouth, and nose. From magazines, her mother, and Graywood, she verified how sun avoidance or employing sunscreen to exposed skin often contained the dramatic discoloration. Her armpits, genitals, and nipple areolae darkened too. A chocolate-colored line, identified as linea nigra by Doctor Lansburgh, appeared where the abdominal muscles joined below the belly button.

Her shimmering blond hair thickened into coarse threads, and manicured nails grew brittle. Frantic, she applied lotions and creams to face and eyelids to tighten skin bloated from the increased blood volume nature decreed necessary for the baby's growth inside her womb. An ugly spider vein appeared where she'd injured her neck in a competitive platform dive.

But greater third trimester complications snapped Maren's tolerance. Her gums reddened. She doubled dental routines to prevent the bleeding and gingivitis that often occurred in pregnant women.

Four pencil-point skin tags budded within skin folds beneath the breasts—three under the left and the largest below the right. Doctor Lansburgh reassured they'd disappear postpartum, but Maren would have none of it. They were promptly frozen off with liquid nitrogen.

Her torment climaxed with the dermatologic condition called pruritic urticarial papules and plaques of pregnancy. PUPPP started as an intense itchy rash along the stretch marks on the abdomen and extended to the upper thighs. Doctor Lansburgh treated with antihistamines and topical corticosteroids to good effect. He explained PUPPP would resolve in two weeks after delivery without adverse effects to her or the baby.

Yet Maren's anger and bargaining over PUPPP appeared on a par with the anguish in patients diagnosed with terminal cancer. She refused to accept the condition as an unwelcomed but manageable part of pregnancy. Mean as a Dixie snake, she peppered Doctor Lansburgh and Graywood on its cause, prevention, and who in what country possessed the most up-to-date therapies.

Both physicians described PUPPP as an unclear relationship between the maternal immune system and fetal cells and how stretched skin may play a role in inciting an immune-mediated reaction. Both repeated reassurances it would end, and the baby would not be affected.

Maren interpreted PUPPP as the repulsive outcome to the intolerable stretch marks pulled beyond limits as the infant increased inside. In secret, she wished for early labor, even if it placed the newborn at risk.

The stress and discomfort levels crowned when the bowling ball sitting on her bladder combined with her fears to push it out. Worse, Maren fretted no man would ever see her as the individual woman she'd been. She vowed never to repeat pregnancy.

On September 16, 2000, Robert Gharrett Graywood gulped oxygenated air and projected a tenacious cry. A full-term infant on the cusp of the new century, he had a father who loved him as precious life itself and a mother who only grieved.

Maren had more than the baby blues.

Postpartum moms' bodies and minds must readjust to the massive changes after childbirth. Critical hormones, estrogen and progesterone, which elevate during pregnancy, fall precipitously subsequent delivery. The mental stress from the recalibration cause over half the new mothers to experience a mild, blue-mood disorder that persists for one to two weeks.

Yet resetting the gravid-altered brain back to its non-pregnant mode could become perilous to a minority of more susceptible women. As many as one in eight suffered postpartum depression, a serious disorder that prevailed for weeks and even months. Maren was one.

Graywood prayed his wife's transition to motherhood would unfold better than the antepartum. She began with courage but withdrew further each day and hinted for help with the infant's care. After feeding Robert at night, she hid in the banister closet and wept. Reclusive, she ate less and slept more … and cradled her cello, not the tiny child.

Maren's mother couldn't leave Maryland, due to her own health problems, so Graywood took a leave from work to stay home. He suspected his spouse had a major mood disorder and scheduled her appointments.

Clinical research had emphasized how untreated maternal depression might harm a newborn's mental and motor development and, as the child matured, was associated with behavior problems, low self-esteem, and poor impulse control. Treatment for postpartum depression positively impacted the family besides the mother. For Graywood it became a slam-dunk, a two-for-one. Even better, a three-for-one.

The latest antidepressant drugs acted as a slow but sustained reboot of the brain with fewer side effects. He confirmed the efficacy in Maren's prescriptions and reviewed every clinical summary archived by the Food and Drug Administration.

Graywood equated treating maternal depression to a parent caught in an aircraft emergency and forced to place on her oxygen mask first. A mom couldn't help her clinging child if unable to breathe herself. Mothers had profound impacts on their children at any age, a no-brainer.

CHAPTER SIXTEEN

Storyteller and Son

Bobby's static room … nothing had changed since the evacuation eight months earlier: turquoise bedspread ajar, saliva-stained pillow, hockey stick propped in its paint-chipped corner, and a bulging closet door hiding its jammed-in disarray. A plastic F22 model jet perched on Bobby's study desk. Piper's glass-covered Rum Tum sketch watched the entrance from above the bed's chestnut headboard.

Depleted, Graywood had to halt the plodding advance toward afternoon's dismal conclusion. For just a short spell, he had to push away the funeral's imploding dread.

Unhooking the frame from the wall, he blew off the dust. Settled upon the rumpled mattress, he ushered a kinder image—a fantasy escape—a coveted father-and-son reunion where he'd tucked Bobby into bed and had spun the first impromptu installment of the tomcat's legend.

"Hey there, Bobby boy, I've got a really special story for you tonight. One that's never been told anywhere in the world."

"Ooooh goodie!" Bobby's blue eyes beamed as the towhead tossed to the pillow and wiggled underneath the covers.

"Ooooh yes." Graywood dangled the suspense. "It's … about … Rum Tum, the unknown Kayak Cat of Alaska."

Comfortable, Bobby mustered glee. "I'm really, really, really ready."

Graywood set the scene: "Rum Tum was a stray cat who lived in Anchorage, which is the biggest town in all of Alaska. Where Rum Tum came from, we don't really know. But we do know for sure that at one time he was a stray cat from our city. One day, he decided he'd had enough of Anchorage, and by accident, he found a way to get passage on a steamship from Anchorage to Unalaska and its biggest town, called Dutch Harbor. The main thing that got him to take this boat was that he'd chased a seagull who'd sneakily stolen the fish Rum Tum had bummed at the dock. It wasn't really certain if Rum Tum was given the fish or he'd beg for it, but either way, he had a fish, and the seagull stole it.

"He chased the crafty seagull to the top of the steamer's railing and saw the steamer's name printed on the side as the *Coastal Voyager.* He didn't know the ship was getting ready to sail to Unalaska, and before he could get off, it had left the port. So he was stuck onboard, whether he liked it or not, and he wasn't known for his swimming abilities, especially in the rough Cook Inlet water, which was way, way, way too cold to swim in anyway. So he took passage all the way to Dutch Harbor. When at last he got there, he was one happy little cat to claw his little paws on dry land because the long passage was quite stormy and dangerous. There had been a gale with howling winds and pummeling rain, which he didn't like at all!

"But he did make friends with all the galley crew on board the *Coastal Voyager.* They fed him some milk, and he REALLY lapped all the milk up when they put a spot of rum in it. They named him RUM TUM, and that became the name he decided to adopt. You never know what cats' real names are, but they do take the names we give them more or less to please us, and Rum Tum did have a hankering for milk with a tiny spot of rum in it.

"As I said, he was a very happy cat to get off the boat. He started his search for a place to live in Dutch Harbor. And he found little Aleutian Girl. We don't know her real name, and if we did, I couldn't pronounce it anyway, so we'll call her little Aleutian Girl. She really liked little Rum Tum because he was such a beautiful looking cat. He had yellow and grey and black stripes and swirls and a big spot of white on his yellow-orange chin, and he also had white hairs on the tip of his tail. Some people might say that he'd dipped his tail in the milk so he'd have some to lick off whenever he needed a snack. But that wasn't true. It was real white fur on his tail and chin. Aleutian Girl was so attracted to him that she really wished to take care of him, and he was so pleased with her that he made up his mind he'd stay with her because he was a true cat, and only a true cat had the final say in all matters with all other creatures. So he agreed to stay with Aleutian Girl.

"Aleutian Girl had a kayak, and one day, she decided she'd take Rum Tum out in it. It was quite a sight to see the two of them because she barely fit into the kayak's hatch, and all you could see of Rum Tum was his little head and furry ears and long white whiskers looking frontward as they went kayaking along.

"Aleutian Girl was very fond of paddling on the Bering Sea coast of Unalaska. Now, Bobby, understand that Unalaska is in the Aleutian chain of islands, and when you're in the water on the south side, you're in the Pacific Ocean, but if you're on the north side, you're in the Bering Sea part. She decided to go out on the Bering Sea side of Unalaska because that's where she had another friend, named Oscar the Sea Otter. Whenever Oscar saw Aleutian Girl in the kayak, he came and swam next to her. This was the first time Rum Tum had ever seen a sea otter … and he was really amazed! The sea otter looked like a little old man. He put his head out of the water and showed a little face with long whiskers, much longer than Rum Tum's. And Rum Tum was totally amazed at how Oscar floated on his back, as if he was sleeping on a waterbed.

"Rum Tum said to Aleutian Girl, 'This is amazing!' Rum Tum wasn't one who liked cold water. 'Oscar,' he asked, 'are you always in the water?'

"And Oscar replied, 'Well, I'm in the water 'cause I like it, and it's where I find all my food.'

"Rum Tum said, 'Well, do you have any food that has milk in it and maybe a little drop of rum too?'

"Oscar said, 'No, no, no! If I ever got some rum out here, oh, I wouldn't know what to do with it.' Then he did a rollover in the water …"

Little Bobby had fallen asleep. And Graywood kissed the boy's forehead, and whispered, "Sleep well, my little one, this long night. I'm going to bed too, and I'll see you in the morning."

Graywood let the fantasy fade. He realigned the blanket to cover the pillow but left the wrinkle where he'd daydreamed the cherished moments.

Graywood searched the room for the yellow-cedar miniature Bearhead had carved. It would be placed on the memento table and then inside the coffin. No success. Vexed, he carried Piper's sketch instead.

An outside brightness swelled and beckoned Graywood toward the window to witness diminished cloudbanks … a hopeful sign for a shower-free ceremony at the cemetery?

He glimpsed the birch tree Bobby had planted the same year of the Rum Tum saga. Kelly-green leaves covered it, three times its height when first planted. The fresh growth drew eyes up and down the white and black trunk.

Somehow the tree suggested Bobby had reunited with Kayak Cat and had restarted their thrilling odysseys with the Unalaska clan.

Such a beneficent tree.

A full smile broke upon the beaten man's chiseled face.

Graywood replenished Brandy Belle's food dish by the kitchen garage door. As she hunkered over the meal, he stroked her and remembered Bearhead's Rum Tum carving had been lodged in the Subaru with Bobby's things retrieved from the hospital.

He discovered and placed it in a double paper bag.

Bearhead had his village, his philosophies, and the Coldsnow sisters. What did Graywood have without Bobby?

If here, Bearhead would listen to Graywood's confusion and mentor toward insights that helped to clear thinking in an instant or jell it opaque beyond four seasons. Bearhead had presented life that way since their first encounter teaching back-to-back Wednesday lectures to the first-year medical students enrolled at the University of Alaska Anchorage.

Brandy Belle licked the dish spotless. Graywood refilled the water bowl and drifted into an oft spoken Bearhead pearl: "What we define today as a thing of beauty or ugliness will change with different eras, cultures, and world views. Obscenity, nakedness, affluence, the downtrodden, the supernatural, old age, and death … they shall vary over time and country."

Yet for Graywood the agonized end to Bobby would never vary. Would he ever make sense of it … the loss of his child? Bearhead had walked in those shoes after he'd lost Sophia. Now would Graywood?

Another Bearhead-ism challenged Graywood's utter enormity of dying: "The morals and myths we create and place in a hierarchy are, for the most part, arbitrary attempts to make sense of the world in order to understand the environment we live in. We create morals to help us comprehend life and death.

"First, we build moral hierarchies out of what we kill to live. Some things we allow to die, some we actively destroy, others we won't dare to, and so we construct the strict boundaries we will not cross anytime throughout our lives. Yet there are lines we choose to cross when we're older that we wouldn't trespass when younger, and the other way around. For example, one person's morals will distribute on the ladder of humanness very distinct places for each of the following five entities: a five-day-old human embryo ordered sacrificed for stem cell research, a first-trimester abortion, a female feticide so her Asian parents may try pregnancy again hoping for a male, a partial-birth abortion, and female infanticide. Each of the five is subjected to different standards of humanity and moral lethality throughout various cultures or subcultures and at different times, past and present. But there are others among us who believe these five products of pregnancy are forever one continuous entity unsplittable, each rightfully sanctioned to live and develop to its full potential. Whom on this ladder would you elect to kill? None, some, or all if need be?

"Let's contemplate two more examples: many countries believe it is morally acceptable and justified to execute murderers while other countries do not. Yet they sanctify thou shall not covet thy neighbor's property or his wife, part of the Ten Commandments given by God to Moses. Please be aware that still today in many countries wives are viewed not much more than property. And a male believer of Islam may have up to four wives, so long as he treats them equally. Depending on viewpoint, wives represented as property are either the morally weaker or stronger components among various societies throughout the world. You students each choose your perspectives on these examples, and I warn you, they may not be ironclad throughout your lives. But consider this: in some cultures you have no choice … particularly if you're female!

"What we term as moral and immoral is, therefore, quantified by our personal and cultural concepts of fairness. For the most part, fairness is a matter of opinion. Your hierarchy of fairness may not be my hierarchy, and so forth …"

Graywood stopped Bearhead's mind-bursting fugue. Those mental imprints had no meaning now. He couldn't cope with the relative amounts of humanness divided between five products of conception or the widespread belief wives were simply property: all unjust cultural directives against the world's women.

No, today Graywood suffered heartbreak—Bobby in a box forever.

CHAPTER SEVENTEEN

Goodbyes

Saint Michael's ring chimes pealed on the cellphone.

"Hi, Raych."

"Did you sleep last night?"

"Not much."

"I didn't rest at all. Gary, do you need any help?"

"I'll always need help."

"I know, dear." Rachel waited. He remained quiet. "Gary, you there?"

"Yeah."

"Cub and I are going to the church in half an hour."

"Rachel … thanks for your help … for everything you've done with Bobby." He wanted to say he loved her for being so loving to his child after Maren had left but couldn't.

She lingered. Letting anguish flow uninterrupted seemed best. But he stayed mute too long. "Gary, Jennelle's planning to pick you up in an hour. Should I call her to come now?"

Jen, the woman who'd left him and had come back. Graywood didn't know what he wanted. Who'd care if he was late? Would Bobby? Where he was at, time didn't matter.

"No, I'll be ready."

"Gary, you let me know if you need help."

"Ah, Raych … I appreciate everything. I'll muddle through."

"We're praying for you and for Bobby."

"I know."

"Jennelle will show in an hour. You want me to come now?"

"No … It's all right. I'll make it."

"All right." Rachel resolved to call when she arrived at the church. "Bye, dear."

"Yeah … bye."

Graywood ascended the stairs to shower and lay out the charcoal suit.

Rachel and Jennelle …

He'd known Rachel almost twice as long as Jen … when Piper and he'd become *Seneca-Sky Woman* partners.

He adored them both, but differently.

"Gary, we're at the church and setting up. I've found a place for the table and picture book."

"Thanks, Raych. You're priceless."

"How you doing, dear?"

"I'll get through."

"Gary, you call me if Jennelle hasn't come."

"I will."

And Maren?

Only an email: "Will try to come."

Will she be there?

Out of a condensed timespan shot the first words Maren had spoken when she joined him in Juneau at the buffet table: "My name is Maren. You pronounce the 'a' like the 'ah' in star … Mah-ren. It means lover of the sea."

For uncountable eons he'd tried to shut her out but failed. Some parts in a person ever loved could never be killed.

Graywood subscribed to societal and religious teachings that a couple should marry to have children. That bedrock supported the other mixed speculations on what a union should be. From his mind-set, there existed no other reason for the institution. He had hoped to father two healthy children when he'd proposed.

He pulled on the suit trousers worn at their wedding rehearsal dinner and brush-shined the black shoes.

Yet odd, poignant memories recirculated: "My mother's a bitch!" yelled Mah-ren. "I blame my obsessions all on her."

Like pop-up screens sneaking past his mental firewall, ageless arguments Mah-ren and he'd bled over replayed peculiar fragments on neural circuits.

Still there had been much of her he'd forgotten. That's the way after divorce.

So why did she accept him as a spouse when she didn't want to be wife and mother? Her thinking and heart mystified and haunted the rest of his life.

Maren had trekked to Alaska in search of originality and found it in Graywood. Convinced, she embraced the richness in him and doubted her doubts before their nuptials. But illusion of romantic love was what she wedded, not the man, not the maturing friendship and habits in a husband or the inherent demands of raising children. She'd married only for one shade of love's multicolored flames.

Bottle-feeding Robert in the dark night voids between sobbing spells, she discovered love had splinters …

From her parents' staying together, she knew of long-married love and wondered how much got chopped from necessity, the rest hewn by fondness. Out of the latter, she concluded little, if any.

Maren adored new-romance love. How could any woman not? She had it once with Gary but lost it with the pregnancy to the point at times she'd rant and wish him dead.

And she'd tried to fit romance into matrimony. It didn't mesh. Angry and terrified, it wasn't worth her sacrifice.

Soul-searching four o'clock in the morning beside the great room's windows, Maren whispered to the city's skyline the lack of maternal love: "Why don't I feel attached? I don't want him to come to any harm. But I can't give myself to him. Am I afraid to see most my history now in him, detest all the time and effort spent on him and regret all I've stopped searching for … for him? Will I confuse him with me? Will Robert become my identity? Can I accept and forgive this tiny child becoming the biggest part of my life and all the controls he'll place on me forever? No … I'm not here or there or anywhere for this."

As New Year 2001 ushered stark snowy landscapes, Maren churned her grim life sentences on becoming a wife and mother. Alaska's harshness coupled to Gary's stolid, classic ways of provider, performer, and protector unfolded as dull, extreme, and too confining. She had to escape the introverted home routines, tedious stifling meals, its pervasive suffocation.

In wedlock, this peculiar wife and husband could no longer be "everything" to each other, nor could she sacrifice self for Robert: martyrdom was such a poor role model for a child born into this young century. Terrorists and saints were pretty much slathered out of the same clay, and she was none of those. She'd find the resolve to force Gary toward another woman who wished to be a mother first, who wanted children.

A hundred times she explored feelings and motivations and would a hundred more. For Gary to plea for her to stay was futile. Her sanity took precedence because all that was Alaska—the marriage, the infant, the disjointed seasons in darkness and light, an ordained future so dominated by home, hearth, and husband tied to expectations for a second child—defined a jailhouse confining her essence away from the exciting, glistening freedoms in Maryland and New York City.

Maren had made two wrong decisions: marrying Gary and having Robert. She lacked postpartum lust for her husband and desire to cuddle the child. Sheer temperament refused to impart emotional juices they both needed and erected limits to face-to-face intimacies. The immense family bonding expected prior and after pregnancy exceeded her capacity to give, and her ego could not accept the doubtless and biting certainty she'd be judged an unsuccessful mother. She abhorred the perceptions of uncaring witch, yet to stay housebound in Anchorage would transform her into a gross, cold goblin.

Maren had read there were no ideal or perfect families regarding the number of parents in the home with children. Some did better with two; others better with one. If staying brought on prison-like despair, then she'd need to break out and seek the shimmering Manhattan canyons and warm Chesapeake summers. Flee to places she controlled and seek the joys there while Gary and Robert diminished in time.

And she'd apologize to no one. Taking the easy road by sacrificing self to unhappiness as countless women had done over the centuries with their passion-sucked-out marriages was farthest from her nature.

The burden of choice was hers alone—as always, what's best for Maren. This would mean Gary parenting Robert solo. If she hurt them, she'd accept that, but it stood better to exit before the baby recognized much of the hurt too. Gary wanted children, and he had earning power to pay for extra childcare. In time, she expected he and Robert would move on.

As the anti-depressants invigorated her, Maren secretly renewed old links with fashion industry associates and searched for work far from Alaska. She drilled for leads on upcoming positions, permanent or temporary, and sent dozens of resumes. The pure act directing her future fortified the primal sense of control. And when self-dominion got coupled to unencumbered singledom, her world would dazzle as before.

Energized, she yearned to organize a spring fashion show pro bono. It propelled her like an insistent cellist plucking concerto strings. She could flirt with delivery boys and cherish the gauzy, liberating, exuberant thrills of the chase in round after round of pursuit, like the huntress Diana.

She restarted her morning face routine with a lighter hand applying foundation. "Made by God, aged by Father Time," she remarked to the mirror, harnessing a wry smile, "but Mother Nature and Fifth Avenue taught me how to camouflage."

The other rock-solid, 100-percent activity with her reflection concerned swallowing the daily birth control tablet with a large glass of water. The method had never failed until wedlock.

Gary so yearned for a boy and a girl, but Maren had forbidden parenthood on short order and insisted they try out marriage only as a couple for three years. Yet she had gotten in a family way a mere four months beyond the wedding. Surprised and seething, she had suspicions her husband had altered the pills. So did the furious river of resentment beneath the camouflaged skin flow.

Maren whitened her teeth, purchased pink lipstick and flower-scented perfume, and wore highlighted hair in bangs. She sorted through the copious apparel racks and overstuffed shoe coop and wrote off over half as useless, including every item bought in Alaska. The survivors were shipped clandestine to her parents in Maryland. Goodwill got the crumbs.

Musical sessions on the resurrected cello quickened recovery from postpartum depression. Maren's thighs and hands embraced the instrument that had provided solace in the bleakest periods. When adolescent classmates had betrayed, she clutched her cello. When scarred by ridicule, she mended and brought to life compositions altered freely to suit impulses. And when she was sixteen, the broad, wooden friend remained the closest confidant as they coped through an abortion. Only the instrument and three others knew. No one else ever would. That oppressive reality, if found out, would shatter her personality, style, and visions of control.

At first, Maren forced the cello's tone: no deft bow landings or booming fervor; no languid caresses or hushed cathedral majesty. Scraping and scratching, she refused to engage showoff maneuvers yet sawed out sections from Rachmaninoff's "Sonata in G Minor" and repeated the adagio tucked in Mendelssohn's "String Quartet in B-flat Major" where the cello sang mournfully with two violas.

As intonation improved, Maren's confidence soared. Stroking easy and natural notes, she lengthened the daily therapy and advanced to surging, modulating pieces, such as Brahms "Trio in B Major" for violin, cello, and piano and the opening to Smetana's "Trio" where the cello's dissonant sound and fury dominated.

By springtime, satisfaction had reentered mind and hardened spine. Emboldened by the selfless instrument and the scores of referrals to follow-up employment queries, Maren emerged from winter's gloom determined to leave spouse and baby.

On the May morning Robert yanked on the great room's couch to stand for his first time, Maren successfully phone interviewed for a fashion design position in support of the opening and closing ceremonies at the 2002 Winter Olympics. She had to start in New York by June.

Illuminated by afternoon's clearest light on the master bathroom's mirror, she practiced the exact facile expressions necessary to deliver the explosive change to Graywood upon his arrival from work.

Wildflowers bloomed from the cedar-wood planter by the double front oak doors. "Maren, I'm home," shouted Graywood in clear baritone. He reached to touch the soft petals.

"I'm in the great room." Ready to chair the break-up talk, Maren's long legs stood apart in top-power mode, and her mane flushed unbroken like a blond battle flag.

"What did Bobby and you do today?" he said matter-of-factly.

"Gary, I'm moving away and going alone. I hope we can remain friends, but I'll understand if you can't."

The room's air congealed. Stunned, muteness masked Graywood's face. The declaration upended him completely.

"I don't believe I was meant to be a mother as you wanted."

"What are you saying?" he whispered, confused.

"I do not aspire to obscurity," she cracked and then waited a beat, "and rarely fail."

"I don't understand," he returned, bolder.

"Understand this!" she snapped. "I'm staying tonight at the Sheraton. I have to be in New York to start a new job. Tomorrow I'm flying to BWI."

"You're not making any sense." Staccato knives twisted Graywood's heart.

"I thought you'd say that." Maren's eyes rolled dismissively. She handed him an envelope. "Read this when you want. It tells how I feel about us."

He took it but remained dumbfounded.

"I fed your son an hour ago. He's napping. Let's not wake him by getting loud. My taxi comes in twenty minutes. Do you have any pressing questions?"

The blazing eyes under high teased hair drained his intestines dry. At last, he said, "Why are you doing this?"

"I … can't … do … this," her voice percussed deliberately as both arms opened wide to indicate the great room and the universe beyond.

"If you mean having our second child, we can adopt."

"Adoption!" She stared back ugly. "You still don't get it. I don't want to be a mother," twitched off her lips. "I will not be treated as if my life is not my own."

Bushwhacked and paralyzed like the initial time seeing her in Juneau, Graywood felt his throat constrict. Deflated, he lacked knowing what to do to save his family from this wicked crisis. He fought rising anger to bargain an equal encounter but got outflanked before speaking another word.

"There are three bags and my cello upstairs. Please continue to be the gentleman and carry them to the front door so as not to wake your son." She stepped forward and nudged him into action. He squinted into her eyes trying to grasp the sudden character change. She'd put in the blue contacts, something not done since Bobby was born.

"You've covered your hazels again," he blurted, half surprised, half confused.

"Yes, I'm going away."

She never looked back. Resolute, she disappeared beyond airport security. Graywood craved a wave good-bye. Not so.

He held Bobby close to his chest. One way or another, he always would.

Still dazed, he opened the note handed to him in the great room.

I have grown tired of you, Gary. I will not swap my glory for the sake of your labels of love.

I am thankful I am always in your heart, sometimes in your thoughts, and never in your debt.

I say for myself, I will only be valued by me, for me. I urge you to understand this.

Suppressing renewed rage, he slammed it into the trash breaking open knuckle skin on the rim. Sucking away the blood, he repositioned shock-faced Bobby in his arms and soothed, "It's not her nature to give, my trusting, little boy."

Anger spent, aided by Bobby grabbing Graywood's reddened nose, the sole parent stepped the opposite way, eyes blinking back tears.

To regain wits, he deployed a medical slant for Maren's behavior: perhaps she had a delayed withdrawal syndrome from the medication. He had monitored her depression drug therapy and its discontinuation for adverse effects. She'd shown no symptoms of anorexia, somnolence, or reclusion that were present before starting the treatment. If anything, she'd displayed irritability.

How much had resulted from residual physiological processes related to pregnancy and childbirth, rather than the psychological aspects of motherhood? Not prepared to accept Maren's change in heart toward him and their child, Graywood refused to sort it out. He loved his wife and would stand by her while she transitioned, however long and far, and prayed she'd come back soon.

Divorce papers were sent to Graywood's office in August.

Fastened to the legal documents was a handwritten letter: Maren boasted her role at the 2002 Winter Olympics in Utah: "Thrilled to be primary assistant to the fashion designer contracted for the opening ceremony …"

On paper, she preferred to remain friends with her former spouse, rather than sparring exes, and wished to co-parent Robert from a distance, although not as partners-for-life. Exuding her steadfast confidence and independence would model those exquisite traits for Robert as he grew.

Utter crap! Graywood tore it to ribbons—written to impress someone else like the New York City lawyer. Maren only followed her own needs, be they selfish, valid, guilt-derived, warped, whatever.

More than five years ticked by before she wrote any meaningful words to her child—a fancy 2006 Christmas card prior to the Graywoods' Kauai spring break vacation.

Graywood draped the suit coat over the kitchen chair closest to the three official condolence cards lying on the breakfast table: one from the medical center's commander at Elmendorf Air Force Base, another by Graywood's boss at the Justice Department in Washington, and the third sent under the seal of the president of the United States. Left unopened, he deferred reading the governmental solaces on his son's death. Yet sympathies received from friends and office co-workers were pasted in a dove-white folder, each mated to the opposite page holding a photo of Bobby selected from Graywood's massive collection. Jennelle's penned compassion started the album, then Bearhead's, Rachel's, Cub's, Piper's, and the rest.

The envelopes mailed by bureaucrats emitted disjointed, foreign-like auras, out of place in Graywood's world. He brushed them to the floor.

He assembled ingredients to make Bobby's favorite breakfast—sourdough pancakes. His mind resurfaced the Rum Tum bedtime story he'd once told to prepare the wide-eyed boy for his initial flight in *Seneca*:

"Aleutian girl missed her daddy very, very much. He worked at a crab processing plant on the Aleutian island that's called Popof. So she laid enough provisions in the kayak for little Rum Tum and her to paddle all the way from Dutch Harbor to Popof, nearly three hundred miles away.

"But her mother found the kayak loaded with food and three canteens of water and wanted to know where she was going. Now Aleutian Girl never told a lie to her mother. She always told the truth, although her mother knew she might have to ask several questions to get all the truth out of her. After much hemming and hawing about the kayak loaded to the brim with food, Aleutian Girl finally said, 'Rum Tum and I are going to see my daddy way out there in Popof 'cause I miss him so and I want to tell him how much I love him.'

"And her mother said, 'Oh, I understand, my dearest sweet one. But I'm not letting you go in the kayak. It's far too dangerous for you and Rum Tum to be on the ocean all alone for such a long way. It's too far.'

"But Aleutian Girl said strong as she could, 'But I want to go, and I'll take kayak kitty, my little Rum Tum, to help me. We're the best team there is, and I know we'll get there, I promise.'

"But her mother said, 'I don't know. It's pretty hard for me to believe you'd get all the way there. It would be safer if we found some other way for you to talk to your daddy.'

"But Aleutian Girl pleaded, 'But I want to see him. I don't wish just to talk. We have no telephone and no two-way radio, and I really want to see him.'

"And her mother said, 'Well, let's go and talk to Uncle Oo-otek and see how he can handle this.'

"Little did Aleutian Girl know that Uncle Oo-otek had a seaplane. And so they went to Uncle Oo-otek, and he heard the story how little Aleutian Girl wanted to kayak three hundred miles across the great Pacific Ocean to Popof Island to see her daddy and tell him how much she loved him.

"And Uncle Oo-otek said, 'Well little Aleutian Girl … I've got a better idea. Instead of you kayaking there, what we'll do is this: I must fly to

Popof in two weeks and deliver a whole bunch of stuff and pick up the mail. So why don't you come along and fly with me?'

"Aleutian Girl's eyes got as big as pancakes, and she said, 'Oh, I get to go! Oh, how can I be so lucky I can go with you!'

"Uncle Oo-otek said, 'It's no problem at all. You can come with me.'

"Aleutian Girl said, 'But I have to take my best little buddy with me, my little friend, my kayak kitty, my wonderful Rum Tum.'

"Uncle Oo-otek said, 'Rum Tum? Who's this Rum Tum?'

"She said, 'Rum Tum's my kitty cat who came to me off a ship from Anchorage, and he's been my little friend ever since, and we've been on lots and lots of exciting adventures together. Oh, Uncle Oo-otek, this will be a wonderful adventure for Rum Tum to fly in an airplane with me. I don't think Rum Tum's ever flown before.'

"Uncle Oo-otek said, 'Well, how much does little Rum Tum weigh?'

"She said, 'When he's fully loaded with milk and rum or when he's empty?'

"And he said, 'Fully loaded with milk and rum. And do you really mean you'd give your little Rum Tum some rum?'

"Aleutian Girl said, 'Oh no, I haven't any rum to give him, but that's the story he told me when he came off the boat. He said he likes to have his milk with a spot of rum in it.'

"Then Uncle Oo-otek said, 'Hmm, I don't know about slurping up spots of rum, but you make sure he's agreeable about flying, and if he is, he can come along with us, whether he's full of milk and rum or not.'

"And she said, 'Hooray! Oh, Uncle Oo-otek, I love you so much!' She threw her arms around him in a huge hug. Then she and her mother ran back to their itsy-bitsy house by Dutch Harbor, and Aleutian Girl went inside and found little Rum Tum and said, 'Rum Tum, guess what we're going to do? We're going to fly in an airplane.'

"Rum Tum said, 'What's an airplane?'

"Aleutian Girl said, 'An airplane … oh … it's like a big, steel seagull we can fly in.'

"But Rum Tum cried, 'Noooo! I don't want to fly in a steel seagull. I'm so fearful of Baron White Gull. An airplane sounds like a really big seagull to me. I don't ever want to get into the belly of a big seagull.'

"But Aleutian girl said, 'No, no, no, don't be scared. I'll be in the seagull's belly with you too.'

"'Why do we want to be in the belly of a giant seagull? I don't really understand,' cried Rum Tum, his little paws beginning to sweat.

"'I'll be in the belly of the giant seagull with you, and we'll be with Uncle Oo-otek,' reassured Aleutian girl.

"'I don't understand why all three of us have to be in the belly of a seagull,' frantically repeated Rum Tum, his little paws shaking and sweating more and more.

"Aleutian Girl said, 'Oh my dear, sweet kitty, you don't understand. This is how we can get from here to Popof Island so I can see my daddy and say hello to him and tell him how much I love him.'

"But Rum Tum said, 'I still don't understand why I have to be in the belly of a seagull.'

"'Because we can get there really fast,' she answered.

"Rum Tum asked, 'What do you mean "really fast"?'

"'We can get there really fast. So fast we can be there in a day. And we can fly back in a day,' she explained.

"Rum Tum said, 'How can we do all that in a day? One time, it took us forever just to get half way round Unalaska in our kayak. To get all the way to Popof Island would take much longer.'

"But she explained, 'The airplane is like a really fast seagull. It's way faster than terrible Baron White Gull. It'll always be faster than him and his evil cronies, so we'll never be attacked by them as we would be if we paddled alone in the kayak.'

"'You mean we won't be bothered by the evil Baron and his crony birds and all his minions?' asked Rum Tum.

"'No we won't be bothered or attacked by them at all because we'll fly really, really fast,' she reassured.

"So Rum Tum said, 'Well … all right. I'll do it. But it may be too big an adventure for me. I've never been up in the sky before.'

"'Well, I haven't either,' said Aleutian Girl, and she tenderly stroked the little kitty's head. 'It will be an exciting adventure for us both.'

"'Okay,' purred Rum Tum.

"So they went to bed and dreamed all about what it would be like in the belly of a giant seagull flying over the sea in the heavenly sky to a far, faraway place to see her father."

Imagining fluffing Bobby's pillow and pulling blankets to the child's chin, Graywood set the mixing bowl filled with pancake batter on the counter. Pretending to smooth blond tangles on the boy's forehead a tad higher, he replayed from long ago the coveted goodnight:

"Would you like to fly with me tomorrow in *Seneca*, just like our heroic Rum Tum?"

Bobby bolted up. "Oh, yes, Dad. Yes, yes, yes!"

"It can get really cold high in the sky, so you've gotta dress really warm."

"I'll wear a coat and sweater, Dad. I will, really. I promise I will."

"Will you do careful and do everything I tell you in *Seneca*?"

"I'll do it!"

"And do quiet and brave when I ask?"

"I'll do brave."

"As brave as Rum Tum?"

"Braver!"

"I know you will." Graywood hugged his child. "Now lie down and go to sleep."

"I'll try. But it's so hard!"

"Just stay quiet and have sweet dreams about little Rum Tum." Graywood smoothed the blankets and started for the bedroom door.

"Dad?"

"What, Bobby?"

"I love you."

"I love you too." Graywood switched off the light. "Now go to sleep. I'll wake you in the morning."

"A chalk-colored, concrete roadblock," reasoned Graywood.

Bobby's casket was not the vessel to return to the earth's womb. The coffin served as a prison, solitary confinement, a slab dropped to a circle in Hell.

A navy-blue suit over a bunched-up beige shirt worn three Junes earlier dressed the cachectic body. Melted down, Bobby's wasted frame had miniaturized a life relentlessly sapped away. At birth, his face had radiated like Apollo's mask. Now forever supine, it still emanated beautiful alabaster, not ivory-grey hues.

The Presbyterian church counted less than a quarter full.

Graywood embodied confused faith, emptiness, and grief. He sat submissive in the front pew on the central aisle's left beside Jennelle with the Coldsnow sisters and Bearhead. Rachel, Cub, Piper, and Mary anchored the row behind. Hillside neighbors, a handful of Hanshew Junior High students and parents, and co-workers from Graywood's office also mourned. The executive officer from the medical center at Elmendorf Air Force Base, Colonel James Sulmasy, represented the Department of Defense.

Hearing few words despite his face pointed to the minister, Graywood fixed his eyes on the coffin. Bereavement gushed memories to compete against the eulogy. Preeminent, his father's Seattle funeral, when Graywood was only age twelve, cast the shadows of missed opportunities the two should have shared. Graywood's dad and son were gone, but Graywood was alive and had missed so much living with them …

Being alone shoved him dreadful raw as had happened before when his mother's ashes were scattered across the Oregon coast near Coos Bay. God had taken her early too, and Graywood missed her more today than any time when Bobby was alive. Raising a child helped to let her go and attach peace to her passing, yet today the anguish for her resurfaced as rock-hard as another concrete roadblock.

Oddly, a different torment evaporated. Graywood had feared Bobby becoming an orphan and worried who'd take care of the boy if he had died. Maren wouldn't, and her father never inclined to visit them in Alaska.

Graywood had swayed between Rachel and Bearhead as Bobby's legal custodian, but once the seizures commenced, he settled on Uncle Roe. Monroe and the Coldsnow sisters willingly accepted the obligation. Still, Graywood put off stipulating the decision in his will—he'd have to obtain Maren's approval. A small hope within him still cleaved to the myth she might return someday to their family. Preserving that pathetic pipedream held more importance than reality dictated.

Last to usurp the pulpit's words were echoes of Bearhead's joy expressed upon Bobby's birth: "Gary, you'll remember days your spirit grows. Now is one. You have a son. May you have wonderful years together as you both grow old."

Beginning, middle, and end, the child had lived one season shy of sixteen years. Had Graywood delved further, something from Bobby's everlasting soul would have danced up to endure this horrendous day as it had done in the final hours when he stood sentinel over the hospital bed. But from the pew, Graywood reverently muffled what he'd exhaled eight days earlier in tandem with the boy's last mortal breath:

"Dying is an art, like everything else. I won't do it as well as you."

A melancholy gravedigger's dusk tinged other remembrances. Graywood's coalesced to granite—desolate and perplexed. With Bobby's death, Graywood had lost something essential … oxygen.

Reaching over the Coldsnow twins, Bearhead motioned Graywood to rise with him and view Bobby for the final time. Next to Bobby's torso, they positioned three mementos—Piper's glass-covered Rum Tum sketch, a paper bag filled with sourdough pancakes, and Maren's taupe-colored slingbacks.

They say love's first learned in a woman's eyes … Had Bobby ever seen it in Maren's? With a single hand aligning the shoes beside Bobby's feet, Graywood wished the precious boy had beheld her love at least once. Graywood gripped Bearhead's carved cat in the other hand.

"Gary," whispered Bearhead, "keep the wooden Rum Tum. It belongs with Brandy Belle. I made this yesterday." He presented a four-inch, scrimshaw figurine shaped and inked as a sitting feline. "It's little Rum Tum waiting to greet Bobby coming home." Cementing the request, Bearhead exchanged the items and bent away to rub off stoic tears.

Graywood's fingers placed the pristine art on Bobby's heart.

But Graywood wasn't ready to go in peace. In silence he voiced the never-ending question bereaved parents have asked since the Book of Job: "This horrible disease, why did it take my child?"

It demanded more than an answer beyond one's faith. Clasping the coffin's side, Graywood's swollen eyes shot to the empty cross above the altar.

"Why?" he cursed, "You ungrateful God! Why my son?"

Astonished, Bearhead interceded, extending a palm to Graywood's chest, and urged, "Gary, please."

"Roe, I have to know what killed him."

"Let it be so, but Gary, pursue without hate, or it'll kill you."

Graywood jerked away and pressed dampness from his face. "It'll damn kill me if I don't know why."

Rejection and torment flooded Graywood from the church to Klatt Road cemetery. A tepid thankfulness for the fleeting calm weather infiltrated the heartache as the casket was lowered. Yet the gravesite ordeal magnified once he scanned for her …

Maren had not come. Not to the service or the burial.

The funeral party retired.

Alone, Graywood remained by the plot. Jennelle was posted at the graveyard's entrance to direct Bobby's mother if she showed. Only rain came.

Hell ache from years past replayed the mother's refusal to meet them in Kauai. Drenched, the torrents pummeled Graywood dumb, his crux forever split.

Closed mouthed, Jennelle drove him to Bearhead's home for the wake. Once they entered, Monroe and April coaxed Graywood to the kitchen after fetching a large towel to dry his soaked body.

"Gary, Cash Goodlette sent an Inupiaq condolence scripted on walrus tusk," reported Bearhead. "It arrived this morning."

"Cash must be somewhere near Point Lay waiting for the research equipment barge from Nome," observed Jennelle.

"He sent a note regretting not coming," said Bearhead, more subdued. "I've got them in the studio for you."

Still lacking grace, Graywood hesitated to move through rooms full of people. Breaking the awkwardness, April said, "Cash sends ivory to Roe whenever in the Arctic. It's a wonder how he does it."

"He's very kind," interjected Bearhead. "When he finds walrus or whale remains, he salvages what's possible and ships it to me."

"Ivory's a fortune," said Jennelle. "I didn't know you were such good friends."

"Well, we write each other about nature and atheism and God, a whole lot of things. Suppose that makes us something."

"More like Internet yelling," corrected April, "ten pages or more every time."

"How long have you been doing that, Roe?" asked Graywood, attempting to forget Maren's searing absence.

"Since meeting him at GB. But Gary, I want to show what he sent."

Graywood, shaking a fretful head, followed Bearhead.

Jennelle witnessed the unspoken tenderness between the two men. Rachel and Cub joined her and April. "How's Gary doing?" asked Rachel.

"He's a strong man who's devastated." replied Jennelle. She surveyed the three and added, "We'll all have to be steady for him."

"Yes, all," confirmed Rachel, eyes narrowed by rage. "I can't believe that Maren didn't show up today of all days. She surpasses even the John Edwards's standard for insincerity."

"Ahh, Mom … who's Edwards?" asked Cub.

"A conniving liar without a thread of authenticity who ran for president," explained Rachel, leaving out the part where Edwards resembled Piper when it came to spousal mistreatment.

"He didn't win, did he?"

"No, Cub, he's just a loser."

June's daylight would linger on Anchorage beyond midnight. Gatherings often plugged along past twilight, regardless the weather.

More than once, Graywood embraced and spoke with everyone but was spent by ten o'clock.

"Jen, I'm ready to go home."

"You look tired." Hooking arms with Graywood, Jennelle walked him to Rachel. "Gary, I need to stay longer and help April and Roe. Rachel can take you home. I'll buzz to let you know when I'm done." She pecked his cheek.

Graywood had no energy to sort out the switch. Jennelle had embarked on a mission, and Rachel apparently had volunteered to take over primary support duties.

To Rachel, he asked, "What's up with her?"

"Jen and April are catching up on Chitina." With prompting eyes, she added, "Come on, dear; I'm taking you home."

Graywood tamped down futile bewilderments on God and women while she escorted him through the front doorway.

The Hillside neighborhood stretched seven miles away. The ride to Snowline Drive fell short of small talk. Not wishing to move even his tongue, Graywood apologized for being glum and quenched the travel time with mental meanders …

He debated a detour to O'Malley Elementary to view the hockey rink where Bobby had excelled. The same O'Malley that had insinuated the child had ADHD and advocated treatment to keep up with classmates.

Graywood shifted to images of Bobby reading to Brandy Belle. The cat extended a clever paw to school books whenever wishing to know what happened next. And if Bobby seemed discouraged by mistakes, she'd whisker the offending hardcover and purr, making him giggle and rethink how fun reading proved.

The excruciating hurt of Maren's no-show made it easier to close her out … again. At the wake, he'd overheard Bearhead to others analyze how her character was flinty and vain, an elitist without a spool of profoundness, someone who'd rather fight or flee instead of compromise. She'd never yield a hair of her independence.

Once he noticed Graywood's craning, Bearhead changed course and urged finding a way to forgive her even if it seemed impossible. Outrageously, he counseled to suspend judgment and attempt to take Maren's point of view.

Like dawn's mist lifting off the Chugach Mountains, a slant layer of Maren had resurrected as Graywood and Rachel rolled up O'Malley Road past the grade school.

Maren hadn't wished to have a child so soon. So distant from Maryland, she'd tried to adjust to marriage and the unknown northland so terribly warped by its strange seasons. Most of all, she wasn't a woman who'd marry first for children. Pregnancy had pushed her beyond coping in Alaska—a place she dismissively called a foreign country. Heading for a cliff, she had to do something radical—leave. A housewife who ran away instead of snapping with a gun seemed the wiser choice.

Could understanding help the forgiving and forgiving help the forgetting? Too soon to know, Graywood concluded …

Damn! Oh, damn Maren! You still should've come!

"Gary, should I come in," offered Rachel, "and fix you something, anything?" From the circle driveway, Graywood stared at the double front door and its years of openings and closings.

"No, Raych, you've been so kind … I need to be alone for a while."

"You're sure?"

"Yeah, thanks." He got out, came to the driver's side, and squeezed her hand through the open window. "Rachel, you're wonderful. I promise I'll never forget what you've done for Bobby and me."

"Gary, I'll never forget him, and I'm here for you," she returned soft. "Just let me know." She had wished to substitute intimate words but deferred.

"Thanks." He straightened and stepped back.

Steadily, she took the Ford around and down Snowline Drive.

He waved goodbye and then about-faced toward the lifeless house missing his son. With a mightiness fused in forgiveness, he resolved to inhume Maren's shadows, but he'd never bury Bobby.

Dear God, what killed my child? Why'd he die? What caused the terrible seizures, the degeneration?

Graywood ratcheted half a decade back to the time the boy's disease had started and went twelve months more when Bobby was absolutely healthy. In those six years, what had passed overt and covert?

Memory is the root of many troubles.

Bobby received neither a birthday card nor call from Jennelle on his tenth birthday. Graywood covered for her and speculated she may have posted greetings from a faraway place, but they were lost in the foreign mail. He dodged the easier lie she'd forgotten because work was too important. He refused to tell the truth about the woman they both still loved: she'd received a marriage proposal from someone else.

Bobby wrote Jennelle a letter telling what might have happened to the mailings from a distant land, but Graywood hid it.

In time, the child suspected his dad had fibbed. Jen would have emailed or wired something. Her absence gnawed all wrong, and he fretted it was his fault.

By his next birthday, Jennelle had still sent nothing. No cards delivered for two years in a row, and his dad hadn't spoken a word of her in months. Something was really bad. In silence, Bobby suffered her loss.

Rachel organized Bobby's parties. Graywood planned to leave early from Elmendorf Airbase to join the boy's eleventh celebration.

Bobby walked slower than normal with Cub from the bus stop. Placidly watching television minutes before the party began, he passed out. Not finding the cause, he was diagnosed with epilepsy.

Epilepsy was the medical term, the label, given to the relentless scarring process within Bobby's cranium. It foreshadowed the cruel brevity to the child's life and the grim vulnerability within his father. As he watched his son diminish, Graywood made decisions, in King Lear-like fashion, which became less sound, less rational, and less controlled.

Clinically Bobby displayed modest losses in higher-order functions, despite five years of unexplained, progressive seizures. Yet CT and MRI scans verified uneven neuronal erosion throughout the cortex.

Bobby retained most short-term recall. His hippocampus continued to undergo necessary self-maintenance to make sufficient connections to build fresh memories. However, serial cerebral scans confirmed an overall loss of bulk there. Because Bobby was a tweener-adolescent, perhaps he produced enough new neuronal linkages to offset whatever had eroded to account for his ability to make and preserve daily mental imprints.

Pitifully, Bobby's prison remained an unknown, merciless, degenerative disorder, shackled to incessant convulsions.

At the child's thirteenth birthday, Graywood prayed the woeful illness would cease its perpetual assault. Then he could recover some of his son … and maybe the boy he'd once been.

CHAPTER EIGHTEEN

Confinement

Fourteen kilometers long and equally wide, Avacha Bay presented a masterpiece of nature surrounded by mountainous ramparts against western winds. Its coast contoured three secure harbors. In the north, Koryaksky volcano towered over Petropavlovsk, the saltwater's dominant city. An eastern inlet, Rakovina Bay, named on account of its many shellfish, occupied the second. Daryesky village, southwest, shored the third natural anchorage.

In spite of customary US State Department complexity, Graywood regularly met with local Russian governmental and health officials: Yuri Komarov, Valery Zaslavsky, and Alexander Nikolayenkoto. At the top for today's conference stood the prison's consolidation into the region's coordinated mass casualty plan.

Their tight agenda centered on collaboration and support integration between Prisontown and local Siberian medical assets. Prior meetings had negotiated first-order logistics that permitted procedures for prisoner debarkations, facility staff rotations, Customs duty waivers, and short-notice shipments of urgent medical supplies and equipment. These relied on air corridor controls between Petropavlovsk's airport and Elmendorf.

Classic ex-Soviet drab enclosed the Petropavlovsk conference venue: a six-story block tower molded from diesel-smelling concrete with chinked exteriors covered with lichens growing on peeling dun paint. From what

Graywood had read on World War II, the structure still projected a better face than the last one standing after the battle of Stalingrad.

Komarov and the interpreter met him outside. Lacking a working elevator, they stair-climbed to the chilled dim room where the others waited.

The Kamchatka peninsula is home to twenty-nine active volcanoes. Ash clouds expelled from a cauldron might extend fifty thousand feet in height and threaten air travel safety across the northern Pacific.

To warn of impending flight perils, a cooperative effort—the Kamchatkan Volcanic Eruption Response Team, or KVERT—between scientists in the United States and Soviet Union was established in 1933.

Graywood advocated the historic principles and operating procedures established under KVERT as a blueprint for the prison's disaster medical response integration within Avacha Bay. If the prison got smothered by volcanic ash, rolled in an earthquake, or hit with a SARS epidemic, so also would Petropavlovsk. Graywood and the Russians agreed to bilateral committees composed of the prison's administrative staff, the onsite prison health-care director, and their Petropavlovsk counterparts to weave the details. They concurred on the first-tier, follow-on emergency support to be provided by Russia and the United States. If needed, additional countries could donate any second-tier relief via the United Nations.

The formal liaison closed with gift exchanges over vodka, samovar-brewed tea, and more vodka. Siberian police escorted Graywood on the hour-long journey to the new prison hospital in time for the afternoon overview with its medical director.

Born in India, Doctor Nayna Pawar spoke English with the cut-glass diction heard on the BBC. The corners of her mouth lifted to draw in and engage whomever she conversed with while intelligent eyes expressed command and purpose. By habit, Graywood noticed physicians' hands—hers opened fine-boned, delicate, and smooth. At length, the two discussed staffing requirements, training goals, and the current budget cycle before they reviewed the health status on the initial incarcerated cohort of banished felons.

From many burdens, past and current, Doctor Pawar's clipped voice sounded old. "These prisoners are people. Always I am wary they have murdered and they may yet kill me or my staff." She pulled up the rogue's gallery on the computer screen, "Forty-eight so far, and twenty scheduled later this month."

"No women," said Graywood.

"The warden does not anticipate them until next year."

"What a shock that'll be," he observed.

"Doctor Graywood, I believe we need to recognize the humanity we all share, even in these prisoners," she interjected. "They are warmed and cooled by the same Siberian summer and winter as the guards and I. They have hands, organs, senses, passions. More than I ever once believed, I find they resemble and suffer in most things as myself."

To Graywood's ear she sounded similar to Shylock from Shakespeare's *Merchant of Venice.*

"I studied medicine to help people, and this is what I do," she stated firmly. "Doctor Graywood, I would not trade places with anybody."

Doctor Pawar had attended medical school in Mumbai where she married her husband Pradeep. She chose obstetrics and gynecology. He trained in general surgery.

In 2002, commercial surrogacy—commonly termed "wombs for rent"—became legalized in India. Doctor Pawar created a premiere clinic to match local women to infertile couples throughout the world. She supervised a team of doctors, nurses, maids, and cooks who looked after eighty to one hundred young women impregnated with the fertilized eggs of childless couples from India, the United States, Britain, Taiwan, and beyond.

She offered one-stop service. The couple provided sperm and eggs, and her facility performed the rest. The surrogate mother, chosen off a waiting list of carefully screened volunteers, was between eighteen and thirty-two years of age, possessed good medical health, and had at least one child of her own. The ready queue of tested surrogates exceeded by far the number needed because the remitted surrogacy fee for completing one successful pregnancy equaled fifteen years of employment as a maid.

The surrogate mother and the potential parents signed a contract that bound the infertile couple to pay all medical expenses and surrogacy compensation to the mother. In return, she would hand over the baby after its birth. Most couples paid an estimated ten thousand dollars for the entire program of fertilization, medical care, and surrogacy fee as compared to eight to ten times that amount for a surrogate birth in the United States or a quarter million dollars should they attempt in-vitro procedures.

Doctor Pawar required the surrogates reside in one of four adjacent group homes throughout their pregnancies. Each spacious house had a matron to oversee the expectant women. These den mothers had been prior surrogates as well: they provided unique experience and emotional assistance to the new mothers once they transitioned into the group facilities after successful conceptions. To soften relocation burdens, the surrogates could receive their husbands and children as visitors during daytime hours.

Critics of India becoming the leader in surrogacy as a viable industry rather than a rare fertility treatment cautioned how human baby farms exploited India's poor women by hiring them at cut-rate costs to undergo the hardship, pain, and risk of labor. Furthermore, Indian health officials had issued only nonbinding ethical guidelines in lieu of governmental regulations to protect the surrogates and children.

Doctor Pawar, her staff, and the den mothers made the surrogates aware of the risks before a contract was signed and again prior to conception. Each mother also witnessed a series of monthly videos on what other surrogates had gone through as pregnancies progressed toward delivery, surrendering the baby, post-partum recovery, and returning home to their families.

As part of her small campaign to correct past sexual discriminations, Doctor Pawar insisted the women study English and computer skills during their confinement. Compared to other countries, the plight of India's women approached overwhelming. On the whole, half the Indian women were illiterate and only 30 percent of girls completed primary school. Once betrothed, the girl's education ceased. Indian law required a woman to be eighteen years at the time of marriage, yet over half the rural girls were coupled into arranged unions long before reaching that age.

What embittered Doctor Pawar utmost was the stark prejudice by some expectant parents who chose to selectively abort female babies. India had outlawed ultrasound examinations solely to determine fetal sex in its passage of the Prohibition of Sex Selection Act in 2003. But within certain prosperous neighborhoods, the girl-to-boy sex ratio had fallen as low as 762 to 1000 largely because of elective female abortions determined by illegal prenatal ultrasounds. Another factor adding to the overall population's decline in girls was female infanticide.

Graywood never pursued the background on why Doctor Pawar and her husband had applied for the onsite medical directorship and general surgeon positions at Prisontown. It was none of his business to delve into their private motivations to leave India and accept work visas for the United States Justice Department facility in Kamchatka. Perhaps smoldering turmoil between India and Pakistan influenced them since their home sat within artillery range of a disputed border.

Both Indian physicians presented stellar resumes and willingness to endure the climate in south coastal Siberia. Doctor Pawar's organizational leadership had impressed Graywood. What cinched her selection for chief medical officer occurred at the end of the video interview: she'd summarized past work efforts as simply trying to assist others with the most natural of desires—to have a family. Graywood knew then she was a kindred spirit. Together they'd manage the difficult medical and social issues derived out of the exploitative clashes of morals, science, and health care inherent within this novel prison community.

Life is unfair and variably intolerant.

As the 767 propelled toward Alaska, Graywood opened the gift bottle of vodka and wandered into the minefields of abortion and capital punishment. From the fetal point of view, society tolerated the ultimate aggression in unfairness with its persistent endorsement of elective abortion. Yet by the 2011 Compromise, America would never again allow the inherent unfairness implemented from capital punishment.

In time, the banished murderers would develop chronic conditions, such as end-stage kidney failure, Alzheimer's disease, and strokes, to leave them bloated, dumb, or speechless. Who'd decide the levels of medical and rehabilitative resources committed to ease their miseries or prolong their lives?

Graywood unfastened the safety belt and searched the galley for a drinking container.

Who says a prisoner with kidney failure shall not receive renal dialysis or a transplant? Who proclaims an Alzheimer's inmate merits no medication to prolong her ability to function with lucidity for another twelve months? Who denies speech therapy to a felon debilitated from a stroke who'll never speak coherently without it?

Into a plastic cup, Graywood plopped three ice cubes. He returned to the window seat and restarted the mental fugue. Bottom line: in Kamchatka they'd suffer more and die much earlier from the lack of current standard treatments available in the States.

But society expected such from those placed on the edge. Next to elective abortion of an unwanted fetus, banishment was the penultimate marginalization.

Graywood poured vodka to cover the frozen chunks and watched the jet's wing pierce the canopy's last cloud layer.

How ironic American society felt ethically enlightened when it had stopped an execution by lethal injection and replaced it with a drawn-out mortality derived from lowered standards of health care. Some might argue it was merely economic and spiritual pragmatism, or relativism, coming into play.

Graywood reclined and nursed the alcohol.

One social guilt lowered but replaced by another.

The banished felon has murdered, but such as it might be, the public would not exact the ultimate justice. By foregoing the murderer's execution, society rather massaged its collective spiritual consciousness—the prisoner lived but must live overseas and die on the cheap.

Graywood's tongue roped an ice chip between the molars and crushed it.

If Congress mandated banished prisoners to bare-bones medical and rehabilitative care compared to the rest of the nation under Alpha-Omega, then that set a dangerous precedent—a damnable double standard.

Graywood swirled the cup. Two remaining cubes collided.

A slippery slope. Health-care standards for other subgroups could get lowered too, once they'd become socially marginalized, but not to the extent of elective aborted fetuses—hopefully.

The bigger cube rested on top of the smaller in the cup. Graywood glared out the window at ultramarine blue without blemish.

How arbitrary that some conceived babies are viewed as convicts who deserve old-fashioned termination while others are beheld as sweet cherubs in the making.

Beyond the aircraft's nose Graywood discerned oncoming darkness.

Is it spiritually pragmatic to withhold treatments for the prisoners afflicted with Alzheimer's as it is reasoned to electively abort unwanted fetuses? Culture selects and massages its spiritual consciousness at different speeds—rapid ripping away unwanted fetal lives yet banishing murderers into much slower deaths. Not so simple, one guilt replacing another.

Graywood drained the beverage and closed his eyes. He'd never make sense of spiritual pragmatism.

He missed his son and dreamed … To glide across the unnamed tarn that drained to Bruin Bay. Made awestruck beneath mountains whose upper halves sported white blouses of snow fastened by crazy granite buttons and lower halves bedecked in cotillions of bottle-green forest gowns swishing in the wind. True Alaskan beauty, wrenching and wise …

Campsite had been good medicine. An innocent, peaceful balm applied on mental wounds—a subtle form of family therapy. It assuaged relentless modernity inflicted upon Graywood and the boy. Flying there in *Seneca*, the kayaking, the fire building and cooking, the storytelling, and wildlife sightings—it intertwined and fortified them to withstand the challenges in ever-changing Anchorage and its hectic lifestyle. Healed and comforted, stints in the woods and fishing on the lake renewed confidence and strength.

The Campsite weeks had been precious. Whenever Bobby slumbered in the tent, Graywood, propped on elbow, admired the child tucked in the sleeping bag. Such days were few, and a father feeling the press of time should make them the most. Like any parent, he'd have to yield to the diverging ways forged out of their destinies … Bobby grown and leaving … he'd have to let him go. Lying supine, Graywood tried not to become older …

The cabin steward awakened Graywood for Elmendorf's arrival.

God blast, another damn headache! Must be the vodka.

Can't wait to see Bobby boy.

The jet landed and paused on the tarmac for rollout lane clearance. Graywood shifted out of brain ache into another spiritual wallow on social pragmatism …

So the condemned murderer was no longer aborted out of America's bosom by execution, only marginalized to third world death in Siberia. Yet he or she was so better off than an unwanted fetus. Fetal innocence was readily sacrificed to cultural whim. Look how Asian ultrasounds altered birth sex ratios: the desire for male heirs over females sharpened thc knives for elective baby girl abortions. Male infants in many Asian countries exceeded females by greater than 10 percent. If one's soul was destined for conception on Earth as a female human being, it hoped for a mother whose culture harbored the least bias against girls at birth.

Bearhead would say there are hierarchies of morals, and they vary within and between societies. And a Martian studying Earth would marvel at how diversely and arbitrarily they operate. Even within a mere city block, morality separates wide when it is attached to stem cell manipulation, waging war, elective abortion, capital punishment, or whatever. It is like saying, "I know morality when I see it!"

The 767 crept toward the terminal, and Graywood drifted from abortion to stem-cell morality.

Depending whom one talked to, a leftover frozen embryo had less, equal, or greater moral status than its adult aunt or uncle afflicted, for example, with diabetes. Applying Bearhead's two-by-two squares, Graywood flipped to the back of his travel orders and scribbled the variables to unearth moral lines that could not be crossed. On "aunt with diabetes" he substituted "father with diabetes," then "child," "wife," and last, "prisoner with diabetes."

The aircraft halted.

In disgust, Graywood concluded the relativism embedded within western cultures insured a fluid morality that lacked absolutes. And relativism absurdly twisted everyone into sophists and pretenders. Regretfully, humanity's main story of historical greatness had reduced to crass hypocrisy; how one dealt with it, internally and externally, unfolded as the prime trial in one's life.

Packing the briefcase to deplane, Graywood recalled a court ruling from Texas in 2007 that epitomized cultural moral hypocrisy and regarded a man convicted on two counts of capital murder for the shooting death of his pregnant girlfriend. He'd dispatched her upon hearing she was six weeks pregnant with his child. His lawyers appealed the conviction because the right to due process had been violated by the prosecution for two homicides instead of one. The Texas Court of Criminal Appeals ruled Texan law allowed the fetal slaying to be tried as murder, regardless of its developmental stage, but the law did not apply simultaneously to abortions. A unanimous ruling declared a fetus an individual with state protections against murderous harm, yet those same fetal protections became nonexistent when in conflict with the US Supreme Court's ruling that protected a woman's right to choose.

Digesting legal sophistry, Graywood fantasized that if this convict could redo the killing, he should confess to having read an obstetrics textbook on the web and to stabbing the girlfriend in the abdomen. He'd present his alibi as a muffed attempt to abort the baby to avoid family scandal. Since he'd horribly botched the procedure, he should be only charged on one count of coerced manslaughter and one count of practicing medicine without a license, not double murder.

Graywood wondered whether this felon was one Texas had punted to Prisontown. Tomorrow he'd email an inquiry to the assistant warden.

The 767 resumed rolling towards the holding bay and then stopped. Scrambled F-22 Raptors had preempted Elmendorf's taxiways and runway.

Graywood resumed the shifting moral hierarchy game and vaulted to the other extreme of gravidity: a thirty-seven-week-pregnant woman scheduled in two days for a partial-birth abortion was killed by a drunken driver. Would there be two counts of vehicular manslaughter or one in Texas? Planned Parenthood had scheduled the baby's termination; it just occurred a couple days too soon by another means.

Shaking his head, Graywood took paper from the briefcase and drew a two-by-two table entitled "Table of the Condemned." The labeled axes were "murderers" and "unwanted fetuses." The upper left square got marked twice with plus signs for legal endorsements for both abortion and capital punishment, the upper right received one positive tick for permitting abortion and one negative for disallowing execution—current American law under the 2011 Compromise, the lower left quarter had a minus for legal abortion and a putting to death plus mark for capital convictions as it had been before *Roe v. Wade*, and the lower right contained two negative signs signifying no legal abortions or murderer executions. Inanimate, Graywood stared at the result.

The aircraft crawled toward the terminal again, and Graywood realized he could subdivide all American adults into the four quarters. He counted himself in the lower right and Bearhead there too. He wasn't sure about Piper.

Yet there existed much more. Graywood could construct similar two-by-two tables and replace the abortion or capital punishment axis with embryonic stem cells or gun control or federal funding for whatever change being emphasized to illustrate the social parameters on any moral controversy. He constructed a half-dozen, two-by-two squares with up-to-date label combinations and anticipated sharing them with Bearhead and Piper. He called them morality squares.

To be pro-life for existing life meant not killing humans, not stopping life's potential buds. Graywood determined residence in any quarter-square was a moral choice from one's self-perceived sense of fairness. An individual viewed the world as most fair within one's own section and was prone to believe the remaining three as unfair, contrarian, or irrelevant.

A person built his moral hierarchies and occupied his own quarters within the two-by-two squares by what he'd kill in order to live and what he'd chosen not to vanquish. That's free will, one's spirit. Rather than trash those not sharing his values, Graywood committed to find and connect to the people who did.

Yet fairness in spirit appeared elusive too, and over time, unfairness was decoded out of such culturally hewn judgments. Slaves can have great spirits and kings little. An individual's spirit, forever present, can change only in amount. One may choose to imprison it or help it grow larger, vaporize it across society or magnify into a Mother Teresa.

The grander spirit that advocated life over death resonated in Graywood: forbid execution for capital crimes and ban abortion. He'd accept the other three morality quadrants' right to exist but never enter them.

The 767's cabin door opened. Graywood stuffed the two-by-two tables into the briefcase and gathered overcoat, gloves, and the reindeer harness bought for Cub. He'd stop by the Base Exchange for the model F-22 jet Bobby wanted.

From the heart-searching treks to Kamchatka, Graywood became the central player in the prison's battle against economic eugenics and its ceaseless collisions with the Alpha-Omega universal health mandate. He lacked the astute answers on how to manage the opposing tentacles of longevity versus convenient termination.

Cultural health restrictions were applied against banished felons and unwanted fetuses. Deemed less socially entitled to the full life, they'd become the initial groups placed at the margin. When would the other subclasses of people bear similar restrictions levied against their access to medical care, or even life itself, in order to better sustain the "more worthy" groups?

Fighting this mega-battle affected Graywood's spirit … and Bobby's.

CHAPTER NINETEEN

Prisontown

The Justice Department selected Anchorage to sponsor the 2015 symposium on recent penal initiatives within the federal prison system. The Beltway bureaucrats chose the March week of the annual Iditarod dogsled race for their conference's time slot. The US attorney general's opening address at the Alaska Convention Center would headline the event. The enactment and current achievements of the Kamchatkan prison campus were designated the featured agenda subjects.

Graywood's boss tapped him to present the overview of Kamchatka's health-care system and moderate group discussions on medical management that blended and contrasted the prison's mission with the guiding principles illuminated under the nation's Alpha-Omega health program.

Since the 2011 Grand Compromise, the perennial assembly had been held in Florida, Nevada, or Arizona. Graywood wondered how the Lower Forty-eight bigwigs would embrace Alaska's cold, listen to Kamchatka's prison biography, and watch a hundred or more sled teams reenact the famous 1,100-mile rescue that sent lifesaving serum to Nome to end a diphtheria epidemic over a century ago. Cub had registered his team. Graywood made sure Bobby and he would witness the ceremonial start.

To prepare for the meeting, Graywood keyed the controlled access codes to enter the restricted archives on the prison's website. He'd mold parts of the confidential business plan, or propaganda as Piper would have called it had he known the details, for background notes.

Graywood reviewed the legislative authority for the prison's derivation from the 2011 Grand Compromise that prohibited capital punishment and replaced it with banishment to Siberia. He recalled whimsical bloggers and television talking heads who'd opined this transition as one of the best examples of outsourcing in the twenty-first century. He elected to omit those comments.

Graywood skipped the treaty preamble with over-the-top platitudes about United States and Russian Federation engagement in yet another joint venture to further their special relationship since defeating Hitler, signing the nuclear weapon test ban treaty, and constructing and operating the international space station. Politicians always seemed too wordy for Graywood's taste.

Within the body of the treaty, he uncovered the sections that specified the prison's land purchase, construction, and operation fifty-eight kilometers west from Petropavlovsk. Sited on the Kamchatkan Peninsula at 53 degrees 19 minutes latitude north, the facility received nearly the same amount of daylight as the township of Ketchikan at the south end of the Alaskan panhandle. For the PowerPoint presentation, Graywood printed seasonal weather graphics.

The fascinating three circles of confinement on the prison grounds comprised a modern version of the vintage inferno and purgatory cantos from Dante's *The Divine Comedy*. At the innermost core of the first circle sat Ground Zero, the maximum security prison-in-a-prison building. Its framework resembled a Saint Andrew's cross. Each three-storied wing had a capacity for 240 detainees, eighty per floor. Prisoners were assigned one or two per cell or detained, when necessary, in the solitary-confinement unit buried within the second floor intersection of the cross. The guards called solitary "ground zero minus."

Meal consumption took place within the cells. These inmates received the bulk of nutrition from eight variations of the US military and FEMA meals ready to eat. Each cardboard-packaged MRE presented a main course of cold ground meat mixed with starches, such as beans or potato salad, a fruit cup, a dessert roll, and a plastic spoon—1,200 calories.

Passed through the cell's metal bar slot, MREs were dispensed twice daily and augmented by one hot meal in the evening served on trays.

Four exercise zones existed, one aligned to each cross's quadrant. Fresh arrivals and the steadfast, full-of-themselves felons were allowed one forty-minute exercise period per day.

Viewed from above, the cross and exercise zones formed a square. A six-meter double fence enveloped the quad and was anchored by observation towers every hundred meters. Ground Zero detainees who demonstrated social progress toward Circle One status got upgraded to two exercise periods each day plus access to a small receiving radio in their cells.

Outside Ground Zero unfolded the rest of Circle One: eight Stalinesque block buildings, each occupying forty-five degrees of the circle's circumference and enclosed with a perimeter of electronic sensors. The structures had four floors and quartered 240 prisoners, sixty per story. Every level provided a large common room and fifteen sleeping bays, each with four or fewer inmates assigned.

Provided in the group area were dining tables, a large microwave oven, juice, milk, and soft-drink dispensers, Prison Library Access Telebooths, or PLATs, and three television screens. One monitor broadcasted news, sports, and weather conditions in English, a second likewise in Spanish, and the third alternated a series of movies and stateside entertainment programs in both languages. Prepared meals were delivered three times every day to each common room from the prison's main food service. Circle One felons organized the distribution from there.

The prison's racial policy stipulated not to segregate room and floor assignments: on each story resided whites, African Americans, Hispanics, and other ethnic groups. The inmates were here for the long haul and had to get used to one another. Sleeping-bay preferences, influenced by individual tolerances, sorted out such that cursory apartheid pockets often cropped up but not to the extent compared to the stateside correctional systems like California and Illinois. Those who could not adapt returned to Ground Zero.

Each building's basement contained a moderate-sized gymnasium, laundry room, and storage area with one designated locker per prisoner. Weather permitting, inmates were allowed outside within their building's established perimeters. A six-meter, single concrete wall, bedecked with laser motion sensors, stood fifty meters peripheral to the structures. The stout barrier demarcated the boundary between Circles One and Two.

Geographically, Circle Two encompassed Circle One more like a large trapezoid. Its expansive compound supported inmate dormitories, the prison headquarters and communications tower, the Central Security Control Directorate, an auxiliary power plant, the hospital and health clinic, the food service building and cafeteria, the library, a small commercial store, workshops, the main laundry, and an indoor sports facility.

There existed eighteen dormitories, each with a capacity to bed sixty inmates. If needed, additional area remained in Circle Two to construct nine more. A prisoner received an individual dorm room whenever he or she socially advanced up to Circle Two behaviors. Most of these convicts labored in workshops, food service, and the main laundry under supervision. A handful performed equipment maintenance and groundskeeping duties. The trapezoid's security border entailed a four-meter fence, abutted on the east by the Itelmen River.

The horseshoe-shaped piece of terrain that constituted the remainder of the 2,880 acres in the penal campus comprised Circle Three. Its area contained the residential quarters of Prisontown, the primary power plant, the penitentiary's farm, dairy, bakery, major maintenance facilities and garages, general store, credit union, education center, cemetery, and a co-located prefabrication factory. Circle Three prisoners could earn wages.

Prisontown village had a grid plot of eight avenues and intersecting streets that formed the inmate's duplex housing. Its central plaza sported the general store, credit union, education center, library/compact disc/DVD outlet, soccer field, and church/mosque/synagogue. Up to eight prisoners, in two sets of four, could be assigned to one duplex. Each duplex half contained four separate bedrooms, a great room, and kitchen for food preparation. Inmates could elect to take individual meals at Circle Two's cafeteria.

Not all of Circle Three's acreage had constructed barricades for perimeter security. Advanced laser detection machinery, superior to equipment deployed on the United States border with Mexico, monitored the gaps. The swift Itelmen River flowed perpendicular to the prong ends of the horseshoe, and old growth forest extended north, west, and south to such an extent that anyone lost within, lacking GPS, could still not be found by three hundred searchers after a fortnight.

In total, the Kamchatka facility incarcerated five thousand banished prisoners. At full capacity, the engineering design specifications had estimated one thousand inmates never progressing out of Ground Zero, two thousand advancing no farther than Circle One, one thousand capable to achieve Circle Two's social status, and one thousand motivated to live their lives up to the responsibilities and freedoms allowed and expected for Circle Three.

The concept of prisoners coping through banishment had produced the widest spectrum of opinions known to Graywood. Bearhead, Piper, and he had had many "trialogues" on potential prisoner behavior stemming out of expatriation. Gazing at Elmendorf Medical Center's parking lot while a flight of C-17 transports droned overhead, Graywood recalled numerous old exchanges.

One might identify the felons who would cope. They'd surprise many by how much they'd change and what they'd do to lead a better life in exile. Perhaps one of five banished inmates would look critically within the self and discover the strength to recognize his or her internal fraudulent behaviors and cease playing the victim and blaming others or circumstances for his or her situation. Sadly, the leftover 80 percent would likely engage the stupid con forever, never to find the needed self-redemption from their flawed characters that had landed them in Siberia.

Vanity swells one's ego, as it did Charles Manson's, to be the center of the universe. For the most vainful, Ground Zero would remain their sole abode.

Yet oddly paradoxical, it was vanity to some degree plus the inmate's will to power that moved them into Circle One. But those who perpetually possessed insufficient insight and self-redemption could go no farther.

Graywood returned to the computer screen and downloaded the warden's welcoming remarks to each prisoner cohort delivered fresh from Elmendorf:

"Welcome to Siberia, your new home. Your past story in America is not important now. You are felons allowed to live here, and only here, until you die. Each of you will inprocess into the prison's highest security block. Once you've completed your inprocessing, wherever you sleep each night from now is your choice.

"Just remember two things every single day you are alive here. Number one, we DON'T buy one drop of your past as YOU see it. Number two, where you sleep tonight, tomorrow, next month, or next year is your choice by YOUR demonstrated BEHAVIOR. You determine that by every minute you're awake. What you say means little or nothing, but WHAT YOU DO each moment says it all."

Graywood wondered if the warden added some dry humor off camera such as, "So sleep on it," or "It's very simple, so don't lose sleep over it."

The fundamental goal was control. Exiting the website, Graywood toyed with comparing Siberian banishment to an arranged marriage within a caste system gone amuck, but then that logic stream got hijacked by his past behaviorist training: "We make sense of the world mostly in concrete ways and rarely by abstract reasoning. To communicate to someone effectively, we express our potent ties to food, clothing, shelter, and health."

The circles leading out from Ground Zero into Prisontown village were concrete enough in concept and scope to motivate some inmates toward Circle Three's benefits. But then an oft-repeated Bearhead admonition resurfaced: "Gary, there's danger in seeing all human relationships in terms of power relationships."

Always, good old Monroe rebalanced anyone's thinking. And he might have said, "In the power game, part of the soul is voided or placed on hold for all, not some, of the players."

Then again, others believed the felons were coddled and given way too much already.

"Use them for target practice," Graywood remembered from a cartoon's first frame on the op-ed page of the *Anchorage Daily News* in early 2012. "Better yet, auction them off for target practice and make a few bucks," followed the second.

Graywood had to quit the sidetracks into tangled, philosophical webs. He needed to concentrate on the pending seminar presentations.

Under the Prisoner Surveillance tab, he opened the "Vp Chip" heading and sifted through tracking and safety procedures that might interest symposium attendees. At inprocessing, each prisoner had a 1.85 mm by 1.2 mm by 1.0 mm beacon chip inserted into the subcutaneous tissue between the shoulder blades. The Vp emitted a continuous identification code to area building and ground sensors whereby triangulation tracked the prisoner's whereabouts throughout the prison compound.

Only Central Security Control activated or terminated the signal. Inmates who'd chosen to sleep in Ground Zero Minus, for example, did not require location monitoring until they returned to Ground Zero.

A felon remained "skin-chipped" until he or she graduated to Circle Three—the locator was excised and replaced by a wallet-sized identification card with an embedded "Z Chip" that relayed a unique emission to the facility's Global Positioning Satellite restricted network. All transmissions employed carrier bands randomly rotated between eleven frequencies to prevent outside jamming overrides.

Graywood perused the related manuals on physical safety procedures. He selected three examples for the talk: no pants belts allowed, the standard inmate clothing consisted of tunics worn over trousers with elastic waists; razor blades shattered into tiny pieces whenever removed from the handle; and dedicated monitors—arrayed throughout Ground Zero, Circle One, and Circle Two—that shut down a cell block or building automatically whenever they detected pepper spray discharged by threatened staff in an emergency.

After scrolling prison census information, Graywood printed the numbers of convicts transferred by year, sex, and state. Zero females and 309 males exiled for 2013. Only 253 males had arrived in 2014, and half that number came from Texas alone—in that year across the United States, there had appeared social sentiments of "buyer's remorse" regarding banishment, except in Texas. For 2015, the Justice Department had planned to ostracize the initial contingent of 38 female felons along with 490 more males. For 2016, 90 women and 678 men were projected to board Elmendorf's flight of no return.

An urgent email from Graywood's bureau boss, Pratt Emrick, interrupted the preparation. Emrick wanted medical modifications to the prison's health-support business plan that allowed Circle Three prisoners to work off campus as seasonal firefighters and tree planters for Tri-P, the commercial wood and prefab factory, co-located within Prisontown.

Whenever Emrick utilized "off campus," Graywood's eyes rolled. Those words resurfaced Bearhead's cutting satire on Kamchatka's prison being akin to a Dakota Indian reservation, rather than Emrick's Ivy League colleges, like Dartmouth or Yale. The term, "prison campus," made the Beltway liberals feel better, yet Graywood shrugged contempt at the insipid irony.

Suppressing smoked-filled forest fires presented a vulnerable set of occupational health hazards. Any communication breakdowns on the firefighting crew when battling a fierce blaze could be lethal. To Graywood, the language barrier for the foreseeable future between the convicts and Kamchatkans remained vast and therefore a dangerous risk.

In contrast, planting saplings to replace harvested trees struck similar to the routines the trusted inmates performed at the prison's farm and dairy. Graywood prepared a short reply to Emrick, closed the prison's website, and opened Tri-P's logo for snippets to round out the symposium's presentation.

Tri-P denoted the American business trademark for Petrov Prefab and Paper in both Cyrillic and English. Tri-P's existence had fostered Prisontown's site selection in Siberia.

Tri-P had formed as a commercial joint venture in 2007 between farsighted Alaskan and Siberian entrepreneurs to manage the extensive Kamchatkan forest resources for sustained timber exports to China and other North Pacific Rim countries. Within a year, the corporation had restructured into the lucrative, onsite manufacture of prefabricated housing instead of simply exporting raw lumber. Backed by investment capital from Alaska's Permanent Fund, Tri-P constructed the main factory beside the Intelmen River—an area brimming with ample water and prime forest.

In tandem with the facility, Tri-P's company boomtown, Petropvolitin, expanded the local job markets. The Siberian government diverted revenues from exported oil and natural gas to construct a feeder railroad line and maintenance road.

In 2011, two events enhanced Tri-P's corporate existence and bottom line. First, it won a hard-fought contract from the United Nations to construct and store inventories of prefabricated houses, schools, and clinics as replacement shelters for the razed, slapdash clapboards and tents at disaster sites trying to recover around the world.

The hit-and-miss global responses to the catastrophic 2005 earthquake in Pakistan's mountains and the post-Christmas 2004 tidal wave engulfing Indonesia and several Indian Ocean countries had pushed into the forefront this internationally sanctioned relief measure. The Myanmar cyclone and the Sichuan quake in 2008 broadened support for emergency housing in the UN General Assembly. The early 2010 seismic destruction of Haiti's Port-au-Prince and that summer's merciless flooding along Pakistan's Indus River crowned the multinational effort to procure ready-made structures for rapid shipment into obliterated areas.

Second, Tri-P submitted its contract bid to the US Justice Department for the banished felon prison site. The Federal Bureau of Prisons had developed selection criteria for the foreign penal location and advertised for bids in compliance with the 2011 mandate. Fourteen countries submitted proposals. Saudi Arabia, Australia, and Tri-P were judged the best.

Tri-P emphasized its proximity to the United States, business ties to Alaska, history of environmental consciousness, and willingness to assist the prison to become fiscally self-sustainable. With intrepid Alaskan political support, Tri-P prevailed over the grandstanding delegation of Texans who'd boosted Saudi Arabia in the congressional backrooms while the K Street lobbyists hired by Australia appeared clueless regarding the intricate logistics and timelines of the great endeavor.

The announcement of the contract award physically and symbiotically linked Prisontown to Tri-P. As time proved, one could not survive minus the other.

Graywood glanced at the clock above the office door—time to retrieve Bobby from disabled day care. Another anticonvulsant dose adjustment had altered seizure frequency from every forty-eight hours to one or two per week. Hopefully none today.

He save-screened Tri-P on the computer and grasped the Subaru's keys.

Graywood and his child, Tri-P and the prison, they'd found their parallel fates.

Graywood completed the symposium's PowerPoint draft and game-planned replies to potential audience inquiries regarding the prison's success with social parameters. He reviewed emails and written notes from conversations with Tri-P's CEO, the prison warden, and the chief psychiatrist at the Bureau of Prisons. He posed a hypothetical question and jotted down elements for its response. Not the stature of a staged presidential debate, he mused, but equal in seriousness.

"Question #1: How will the prison's existence affect the criminal justice system in the United States?"

"I'll offer a three part answer:

"The standard feel-good reply is that crimes of first-degree murder will decrease once the ironclad banishment penalty permeates the penal codes in all fifty states. Why is that you might ask? I speculate that compared to the death penalty, the chilling immensity of lifelong banishment may influence, overall, less murder. That's because perpetual stays of execution—so common before the 2011 Compromise, which had helped felons beat their raps for decades—will no longer have a moral basis. With banishment, instead, the sentence of execution and its ever-encircling delay upon delay is pulled out from under the convicted murderer. Now the potential criminal will think one more time not to kill in cold blood.

"Second, federal and state sentencing guidances could inflate to make banishment the most severe punishment for heinous crimes that do not involve first-degree murder, such as multiple counts of second-degree murder or child molestation.

"And third, other English- and Spanish-speaking countries, like our North American trading partners, may wish to negotiate places for their own felons at Prisontown, if space is available."

Graywood bet no one attending the conference would have imagined international trade in felons.

He continued with the hypothetical questions and responses. "Question #2: Why are terrorists who are American citizens not sent to Kamchatka?"

"The two-part answer: first, there is no desire on Capitol Hill at this time to repeat Guantanamo, and second, the Russians don't tolerate terrorists one bit. You get my meaning?"

"Question #3: Can you summarize the psychology employed in the rehabilitation processes from Ground Zero to Circle Three?"

Graywood lingered. Out the frost-rimmed office window beyond the parking lot stood a naked birch grove in yard-deep snow—not burled and crooked as in Kamchatka. Feeling embarrassed with the self-charade, he chided himself for being the flimflam, carnival barker found in every twisted politician. Whoever summarized the psychology for the criminal justice system was either a god or a fool, yet Graywood tried to comprehend this soft science, this religion of selected speculations and biased reasonings, this dogma of subconscious denigrations that masqueraded for facts …

There were really four prison communities contained within the Kamchatka facility—Ground Zero and Circles One, Two, and Three. The working theory recognized how individual exiles in Kamchatka varied in their abilities to engage in reciprocity and social cohesion: Ground Zero felons displayed the least, and Circle Three denizens had matured the most. In essence, the prisoners sorted themselves by their behavior choices that reflected their capacities toward long-term displays of these two qualities. All of them had killed others, the extreme antithesis to humanity's kindest traits. How far the malefactor might grow away from the baseline of murder was his or her choice.

So what motivated the inmate to reciprocity and social cohesion? Raw hedonism or the game of less pain, more gain?

Homicide was not a Hollywood cartoon. Banishment was its justice through isolation. It was THE major life change for any person short of execution. Depression, exhaustion, and ennui—even if denied—accompanied exile. Might Ground Zero approximate the frauds and voids of souls cast down to Dante's Inferno and the three circles represent the first half of the seven-storied mountain of redemption in Purgatorio?

Graywood gazed at the ceiling's acoustic particle board pitted with tiny holes and crevices. Why should he even care for convicts? Why should they receive a dram's worth of redemption? Back and forth, he considered the felons' behaviors until he slanted into Bobby's terrible illness, his boy's prison, the mysterious unfairness wrecking his son's short life.

He clung to the hope Bobby might recover like the birch trees showing their green announcements of oncoming spring. Reclined in the desk chair with closed tired eyes, he reasoned by semi-dreams in the dark …

Was it fair to offer prisoners like these a chance to return to humanity, to go beyond the absolutes found in Ground Zero's warehouse and demonstrate true reciprocity so cohesion might exist? Was it honest to provide an inmate the opportunity to attain a bit of the human family after wallowing alone in long winters of discontent? Graywood tried to walk in their shoes:

"Call me Martin.

"And when saying my name, emphasize the second half, 'TEN', as 'Mar-TEN,' like the number ten.

"If I'm banished to Siberia, how should I battle the stress, the dislocation, my pervasive anger? I've lost control. I've lost respect. I've lost love. I could choose Ground Zero isolation or seek out measures of fellowship. But whom can I trust? Who's my friend, my enemy? What's a friend here, and what's not? What's the best agenda for me? How will this prison hurt me? Help me?

"If I stay in 'me' mode, I'll never leave Ground Zero. When will I realize the pride in 'me' must morph somewhat into a pride of 'us'? And who are 'us' in Siberia?

"Maybe one inmate, a group of inmates, or someone free outside the cell wall. All of them, perhaps? Will the pride in 'us' become pride for the prison? Could I ever accept that? Believe that? Label it brainwashing or, at best, Marine Corps boot camp?

"The warden warned where I sleep is determined only by the behavior I choose, always determined by my actions, never my words. My deeds are judged pretty much in good and bad flavors. Good generates trust, and bad takes it away. So I'll control my actions and select the ones that benefit me. Ones I trust.

"But what if I chose actions that benefit someone else? They might help me even more to get out of Ground Zero because I'm growing their trust too. Out of this, I build my self-esteem, and that might be the best antidote for the burdens of banishment. It's so simple—help others, and I help myself. And I get to enter Circle One.

"So where do I begin?

"Find out how the prison staff can help me do one or two things each day that they and I would be proud of. They'd tell to start owning up for past actions of fraud and avoid recommitting them. And I'll find those who believe in me. In return, I'll truly believe in them. Truth displayed in action, over time, will generate trust. Then we'll advance to the circles and start coming back to family, into community."

With reopened eyes, Graywood clicked the prison website to its photo section. Felons witnessed a bold-lettered sign screwed over the entry into each adjacent, higher circle. Graywood located the picture he wanted: TRUTH + TIME = TRUST. The best response to the rehabilitation-psych question punted earlier and perhaps the answer for living and growing faith for all. He pasted the image into the PowerPoint presentation.

Residing at Ground Zero or Circle One need not become a permanent choice. The prison had created layers of cohesiveness. It emphasized extended families in Circles Two and Three, akin to Sir Thomas More's Utopia.

In his mind, Graywood scrambled together TRUTH, TIME, TRUST, Purgatorio, and Utopia. Someday he'd blow their four-square combinations by Bearhead for comment.

Yet he stubbed into a hard-nosed question: Who's conning whom here? Bobby's condition brewed so ragged it created semi-hypnotic head games where murderous exiles worked trust into the privileged circles at a Siberian prison. Knives from a dozen skeptics could fillet such goody hockspit.

Drained, he exited into the night.

A Bureau of Prison's reckoning after thirty years revealed for every nine felons banished, two had chosen the pathway to Circle Three fugued in Graywood's semi-dream.

By the Memorandum of Agreement between the Justice Department and DOD, Prisontown's pharmacy was designated an outlying component of the Elmendorf medical center. Twice each week, Air Force flights from Alaska supplied drugs, medical supplies, and vaccines.

But Graywood faced a dilemma: two standards of health care existed within Prisontown. The penitentiary's staff received the medical and pharmaceutical access and quality equivalent to Alpha-Omega in the United States. The inmates, however, were provided only care rooted at mid-twentieth century levels.

The Department of Justice had interpreted the 2011 Compromise legislation to specify no heroic health treatments for an exiled prisoner. DOJ reasoned the felon, at one time, had resided on America's death row destined for execution for taking a life or lives; because of banishment, he or she had been granted a natural death instead, but ONLY a natural death. Extending such lives by all possible medical means was deemed counterproductive and financially unsound to sustaining the prison. Ending capital punishment was a great moral leap forward that reset America's social boundary, but Cadillac health care for murderers pushed it too far.

When Bobby's seizures emerged in 2011, Graywood took as many piecemeal absences from work as necessary to insure everything possible was performed regarding his son's medical evaluations and therapies—preeminent clinics, finest pediatric consultants, all the components of care. Graywood's spotty unavailability had forced the Bureau of Prisons to draft the prime medical guidelines without his input: The Beltway bureaucrats had codified the access and quality limitations for the expelled prisoners. Bobby's deterioration magnified over the ensuing four years and diverted Graywood from moderating the manual's initial Spartan fundamentals or its annual revisions from Washington.

Graywood decoded the 2015 edition, "Medical Directives for Prisoner Health." Simplified, the three hundred pages had winnowed inmate care to first aid, mental health support, addiction treatments, and pain control. In sharp contrast to the pharmacy benefits accessible for the penitentiary's staff employees and guards, only generic drugs were listed in the prisoner's formulary. A double standard of care existed within spitting distance—a first-class facility and a third world aid station. The discrepancy gashed Graywood's ethics for fairness. He obligated himself to patch the gap.

Kicking the sides of the office desk, Graywood thumbed the manual ready to tear it apart. He stopped at the section for the management of elevated cholesterol: "Treatment of hypercholesterolemia shall be restricted to dietary changes and exercise. Prescribing statins to lower cholesterol not allowed."

He leafed to the introductory page on heart attack care: "Treatment standards for myocardial infarction are centered on making admitted inmate patients comfortable in the prison hospital. Generic beta-blockers, nitro-glycerin, digitalis, diuretics, and aspirin are available. Not allowed are bypass surgery, angio-stints, cardiac pumps, pacemakers, heparin or heparin derivatives, or other vascular amendments commonly administered to Alpha-Omega and Medicare beneficiaries. Cardiac failure, with or without pulmonary congestion and/or rhythm abnormalities, shall be allowed to progress on its natural course without mitigating medical or surgical interventions."

Graywood snapped shut the volume.

Without mitigating medical or surgical interventions.

How could a medical colleague write such draconian bull? The prisoners were human beings too.

Graywood backtracked and reviewed spreadsheets on the budgetary health parameters he had to implement: personnel compensation, staff continuing education, medical supplies and equipment, pharmaceuticals, electronic consultations, equipment maintenance and depreciation, and the eight other major categories that pressed against his fiscal bottom line. The Department of Justice paid him for executive leadership, paid him to divide and balance the annual financial plan into the best possible prison health system. Yet Prisontown's operation manifested worse than the most severely flattened, cost-quality-access triangle he'd ever seen depicted for Alpha-Omega, Medicare, or Alaska's Medicaid. How much should he allow the medical staff to treat the prisoners, and how much more must remain undone to keep the medical department on track with budget restrictions dictated by Department of Justice?

Tackling the double-standard in drug access, Graywood switched to Tri-P's occupational health formulary and reviewed its onsite support plan for the factory workers and their families. Like any major company, Tri-P took a proactive approach. It recognized that any disabled employee, on the job or off, would lessen productivity and subtract from the bottom line. With a prevention emphasis, Tri-P provided a full medical package for the workers and their families: smoking cessation, musculoskeletal overuse injury interventions, drug and alcohol rehabilitation, mental health support, referred triage care at Petropavlovsk, and more.

Graywood reviewed the formulary that bolstered Tri-P's medical care and studied its two most expensive drug categories—cancer treatment regimens and state-of-the-art cholesterol-lowering meds. He concluded they were rather equivalent to Alpha-Omega's. Tri-P also placed an overall premium on meeting the wellness requirements of its employees and their families and planned to continue services into their retirement years. It made sense. To attract and maintain a reliable workforce at an isolated location required, in part, a good health benefit.

By Graywood's assessment, the prison guards and administrative staffs received modestly superior health care to that for Tri-P's employees. But twenty-first century medicine remained elusive for the prisoners. The moral morass fogged Graywood's ability to lead. Two different standards existed side by side: up-to-date medicine advocated for the facility employees and nearly the same for Tri-P, but Sputnik-era care for inmates.

"What would Abraham Lincoln have done?" he pondered. At the close of America's Civil War, Lincoln had envisioned a great healing of the nation after it had murdered itself. "Malice toward none and charity for all."

And Thomas More's impression regarding guards getting better health upkeep than prisoners? His *Utopia* had championed abolishment of social status to determine access to goods and services, and that applied to medical care.

Social change took time. For Graywood, Tri-P's health program had set the medical baseline to achieve for the prisoners in contrast to Washington's sparse directives. Once accomplished, he'd lobby to elevate everyone to the Alpha-Omega levels that the prison guards and employees received.

Tri-P staffed a small health and emergency aid station at the factory and contracted the more complex treatments to Russian doctors in Petropavlovsk. With Prisontown's medical department hardly two kilometers away, fully operational, and web-linked into Elmendorf's medical center, Graywood brainstormed a plan to usurp Tri-P's Petropavlovsk medical connection. He'd negotiate leveraging Tri-P's health-care costs with the prison's expenditures. With Tri-P as a major customer, he'd capitalize a portion of the added revenue stream toward improved access to better therapies for the prisoners.

Graywood contacted his boss in Washington on the secured webcam to discuss the double standard debacle and his solution …

"Gary, I understand the difficulty that two juxtaposed standards of health care make," oozed Pratt Emrick, Graywood's round-faced, bifocaled supervisor with thinning, clove-brown hair.

Unctuous in the leased federal offices at Tyson's Corner, Virginia, Emrick worked overtime in Beltway group-think mode as the government's working mouthpiece for whatever smarmed toward the Federal Bureau of Prisons.

"Remember, Gary, the implementing guidance from the bureau and DOJ is pretty clear not to overextend these felons' lives."

"I know that," clipped Graywood. "I just want everyone to know at Justice it's gonna be damn hard to hold back care to someone we could've helped."

"Gary, we know that. But do I have to repeat all the compromise bull-carp about murderers getting death sentences commuted so they'd die natural deaths?" huffed Emrick. "Remember, 'natural' is the glorified word in the Grand Compromise. Given our history on capital punishment, that's a sure damn shift our country's now committed to."

Graywood sat motionless.

Emrick soothed, "Recall, Gary, other countries that forego death penalties really don't go out of their way to keep their lifers alive either. That's the dirty little secret we now get to share with them. So we'll politically trumpet to everyone we've got no more death penalty, and we'll let the convicts die at their own pace, slowly, naturally, whatever."

"Well, that naturally says a whole hell of a lot about our world," returned Graywood, in bitter tones.

"Yeah, it does," hastened Emrick. He paused to oil another tactic. "I've been reviewing medication costs by diagnostic categories. Did you know last year was the fifth time in the past ten that prescription drug sales for cancer drugs exceeded the amount spent on statins to lower blood cholesterol?"

"I'm not surprised," said Graywood. "Once Alpha-Omega gets up to full stride like Medicare and we get older as a nation, cancer will kill off more of us every year than heart disease."

"Did you ever think new cancer drugs, being as expensive as they are, might break the country's health budget," countered Emrick, "as more and more patients get them?"

"Why not!" bellowed Graywood. "There's never enough money to pay for everything."

"Just between you and me, Gary," softened Emrick, "HHS is talking offline to POTUS about upping the VAT and Medicare part of FICA to cover the ballooning costs of treating cancer. It'll be a hard sell for the country to accept more taxes."

"Pratt, I know where you're leading," conceded Graywood. "If Alpha-Omega is running out of money, then there's going to be restrictions placed on availability of cancer drugs, and for damn sure there won't be any for prisoners dying of cancer in Kamchatka."

"Well, Gary, it's hell to sell voters on spending scarce funds to treat an exiled killer with lung cancer most people think should've been executed in the first place," maneuvered Emrick, "especially when others back home need help like the innocent little girl with leukemia on Medicaid or her kindly grandmother with breast cancer who barely survives with Medicare."

"I know, I know," Graywood coughed.

"It's just a matter of perspective," said Emrick. "Gary, you're supposed to see the world your way and do what you think's right. You advocate for those you're responsible for, and let me say, you're doing a heck of a job. I really admire you for that. But I'm afraid you've got a group who don't carry a shred of political clout."

"Fine," concluded Graywood tersely. "I've got my marching orders. Talk to you at the weekly videoconference. Goodbye."

"Gary, wait, one more thing," shot Emrick.

"What?"

"Your request for leflunomide to be added to the prisoner's formulary to treat rheumatoid arthritis will be denied."

"For Christ's sake, Pratt, that's not a bioengineered drug costing thousands; it's dirt cheap."

"I know, Gary. We can get it from the manufacturer for twenty dollars a month, but that's still a couple of bucks more than sulfasalazine, and I had to fight like hell to get you even that little gem when there're two other generics you've also asked for that cost even less."

"So I've approval to include sulfasalazine and the other two on the prisoner's formulary to treat their rheumatoid arthritis?"

"Yes, and for now, three drugs for rheumatism are enough.

"And for the guards and prison staff?"

"Well of course, they get access to all the anti-rheumatoid drugs approved for Alpha-Omega use, same as anybody else."

"Including the new bioengineered drugs?"

"If they're on Alpha-Omega's formulary, they'll definitely be on yours for the employees. The bureau takes care of its own."

"Pratt, we're back to where we started. Two standards of access, two standards of care."

"Yep, that's the bullshit way it's gotta be, Gary."

"It's rationed care!"

"Yeah," agreed Emrick. "You're the fuckin' poster child for it."

Disgusted, Graywood reached to shut off the webcam.

"Oh, one more thing," added Emrick.

"Christ, what else?"

"Gary, you need to know any drug or therapy you request to treat a prisoner with a chronic disease costing over twenty dollars a month will probably be denied by DOJ."

"Well that pretty much ties my staff's hands to just dishing out first aid and methadone."

"I know it sounds ridiculous, Gary, but it's the Grand Compromise."

"Yeah, Pratt, nice to have that as our new morality. By the way, isn't next month your birthday?"

"Yes, why you ask?"

"You gonna make Alpha-Omega's weight standard or lose half your tax exemption?"

"Gary, my cellphone's buzzing. Got more hot issues to tend to," said Emrick, faking distraction. "See you and your staff at the videoconference."

Graywood felt glad Emrick had lied about the cellphone. Terminating the webcam saved Graywood from hearing Emrick's stock muddle for political compromises couched in policy standards linked to evidence-based medicine that delivered the best health program possible.

A waste of time. Price constraints always remained huge modifiers in providing efficient medical care. Graywood repeated that concept to the first-year medical students. Before Alpha-Omega, health expenses were controlled by access barriers that denied claims, created payout limits, employed co-pays, plus had a host of other gimmicks. Private insurers and all levels of the government deployed them to delay, avoid, or shift costs to each other. After Alpha-Omega arrived, price controls became more gussied up, transparent, and connected to fancy terms, like evidence-based medicine, health promotion, and waste reduction. Consensus recommendations from authorities and selected consumers further camouflaged the fundamental intent to taper all spending by dressing up or down the access and quality components of care. Yet a biased "expert consensus group" could mobilize at any time and recommend or prohibit the provision of a therapy. Nothing commercial within the medical-industrial complex bore immunity against interference by various political and trade interests.

Bottom line, Graywood had to acquiesce to the medical bureaucracies rationing care. There existed a set amount of money to fund everyone's health programs, and always there would be more demands than available funds. Otherwise, the American quest for universal immortality would break the bank.

"Choice with limits," he mused. "Why can't Washington, DC, just say limited choice out loud?"

Alpha-Omega sounded so comprehensive at its beginning, but its access had to be controlled, or costs would fly up the chimney. The double-talking tongues dueling in every politician's mouth would never speak the truth.

And the amount of health care rationed to beneficiaries might be further diminished or negated despite an individual's most dire needs. Advanced cutting-edge cancer medicines demonstrated a sour example: higher in price compared to older, generic drugs; alluring promise of potential cures or improved quality of life; yet debatable benefits whenever viewed through the lens that they only prolonged life three months on average with a host of side effects, many toxic. How to balance society's expense against a patient who might benefit a lot, somewhat, or little from the new anti-cancer medication? The rare cure versus the usual six months, three months, or even one month more of life—was it worth it?

Graywood thought of Bobby and his terrible, ravishing disease. The deterioration molded Graywood's perspective on life. He'd cling to every shard of hope, never giving up on Bobby as the relentless illness diminished him away. As with cancer, that focus made the most sense. That's what it's all about, living.

"How did he do today?" asked Graywood.

"Bobby's a pleasure to work with," enthused Kara, the childcare assistant at the special education facility on Dowling Road. "Today he did numbers and picture book perfectly."

They lifted Bobby from the wheelchair into the Subaru.

"He score a ten?" asked Graywood.

"This morning he got seven correct, and eight on the second try, then a ten this afternoon," she confirmed.

"Ahhh … ten, taah," slurred Bobby, holding up ten fingers, right hand higher. Bobby tried to form a meaningful whole out of the sensory information incompletely perceived or integrated by his dysfunctional brain. Today's summary was good.

"Any problems eating?"

"None," she said. "And no blackouts of any kind."

Relieved, Graywood grinned and stroked the boy's head before buckling the seatbelt. When Bobby suffered a seizure, Graywood compared it offhandedly to corrupting his internal browser. As each updated medication regimen prevented all or most of the disruptions for a month or two, the repairs and reconnections of his neural circuits could proceed.

"Bobby, you ready for home and little Brandy Belle?"

"I seeh, ah …Brana Bell … gooh!"

"Good! Me too!" encouraged Graywood. He'd stopped correcting misspoken speech months ago.

Mute, Bobby watched the passing window's world on the way to Snowline Drive. Doctor Timm and Graywood had no explanations for his dearth of expression other than disease progression, an undocumented side effect of the ever-changing anti-seizure combinations, or Bobby's sheer preference to feel uninterrupted road vibration. Lacking dialogue, father and son drove across Anchorage as Graywood mixed thoughts of Bobby and the Kamchatkan prison—a tandem confinement more and more shackled.

Doctor Timm had categorized Bobby's malady as progressive degeneration of the nervous system that impaired speech and coordination, similar to Friedreich's ataxia … yet with a greater contrasting scope. But Bobby's disease had manifested as hard-to-control seizures, a sign that matched poorly to Friedreich's and its complications toward heart failure, often late in the course. Regardless, the mysterious disease withered Bobby's brain and body and shrunk Graywood's pitiful hope.

At a recent appointment, Doctor Timm broached Bobby's full-time placement in a nursing facility. Although not spoken, both physicians acknowledged the slow death march and the requirement to designate advanced directives for end-of-life care.

A southbound accident on Glenn Highway thickened traffic to a crawl. Trapped two miles from the off-ramp, Graywood reckoned Kamchatkan banishment with the lifetime health-care needs of those liberated out of death row. Exiled felons who lacked sufficient medical care were sanctioned to a plodding death over an executioner's instant one, certainly a cost shift and an unintended consequence never addressed in the heady days of the 2011 Compromise. Clueless politicians who led, or pretended to lead, had left the critical details to the bean counters and frontline providers to resolve.

Graywood recalled episodes where one people had branded another as unworthy for equal rights and respect and then viewed these others with contempt. Once ingrained that the others were something less, all imagined horror followed. To Graywood, the Kamchatka inmates were not unworthy of modern health support.

The traffic snarl speeded up. Graywood planned the evening at home. For dinner, chili puree with melted cheese topped over spaghetti squash with milk … an hour of television followed by Bobby's passive and active range of motion exercises … ice cream treat, son's sponge bath and bed. Thereafter he'd migrate to the den and troubleshoot the Kamchatkan care dilemma.

Blanket-wrapped, Bobby slept safely.

Rotating the den's chair, Graywood viewed the dimmed backyard. Moonlit shadows fenced the markers of Bobby's outside play area from years ago. Much had happened since.

The prison work beckoned.

Attempting to crack Prisontown's supply-and-demand health puzzle, Graywood swung around to sort his racks of bygone movie DVDs. He settled on *A Night to Remember* and *Titanic,* two commercial versions where lifeboat supply proved inadequate to meet rescue demand once the unfortunate vessel struck an iceberg. First-class passengers got better access to safety because they were rich, important, and had paid more for boarding tickets.

Graywood equated the *Titanic*'s elite to the prisoners in Circle Three. Should Circle Three inmates receive better health care than the others because their labor mitigated the cost of running Prisontown? Splitting hairs that way might solve the prison's maze of mismatched medical care.

Through their rise from Ground Zero, they'd proven themselves "first-class" prisoners. They'd become less "other-like" and closer to the non-felon population in the United States. If the prison health budget could find the money, a Circle Three prisoner ought to have higher priority for a pacemaker, whenever needed, than a Circle One … or receive heart-valve surgery to repair a debilitating defect and hasten the return to work in Tri-P's factory.

Yet Pratt Emrick posited there was only so much money for prisoner treatments. Graywood had to triage the most bang for every buck. He also knew Emrick viewed Circle Three inmates as more valuable to DOJ's bottom line. So it made financial sense to allocate a medical resource to Circle Three first, then Circle Two, and so on until it vanished. But how to do it morally?

Graywood held a DVD in each hand. The night the iceberg gashed the *Titanic*'s hull, all on board were condemned, both the passengers and crew placed in the lifeboats, as well as the rest who drowned outright in the frigid waters. The following morning, the ship, *Carpathia*, fortunately rescued those in the small boats who'd shivered through the calamity. Otherwise they'd have been doomed too.

A capital crime conviction paid for a prisoner's ticket to Kamchatka—the equivalent to boarding the *Titanic.* And the iceberg equaled death's looming assault from Prisontown's inadequate health program. Only a matter of time until everyone drowned.

Critics railed against Prisontown providing too much inmate medical support or not enough. No one proclaimed it gave the right amount. The same harpoons also impaled Alpha-Omega stateside.

It had happened prior to and after Alpha-Omega's advent—the noxious cost shifting of payments between the insurance payers—the primal game played in financing any modern health-care system. It had to be done because public and private demands for access and quality invariably exceeded the available funds for services. Cost shifting remained the covert form of rationing.

As Prisontown's health administer, Graywood's greatest problem was also the basic—he had only one payer, the Federal Bureau of Prisons, his *Titanic.* He needed more payment streams to shrink the gap between the two standards of treatment. He wanted a *Carpathia* or two or three to rescue his overfilled lifeboats.

And he found them.

Foremost, he'd underbid Tri-P's occupational medicine contract with Petropavlovsk and champion access into the comprehensive care component at Prisontown. He'd collect Tri-P's revenue and leverage its medical care requirements with Prisontown's. With funds left over, he'd add a handful of services for some of the prisoners.

Graywood still needed more payers …

"Jen, how's the setup for your hep C trial coming?" Graywood inquired from his Elmendorf office.

"Gary, it's nice you called," she replied. "It's on track, but please tell me how Bobby's doing."

She'd thrown him off his goal. Frustrated, Graywood retooled a response. "Ah, there's not much, Jen, I'm happy about."

"Oh, I'm so sorry."

"I mean he's seizing as much," his voice quavered, "but there's so much less of him." Graywood paused to regain control. "He can't walk on his own, but the speech therapist says he's stopped his language slide."

"Gary, what may I do to help?"

"I don't know … I'm sure he'd like to see you again."

"Let's do it!"

"So, which evening can you come over for dinner?"

"Sometime next week. I'm swamped now and leaving for the panhandle early tomorrow."

"Tuesday next week?" he offered.

"Thursday's better."

"Ah, okay. Thursday ... say six p.m."

"I'll be there. Say, Gary, I'm running out of time. I've got groups of town and village project arms to set up with my people before tomorrow. If it's all right, I'll give the situation on the field trial to you after dinner next week."

"That's fine, Jen. See you."

"Bye-bye, Gary. Tell Bobby I'm coming."

What compelled Graywood to extend these felons' lives? They were humans who'd killed other humans. What good would come from shedding scarce health dollars on them? There were others in the world more deserving, who hadn't murdered.

But there had been millions who'd taken lives in all the grand causes mandated and glorified by their countries, all the fought wars and horrendous slaughters of other peoples—bayoneted, gassed, shelled, bombed into oblivion.

Graywood ached for the innocent babies aborted out of preference, especially those identified by ultrasound as females, instead of males. And honor killings. Wars, abortions, family esteem ... who damn well decided who was more deserving? How were they so right?

And Bobby and his enduring hell, imprisoned by an unknown disease stripping him away piece by piece.

"God, this is terrible, terrible, terrible!" declared Graywood in silence whenever he left the boy in another's care. "It's the worse prison possible. Oh, please God, please help me to help my son."

He cursed medicine's inability to stop Bobby's destruction. He railed against the unknown illness wiping out neurons faster than the brain's adaptive ability to reroute internal connections to maintain or even regain the proud little boy, the human dynamo, he'd once been.

Ironically, both Bobby and the banished inmates had been confined to health-care hell. Everything Graywood had done for Bobby made not one dram of difference: The world lacked the knowledge about the brutal condition decimating the child.

In contrast, with an extra thousand bucks annually per prisoner, Graywood could redesign the medical home in Kamchatka to insure for each, on average, seven or more years of additional life. If given that time, some might grow more capacity to reason and sprout a bud or two of compassionate spirit. But they had access only to a harsh health facility—a piecemeal shack of triaged, bare-bones rationed care.

Graywood resolved three things: concentrate on life, someway fill part or all the nebulous void surrounding Bobby, and eschew the medical scraps dispensed by the Justice Department. He could never rationalize down the social duty that banished inmates had to die quicker than their guards. The implication they were to expire out of sight from the rest of the United States had crossed a crass line into economic eugenics. If it happened to them first, who would be next? Graywood could not socially accept such a corrupted ending.

Morality always vexed him. It appeared natural and supernatural, biological and theological. As a willing child, he learned human and divine righteousness together, but as an adult, he questioned the myriad splits within both the common and sacred interpretations.

Cashel Goodlette had preached that all religious dogmas were human-derived and solely composed from underlying, cave-dwelling motivations which, more often than not, clashed hammer on anvil.

Yet for Graywood, there existed primal justifications that bound social decency. He'd read Adam Smith, Immanuel Kant, and Schopenhauer. And Bearhead had pointed to Mencius of China. The philosophers had argued humanity naturally inclined toward compassion and kindness.

But a sense of power also lurked in brotherhood displays of sympathy and benevolence, especially whenever framed by the Kamchatkan medical dilemma. To give anyone something such as quality medical care made Graywood feel superior—it recreated a sense of control within him that had been extinguished by Bobby's savage illness.

The potential opposite also showed prevalent—to take something away asserted one's personal dominance as well. Whether one acted out of spite or pity, envy or love, gluttony or sacrifice, the motivation to showcase primal control persisted. Through all sizes of governments, past and present, notorious power plays always happened.

Within Graywood, the prisoners' fate wove into his child's. Impotent to his own son and hellish mad, he'd anchor his desperate sanity by fighting the prison's double standard of health care.

"It's an insane world I live in," Graywood said the evening he embraced Jennelle good-bye at the front door.

"We live in," she gently empathized. "Gary, thanks for the grilled salmon. You made a delicious dinner."

"Well, thanks for extending your hep C trial out to Prisontown."

"I'm confident CDC will permit it since it allows them another political angle and—"

"And it means more funding control for them," Graywood completed. Both laughed.

"Tomorrow I'll massage them into adding Kamchatka into the Alaskan trial's arm." After adjusting her coat, she grabbed his hand. "Gary, dear, call me if you ever need help with Bobby. When I'm in town, I can watch him and work out of your den."

"I will."

The evening was successful, despite Bobby vomiting twice after dessert. Graywood cleaned the floor while Jen assisted Bobby with range-of-motion exercises.

Prior to dinner, Jennelle had summarized the Alaskan component of the worldwide hepatitis C vaccine field trial. Using the den's computer, she displayed the map of recruited cities, towns, and villages tagged to their supporting clinics.

"You've signed up Chitina and Glennallen," observed Graywood.

"Sweet Roe insisted," Jennelle confessed. "He didn't want them forgotten."

"Did you know his first wife died from liver cancer?"

"Yes, Roe told me. He wanted me to know he'd read the hep C literature and it caused liver cancer and hadn't stopped spreading among Alaskan natives."

When pitching to Jennelle to extend the trial to Kamchatka's Prisontown, Graywood remained upfront on tapping her funding stream to augment the prisoner's primary care needs. He detailed the flat tradeoffs between the two standards of care provided to the employed staffs and the banished inmates. If Graywood could not outright treat the convicts at the same level as the guards, Jennelle's hep C trial could narrow the gap.

He reviewed the three circles of felons and implied most trial volunteers would come from Circle Three. He'd cost-shift into Jen's vaccine trial a portion of their annual medical expenses, such as screenings and abnormal test follow-ups. The meager money that freed up would be reprogrammed to fill the holes in care for other Threes and some in Circle Two.

Guard and staff volunteers were anticipated from all Prisontown sections. Likewise, part of the costs of their health-care benefit would be shifted to Jen's trial, and the saved resources would then be designated for the less fortunate prisoners.

In return, Graywood committed to impeccably train Prisontown's medical staff on the trial's procedures and assist Jennelle with data processing and analysis for Alaska.

She agreed to cover the treatment costs for participants who developed any form of liver inflammation as a potential vaccine side effect—be it from alcohol, fatty infiltration, infection, medications, or other conditions not related to the trial. And she insisted everyone, the prisoners most of all, sign full-informed consents to negate any possibility for what had occurred a century ago when unaware Alabama prisoners had enrolled into a dangerous syphilis study at Tuskegee.

At the negotiation's conclusion, Jennelle shared an impression of the three prisoner circles: Graywood's description oddly reminded her of Alpha-Omega's weight classifications she'd heard him explain to medical students years ago.

"You're kidding!" he blurted. "I don't get it. You're saying the weight cutoffs for us are like the prison's circles for the inmates?"

"It's just amusing how the bureau and you split up the prisoners," she smirked.

"What do you mean?"

"You described Circle Three as a much better place to live than Circle Two and way better than One."

"Yeah, well, that's the way it's designed."

"Perhaps ... So Alpha-Omega splits all of us into normal weight, overweight, and obese, and the normal ones get to keep their tax deduction but the others lose half or all of theirs," she clarified. "They get it back only once they reform themselves weight-wise for the common good and come down to normal."

"Oh, I get it," he said. "You've connected the obesity level to Circle One's confinement, overweight with Two, and normal weight and Three. That's clever, Jen," Graywood added, smiling. "I'll have to use that in one of my lectures."

She giggled. Part of him hadn't changed ... Doctor Triangle.

Graywood checked on Bobby after Jennelle left—asleep with Brandy Belle nuzzled beside him. Graywood stroked their heads. She purred.

He heated water for tea. Sipping down hot tannic acid coated his bottom-line thinking and encouraged his mind to run sprints around ethics. Carrying two large mugs of Earl Grey, his feet coasted to den and computer.

What should be the new medical home for Prisontown? Graywood commenced with the premise of equal standards of care for the guards and prisoners, and the services provided should reflect, at least, those available in a rural stateside location under Alpha-Omega. But Prisontown's current medical home presented a house divided: first-class occupational medicine for guards and staff; third world support for inmates centered only on first aid, mental health, and substance-abuse rehab and juiced by a few ounces of primary and chronic care he'd rammed past Emrick and the Beltway minions.

Too many underfunded components forced prioritizing disease treatments out of the dollars earned from Tri-P plus the money garnered from cost-shifting into Jen's vaccine trial. Drawing on his management of a stand-alone clinic twenty years ago in Bethel, Alaska, Graywood inclined to commit more resources toward mental health and substance abuse.

But he needed input from the prison's onsite medical director before finalizing priorities. Yet whenever he contacted Doctor Padwar, she recited two or more pages of unfunded requirements, followed by requests for nursing home and hospice care—both long-term necessities. Graywood had to organize those as well but wouldn't.

His ambivalence toward terminal medical care was pooled by his son's dismal condition. Doctor Timm had gently pushed at their last appointment to consider nursing home admission and modifications to Bobby's advanced directives. Graywood wasn't ready: His internal battle raged between denying the child's pernicious decline and accepting his wretched fate.

He recharged mugs in the kitchen. Tonight he'd swap the cart and horse and think hard on Prisontown's nursing home and hospice needs instead of Bobby's.

In time, minds and bodies break, and organic shells become empty. Not many policymakers had reasoned the legacy costs of inmate elder care, particularly felons with unabated chronic diseases.

Banishment had replaced execution under the 2011 Compromise. In two decades, perhaps sooner, a significant number of inmates with chronic impairments, such as vision loss, depression, Parkinson's disease, and heart failure would populate Prisontown. They'd require more humane assistance as they physically and mentally deteriorated like the destitute elderly residents stateside confined to a nursing home, albeit a Kamchatkan nursing home with high fences and armed guards.

Attempting to devise a final-care business plan, Graywood scoured the web and centered on Oregon as a prototype. The Beaver State had done a decent job in caring for its elderly poor and disabled. Oregon preferred in-home assistance over nursing home placement and boasted its system had equivalent support levels at just one-seventh the cost.

For each cohort of aging inmates in the coming decades, Graywood outlined an implementation blueprint that met the prison's requirements for assisted living and nursing home care. He focused on building modifications before tackling staff augmentation and training personnel. Fleshing out the options, the obvious need for a hospice facility within the prison campus loomed.

Another web search discovered St. Christopher's in London, the first hospice created in the 1970s. Medicare's current hospice qualifications and how they'd changed from the past were reviewed and compared to the palliative approaches encoded within the European Union.

In Doctor Triangle mode, Graywood divided the long-term care support into three elements: assisted living, nursing home, and hospice care.

It also occurred to him to include a mortuary element. Would deceased inmate remains stay in Siberia or be shipped to America for burial or cremation? Graywood needed Emrick's clarification. Meanwhile, he'd mold all the parts into a continuum.

Graywood linked degrees of physical and mental feebleness into the assisted living sub-plan. Each elderly inmate's cognitive capacity and ability to self-perform activities of daily living became the main parameters that fed decision trees for placement. Graywood worked out grids for states of mindfulness and activities, such as bathing, feeding, toilet skills, dressing, and transfers from bed to walker or wheelchair.

Progressive accumulation of physical impairments or increasing disabilities from diseases, such as Alzheimer's and AIDS dementia, booted the inmate from assisted living into the nursing home sub-plan. Chronic illnesses that entered terminal stages, such as severe kidney failure, stage four heart failure, or metastatic cancer, placed the prisoner in hospice-mortuary.

Graywood considered building modifications and concluded a two-winged facility for infirmed felons appeared best constructed in Circle Three: one part designated assisted living; the other nursing home care. Prisoners posed no escape risk hobbling on walkers or hand-propelling wheelchairs over the Itelmen River and through the woods. To complete the breath of support, he cordoned a handful of beds for hospice within the nursing home.

He'd pitch the design idea to the engineering staff for input and suggest Tri-P fabricate a module for potential export—after a natural disaster, a structure like this would be necessary to care for survivors with serious chronic disabilities. If a catastrophe devastated a megacity in the developing world, like Port au Prince, Haiti, the debilitated would not long survive without such a building.

The greatest expenses in Prisontown's chronic-disease care plan comprised recruitment and training of the staff personnel. To stay within the bureau's budget, Graywood elected to educate healthy Circle Three prisoners as aides working under the prison's nursing staff. They'd provide the bulk of daily assisted living and nursing home support: meal preparation and service, cleaning, bathing, and helping the frail to ambulate. A few might even augment the hospice care.

By prisoners supplying and receiving care, perhaps seeds of compassion would sprout among them. Wisps of unselfishness might permeate places, bodies, and souls.

Convincing the bureau's decision makers about how exiled Kamchatkan felons would make a positive difference in assisted living and hospice care appeared pushing boulders uphill. But if some inmates were amenable, it seemed absurd not to engage them as a resource instead of warehousing. Their labor would help the bottom line, and for the bureau, that should be enough.

Regarding mortuary services, prisoner remains not returned stateside, ironically, might be outsourced to Petropavlovsk. Graywood postponed that sub-plan's further development until Emrick and the legal staff sent guidance.

He turned off the computer, checked on Bobby, and went to bed.

"Gary, you've conceived programs with loads of merit," concluded Emrick at the webcam's end concerning the hepatitis C trial expansion into Kamchatka and Graywood's assisted living, nursing home, and hospice proposals. "Inmates are last to suck the prison's tit," mused Emrick, "and it makes sense to mobilize human capital out of the three-circs."

Peeved whenever Emrick called them that, Graywood grimaced and asked, "So you're giving me the go ahead?"

"Sure as hell am, and I'll back you 100 percent," confirmed Emrick. "Send me details so I can play them to DOJ."

"Will do," Graywood answered with gladness.

"But I've got a problem with your intent to reprogram funds saved from costs shifted to CDC," cautioned Emrick.

Graywood turned stony faced.

Emrick clarified, "The bureau will want you to program the money first to train three-circs for the nursing home. Whatever's left over you can use to supplement their health care."

Grinding his teeth, Graywood probed, "What about helping some inmates in Circles Two and One?"

"Those people have no right to be in society," deduced Emrick, sliding his chair from the screen. "The miscreants who've gotten into Circle Three have common sense and deserve a few benefits. But two-circs and one-circ jerks pretty much do squat to nothing for the common good. If there's any wheat to be harvested, it's growing in Circle Three. The rest, Gary, just chaff."

Wanting to smack his boss, Graywood countered, "Listen, Pratt, I think I can find more outside sources to leverage prisoners' health-care costs and improve all circles of care."

Emrick's animosity surged, enemy-obsessed. "It's a tough jungle, Gary, winners and losers. You and I are forced into hard-headed practicality." Oozing, Emrick intertwined fingers behind his skull. "We've gotta get more comfortable with all the limitations placed on Prisontown."

"There're skilled prisoners working in Circles Two and Three, defended Graywood, "who lighten Prisontown's bottom line. They're worth a lot. And you won't have to send me funds to recruit nursing aides from the states."

"Gary, you can't goddamn build the Mayo Clinic out in Prisontown," half-sneered Emrick.

"But that's my goal," muttered Graywood.

"We scorn them, but some have a use as helpers," scoffed Emrick, eyes smirked to obnoxious. "The bureau supports the hep C trial, but any money saved there goes only to three-circs."

Futile to fight Emrick's declaration, Graywood scrutinized the Air Force-blue carpet beneath his desk and said, "Mission understood."

"Have you thought about using one-circ jerks and two-circs in some drug trials?" half-offered, half-goaded Emrick. "That'll make sense to me."

Holding back disgust, Graywood's head shook no, and he added, "Talk to you tomorrow at the teleconference."

"Oh, one more thing, Gary, before I switch you off."

"What?"

"We don't fly back dead murderers. They're *persona non grata.* Bodies stay there. Add disposal to your Prisontown plans."

Death had screwed tight into Emrick's mouth and shot out both nose and ass.

One question dominated when Graywood prepared the full proposal for Pratt Emrick: How much long-term and hospice care would Prisontown require?

Like any aging population, inmates who were impaired due to chronic illness, injury, and cumulative disability needed assistance to perform daily living tasks. The aid might last years, for many banished souls might live into their ninth decade or more. Alzheimer's disease afflicted half the seniors over age eighty-five. In time, the number of trained aides deemed essential at the Circle Three nursing home might surpass even the hospital.

Regarding infirmed Circle One and Two inmates, Graywood proposed a long-term care facility connected to the hospital by heated walkway in the upcoming five-year construction plan. He'd revamp duplexes for those living in Circle Three into resident nursing homes as needed. Providing their care in familiar surroundings made sense, as he attempted the same for Bobby in Anchorage.

For the prisoners' final days, there stood no alternative to the hospice approach—terminal illness, softened with palliative care. The felons dying in Kamchatka had physical, psychological, social, and spiritual aspects of suffering identical to aging stateside Social Security pensioners. Hospice was a philosophy, not a specific place. If done in patients' abodes, nursing homes, or hospitals, so be it in Prisontown.

Graywood assessed the hospice requirements for manpower, personnel training, facilities, equipment, and drugs by employing customary quality assessments, physician and nursing protocols and procedures. He adapted guidelines from the National Hospice and Palliative Care Organization and incorporated their baseline eligibility definition: "a patient with a terminal illness and estimated prognosis for less than six months of life." If a convict lived a few extra while the disease ran its course, so be it in Kamchatka. Graywood downloaded the Karnofsky Performance Scale, the Palliative Performance Scale, and the Palliative Prognosis Score to determine whether a terminally-ill prisoner had a life expectancy short of six months.

He reviewed mortality data from state and federal prison systems to derive numbers of hospice-eligible prisoners by age brackets and recalculated the potential with debilitating diseases, such as Alzheimer's dementia, congestive heart failure, HIV infection, and emphysema. He estimated frequencies of who'd develop cancers of the lung, prostate, breast, liver, colon, rectum, cervix, throat, and mouth.

Out of these sets, he forecasted one-third of a hospital wing, or the equivalent in the proposed long-term care facility, could manage the hospice prisoners coming out of Circles One and Two. For Circle Three prisoners, he'd advocate hospice care in the inmate duplexes. A Circle Three individual could choose support in his or her own quarters, in a modified duplex reserved for terminally ill prisoners, or in the hospital.

Medicare regulatory guidance yielded wide latitude on what might be offered for palliative treatments. They often were determined by hospice size and financial reserves. In smaller facilities, expensive therapies, such as palliative radiation or chemotherapy, were uncommon. Due to funding shortfalls, the bulk of Prisontown's hospice care remained limited to assistance in activities of daily living, emotional care, and the control of nausea, pain, and other distressing symptoms.

"Booties," chortled Bobby, coming out of a vivid dream skimming over snow in Cub's dogsled. Wheelchair strapped, he rocked to and fro whenever alert. Paper-loose skin from anorexic shoulders hung to gaunt hands that projected ten pencil-knobbed digits eager to caress Brandy Belle. Hollowed-eyed with palms stiff as paddles, he patted his shirt or pushed balloons tied to the restraint bar. The sallow face, never still, tumbled rapid-fire expressions of cold staring, astonishment, suspicion, and playful verve.

Despite heroic efforts by teachers, Bobby's special education ceased. The relentless, four-year progression had reduced body and mind and shackled him in sleep greater than eighteen hours each day.

Graywood placed him in a skilled nursing facility located one block off Lake Otis Parkway. For the workweek, Bobby spent days and nights there with his dad visiting until midnight. Graywood brought the boy home on pass every Friday to live out the weekends … clinging to whatever remained alive in the child.

Initially, Graywood had wished to keep Bobby at Snowline Drive with caretakers while he worked at Elmendorf, but fears of inclement weather disrupting everyone's schedules ruled that out. Dividing the week with the care facility enabled Graywood to tolerate work pressures and his crushing angst. Vodka diluted both. Swallowing an antidepressant helped.

On the Saturday before Thanksgiving, Bobby succumbed into never-ending seizures—a crisis where the brain shorted out like an overstressed electrical grid rolling brownouts, blackouts, or both. Evacuated to Providence Medical Center, only an anesthesia-induced coma terminated the mashing malice within. After eight days, the hospital specialists had maneuvered Bobby onto a successful seizure control regimen of five medications.

But the doctors uncovered a new complication: hyperviscosity syndrome. An unknown reaction, perhaps triggered in part by Bobby's altered brain cells, had caused his immune system to produce excess immunoglobulins. These proteins, in turn, coated the red blood cells to increase the serum's viscosity. Without treatment, Bobby's plasma sludged as heavy oil and poorly perfused oxygen to the tissues. Advanced signs, such as spontaneous bleeding or vision changes, had not yet developed. Periodic plasmapheresis—straining the blood through a machine to reduce the immunoglobulins—treated the condition. With each filtrating purge, Bobby mentally improved, but his body wasted away.

CHAPTER TWENTY
WHO

Jennelle scrolled the email backlog once she'd verified the March 2016 software upgrade. An automatic CDC alert flashed:

"International experts from the World Health Organization (WHO) admitted they were baffled by an unidentified disease that had killed fourteen children and young adults and had hospitalized 109 in Senegal, Western Africa. Victims were between twelve and twenty years. All had developed seizure disorders and complained of sleepiness, dizziness, and difficulty in speaking and walking. The most prominent sign was profound physical wastage.

"WHO ruled out viruses as potential causes since the condition appeared not transmitted person to person. The unknown malady was believed to have begun two years ago within villages on the fringes of Dakar, Senegal's capital. No one in the outside world had noticed the outbreak until French television aired parents' angry pleas for more assistance.

"The deaths occurred one after another over fifteen months. At first, local authorities suspected malaria or tuberculosis that preferentially infected the brain. Yet doctors at area health clinics continued to see the same symptoms without responses to treatments. They ran additional tests but could not determine the cause of death. They notified WHO to send experts to investigate.

"WHO did not find malaria, AIDS, or any of the diseases that killed the African poor. WHO deployed recent developed tests on relatives of the dead children and young adults for a mutated HIV-like wasting syndrome that earlier had given false-negative results on standardized ELIZA and RIBA detection kits used to screen blood transfusions for HIV. The negative results obtained from the cutting-edge technology, however, ruled out this theory.

"WHO also tested for toxic-lead exposures on speculation an epidemic of environmental lead poisoning had taken place, similar to the 2007 tragedy in the neighboring township Thiaroye Sur Mer. But blood-lead levels were not elevated.

"The investigation continues, and consensus posits the outbreak as an unknown toxic exposure.

"For complete report, upload //0000045epicon@NIH.gov // 00000337 - WHO2016//r/ns."

Jennelle clicked the address and located the website's primary manager, Nicholas Severstal. She knew him well as a professional and admired his reasoning skills.

Nick had bounced for two decades between the Food and Drug Administration and the National Institutes of Health. As a reviewing investigator in 2002 for the FDA, he advocated halting the Prempro clinical trial that assessed health outcomes in an estrogen-progestin combination drug prescribed to postmenopausal females. For twenty years prior, physicians had prescribed these hormones to women in the belief they provided protection against heart disease and prevented bone fracture.

But the docs were wrong—the combination caused more harm than good. Participants who had received hormones developed higher risks for heart attack, breast cancer, stroke, and blood clots. The clinical findings disproved the medical community's longstanding adage, and they forced the development of fresh, evidence-based practice guidelines for the management of hot flashes and bone loss that occurred with menopause.

"Nick, hey, it's Jen Daniels calling from Anchorage."

"Well, Jen, how are you?" said Nick, surprised to hear an old colleague. "What's going on with you up north?"

"I'm up to my cheeks with this hep C vaccine trial. Someone could say it's boring, but it's doing fine." She'd read his entire report written in bland, international correctness. "I saw the Senegal alert and wanted to get all the hoops, loops, and fruits behind it."

"You sound as if you're saying I sugared the investigation's status," said Nick, half-amused.

"Damn straight not so, Nick," she kidded back. "I know how NIH loves to look into weird diseases, so give it up."

"Well, right now we and WHO don't know squat about what's going on. How's that?"

"Ooooh, way too brief, Nick, and not sounding too good."

"You got that right. We could sure use a sparkplug like you."

"I'm half tempted, but I've got everything up here at critical."

"Yeah, suspected as much, or CDC would've punted you to us a couple of months ago."

Still suspicious, Jennelle asked, "Dear Nick, please come clean. Why's NIH really involved in a strange African disease?"

"Okay. When we first heard it, we followed procedure and crunched a preliminary web search from the national e-med record bank for any sentinel events reported out like those in Senegal."

"What turned up?"

"Nothing except a random geographical distribution that plotted out twelve cases entered under seizures with chronic paralysis, and epilepsy or seizures with residual hypophasia, cause unknown.

"And you just couldn't leave random alone, could you, Nick?"

"Well, no, I really couldn't because the cases were all on the young side."

"Really, what ages?"

"Oldest was twenty-six, youngest ten and a half."

Jen paused. The e-medical record bank had been established in 2012, but not all medical practices across the country had fully converted to it. With an Alpha-Omega payment incentive, doctors' offices electronically entered each new patient encounter, yet their staffs scanned in the handwritten, pre-2012 sections of each medical file only whenever time permitted. Commonly, that meant never since there existed no financial gain.

Coding in 2012 also had changed to add cumbersome illness categories intimately tied to the tiered payments for health care. Jennelle swiftly surmised how the fiscal complexities had combined with incomplete data capture to underreport the country's number of suspected cases.

"Any reported from Alaska?" she asked.

"Nope. One out in Hawaii, the rest in the Lower Forty-eight. Ah … you still call us the Lower Forty-eight up in Alaska, right?"

"I'll call you that if you like, Nick. There are others here who'd call you people down there something much worse."

"Oh … let's not go there."

"So how are Amy and the girls?"

"Toni's discovered the awesome power she has over boys in her seventh grade class, and thank God Connie's not hormonal yet," he summed smartly. "Amy's got a super position at the Smithsonian."

"Wow, Nick, wonderful. So … better let you get back to work. Tell Amy hello and give 'em all my best."

"Sure will, Jen. Take care up there."

Jennelle scanned the remainder of the new emails and opened an urgent one from Monroe Bearhead. He'd asked to see her about a potential problem with her vaccine trial in Chitina.

The lecture order for the medical students was reversed at the start of the New Year: Professor Bearhead preceded Doctor Triangle to better accommodate Graywood's intensified obligations to Bobby, the Justice Department job, and the management of the Kamchatkan portion of Jennelle's hepatitis C immunization research. Bearhead often remained to hear him instruct.

As best he could, Graywood masked the rising desperation in his voice. Baneful change had swept him to where he rethought what mattered. More and more, fiscal expressions such as "the bottom line" and "human capital is equivalent to income and directly linked to productivity" permeated his edgy delivery with the phrases stolen from Cashel Goodlette: "Money is power, so follow the money."

When the students left the classroom to enjoy a rare sun-splotched afternoon that hinted toward spring's snowmelt, Bearhead offered, "Say, Gary, want to head down to Starbuck's by the library and catch up?"

"I'd like that, Roe."

"How's the effort going in Prisontown?"

They descended the stairs, and Graywood summarized the training program for Circle Three prisoners who helped control the legacy costs inherent within Prisontown's health-care system.

"The inmates who assist you, they're the ones with the better living conditions?" asked Bearhead, as they approached the barista.

"Yep, they are." Breathing the liberated aromas, Graywood ordered, "I'll have a grande, non-fat mocha."

"For me," said Bearhead, "one regular Sri Lanka tea, extra-fizz, with peppermint and nutmeg, please."

"Nutmeg?" questioned Graywood.

"Helps me smoke less." Bearhead's kinetic hands rubbed together to negate the desire for tobacco. "So, Gary, they get the better health quality than the inmates confined at the lower circles?"

Ceasing the crusade to eliminate the disparate standards of care in Prisontown, Graywood had accepted partial victory and acquiesced to Emrick: Circle Three prisoners earned an upgraded medical benefit because of their positive support to the prison's overall mission. Through Graywood's relentless efforts, their level of therapeutic access approached the guard's and only lacked tertiary referrals and advanced rehab, such as robotics and organ replacements.

"I don't like to say it, but yes they do," said Graywood, staring at his scuffed shoes.

"You've got a dilemma," cautioned Bearhead, forehead skin furrowed rock hard. "Your creation of a hierarchy opens the door to some prisoners and denies it to others. It assigns worthiness and unworthiness."

"With Circle Three manpower, Roe," countered Graywood, "I can do a lot more for all of them." His body jerked, irritated, yet he avoided Bearhead's eyes. "And they'll have the chance to do something to regain self-respect as well as help the prison." He paid for the tea and mocha.

"Don't you mean help the Justice Department with its budget?" cajoled Bearhead.

Graywood refused the bait.

Bearhead fought the urge to exit and smoke. He needed to figure how to explain money should play as a neutral, tangible surrogate to a person's will, indeed, to one's spirit. And the same for cultures too. How money was acquired and spent within a society signaled green or red flags on community growth or diminished heart.

The barista delivered the order, and the Ravens moved to a corner table.

"My first take on your program is this," resumed Bearhead. "It's gratifying some Circle Three prisoners get an opportunity to aid others by providing their care. You're right that when they help others they help themselves. But permitting their access to superior health care because they sustain the prison's budget ... ah, borders on eugenics."

Bruised, Graywood declared, "It is responsible sustainment, Roe, not eugenics. No one's being sterilized."

"It brings you right to the border of eugenics," said Bearhead, plucking back his head. "You're selecting prisoners into different standards of care by what they do. Why does "Arbeit Macht Frei" wish to now echo loudly in my ears?"

Simmering between his confusion and Bearhead's explanation, Graywood said, "The inmates took someone's life. That's a helluva difference from state officials rationing out care or, even worse, sterilizing the mentally impaired."

"Gary, please ... by what you're doing you're seeing Circle One and Two prisoners as only having less value. You go beyond patronizing them; you discriminate against them."

"Damn it, Roe."

"Play the game of hierarchy, but don't lose your compassion for the others, all of them," pressed Bearhead.

"Don't be ridiculous."

"What about your son, Gary?"

"Huh ... what?"

"At age six and a half, the school system labeled him deficient. Remember how hard you slammed down ADHD then? Should Bobby's learning impairment lead to sanctions like sterilization or less access to health care?"

"Don't you dare bring him up that way, you half—just forget it!" Hellish mad, Graywood shot dagger-eyes that he'd heard enough.

"I'm sorry, Gary, I didn't mean it. I stretched too far with my—" A coughing bout stopped Bearhead. Forcing his chest to clear, he thought the only good attribute in anger was how it undressed hidden truths to quickly come out.

Graywood brought a plastic cup of water to his friend. The void in the debate was necessary; the golden minute of calmness indeed welcomed.

Regaining some lung power, Bearhead's faint voice concluded, "Our very humanity rests on our reverence for all life, Gary. Don't you agree?"

"Don't go quoting Albert Schweitzer on me, Roe," Graywood said with a soft smile. "It's marvelous how you've gotten high opinions for all people."

"I'm asking you only to move your heart forward, Gary."

With bone-deep disillusionment, Graywood scanned the suspended ceiling. When his head wavered sluggish back and forth, he uttered, "I don't have much heart left to move."

Bobby's arduous descent had set Graywood adrift.

Waiting, Bearhead said nothing.

"I know, Roe, I've rationalized down prisoner health care into tiers because we can't consume and spend beyond our capacity to produce. Circle Three prisoners increase the capacity of long-term health care for all in the prison. Any money saved and benefits created by their work should go to them first."

"What happened to the right to equal life for every human being from conception to natural death?"

"You sound like Rome's pope," Graywood groused. "What's a natural death?"

"You … tell me," Bearhead wheezed. "Please, Gary, don't … speak the language … of snakes and sophists. I … smell the evil act in all its good. It's a matter of economic … malice cleverly disguised by … Justice Department's coven of lawyers."

"You gonna be okay?"

"An inside twinge … passing," said Bearhead, lips pursed to aid breathing. "I'll be fine."

"Spare me some slack, Roe. Emrick and the bureau really embrace the program." Graywood's eyes turned fiercely tragic. "They're gonna give me an award," he mumbled. "Can you believe it?"

Graywood had been captured by Washington's domain to divide, denounce, and deny. He looked at the wood-worn floor and wished to escape. "I really don't like that where you live in Prisontown will determine how long you'll stay alive when diagnosed with some sort of cancer or organ failure."

"Yes, Gary," encouraged Bearhead. "You're made for much more than that."

"Oh, good God," said Graywood, peeved, "You want perfect, and perfect's the enemy of the good. Trying for medical care perfection in Prisontown will amount to paralysis."

"All I'm saying, Gary, is when you intercede to delay a natural death for some, you've got to offer the delay to all."

Graywood's temper flared at Bearhead's insipid words. Curling a lip, he snapped, "No one likes a know-it-all, Roe." He placed both hands around the mocha and sulked. "The only sure thing I know is I don't know it all."

"No one does; no one ever will," said Bearhead. He watched Graywood peel off the plastic lid and down the contents.

Graywood slid back, ready to leave.

Bearhead leaned forward hindering Graywood's attempt to end the encounter and said, "Do you recognize you're designating worth by the relative lack of need or by the increased ability to contribute to the prison's bottom line? It's like saying needy children are less worthy of care."

"Don't bait me with kids! You and I agree every child has equal worth, born and unborn. We're talking about murderers here, Roe. The ones who damn well make it all the way to Circle Three have shown some growth and insight, and they deserve some benefit for that."

"Gary, it's still a financial hierarchy. Don't let selfish people convince you that condemned prisoners, unborn kids, or whomever else society chooses to denigrate are worthless. They all have spirits. Reach out to the least of these … the most gracious act of spirit is to demonstrate mutual growth, yours toward and with another's."

Exasperated, but punctured, Graywood audibly sighed and turned away from his guide.

Into the fellow Raven's back, Bearhead burned acidic tones he'd never said before. "Gary, your prison hierarchy is a barrier that creates isolation through successive levels of human intolerance and division. It's not fair. How could you forget that, Gary? Your Circle Three health care codifies some people more equal than others. It's like saying some babies are more equal than others. Those who advocate these slippery slopes have very small souls. Gary, please don't ever forget that. Don't ever accept it because once you do, you'll have a smaller spirit too."

"Don't talk to me about being fair," said Graywood, sweat boiling from his head. "My son's entire life is nothing but unfair, and you know damn well I curse God for it!"

"Oh please, Gary, unfairness is relative," said Bearhead, generalizing to avoid slicing Graywood's jugular with Bobby's pitiful existence. "Please don't pepper sacred life with Washington's economic fraud or your unholy anger. Taking life is absolute. Partially withholding care is right behind it."

Graywood squared to his confessor but avoided his face. "We're not withholding care; Roe, we're adding it on."

"Only for some. Having Circle Three deemed better than Two and One and tied to better medical care is eugenics. When giving rankings to groups, you're in the devil's playground."

"Oh Jesus crap!" Graywood's astringent eyes shot to Bearhead's. "Damn, Roe, there are mentors and there're tor-mentors. Where should I rank you?"

The verbal thrusts welled up Bearhead's emphysema. The parries robbed oxygen and constricted his torso. He wanted to avoid a brutal exchange.

"I'll agree to any … rank you give me, Gary," Bearhead said, mouth puckered. "But I agree, too, that … one of us is ridiculous, so let your heart … tell us who it is."

Graywood remained stone silent.

"As you think … my question, please consider another," Bearhead said, almost inaudibly.

"Phhtth … Oh, on what, Roe?" Graywood leaned closer to hear Bearhead's parsed breath.

"I listen to your lectures … What you're going through at Kamchatka is prelude … to what our country will do to sustain … Alpha-Omega and Medicare. Claims triaged … and care rationed unsparingly. For lack of money, it will become the norm. I've heard you say it … to the students."

Graywood's eyes confirmed.

"What's it you say, Gary?" pushed Bearhead, air sacs regaining volume. "There can't be unlimited access and quality because there's not unlimited money to pay for everyone's health. Those who do more for society, however that's judged, will get more health care so they can do more for society. It's the cycle of the haves sustaining themselves at the expense of the have-nots. Once you're a have-not, you're expected to die gracefully like Circle One and Two prisoners. Even though we're all human, some of us, economically speaking, are judged more human than others."

Graywood recognized Bearhead's counsel—a fair partial solution didn't exist because hierarchies caused harm. Pratt Emrick and Washington excelled in choosing winners and losers.

Embittered by Bobby's deterioration, Graywood had trespassed into making other people's spirits smaller. His mind groped to conjure a near-term health benefit that might not exclude or injure anyone at Prisontown.

"Well, Roe, thanks for the summary on my lectures. Sounds as if I've strayed from our path where all humans are precious."

"Yes, Gary," Bearhead's voice enthused. "Don't let the bureau become your religion." Bearhead perceived their argument might have been an offshoot of the longstanding quarrel Graywood fought with God over Bobby's fate. "You have a life with purpose. Don't waste it."

Absolved for the moment, Graywood rubbed both hands in circles over his forehead. "Say Roe, have I mentioned we're funding a heated swimming pool as water therapy for the prisoners?" He now scanned Bearhead's face as an equal. "Kamchatka is loaded with arthritis, you know. After a winter or two, it's pretty easy to come down with it."

"Missed hearing that, I think."

"I probably didn't say it. Anyway, it'll be available for all circles … I'll see to it."

"Outstanding, Gary," said Bearhead. The old Raven looked heavenward. One was blessed whenever he watched someone else grow and twice blessed if he'd helped the transformation.

"There're natural hot springs all around," finished Graywood, grinning. "And it's time I get back to Elmendorf."

"Gary, when did you last spend some time at Campsite?" asked Bearhead, trying to add a layer of spiritual healing.

"Don't remember."

"When you go, I'd like to go too."

Afraid the wounded years suffered with Bobby might supplant the happier memories if he'd return, Graywood muttered, "I doubt I'll ever go back."

"Allow to be calm and go there. It'll help you."

Stepping away, Graywood grabbed his coat and said, "Allow yourself the same, my friend, and quit smoking. It'll help you too."

Alone, Bearhead's cellphone chirped a texted message: dr j daniels 2 c u.

Jennelle raced to Grace Hall after the meeting with Bearhead and initiated an incident probe into Chitina. Theo Nowell's son, Frankie, had died.

Aware many, including Frankie, had been recruited into Jennelle's hep C trial, Bearhead had shared his trepidation: Frankie's unexpected death would negate the village's willingness to prolong her study. Theo had preeminent influence in Chitina. All feared crossing him. Bearhead wanted Jennelle's face-to-face reassurance the vaccine had no part in Frankie's death.

Jennelle scheduled a dawn flight with Piper. She uploaded Frankie's enrollment data and compared it to the e-medical record. Nothing unusual: born April 6, 2000, recruited to the trial August 2014, parental consent scribbled in Theo Nowell's hand, negative medical review of systems, normal blood pressure and liver panel. Body weight: 63.5 kg., adequate for the three-dose, adult inoculation series, each given a month apart. Initial injection administered September 10, 2014, eighteen and a half months ago. No second dose recorded—a protocol violation not brought to her attention.

Blank. Frankie's e-medical record lacked entries other than identifying information.

Jennelle elected a detour to the Glennallen clinic to review Frankie's old, handwritten health notations. Having them faxed to Grace Hall required lengthy coordination and another round of long-distance parental consent, not ideal in a dreadful crisis. More important was supporting the grieving Nowell family in person.

The two women wove between a half-dozen coeval dwellings plopped on the ruddy clay path from Nowell's lodge to Bearhead's longhouse. Melting snow uncovered kelly-green moss mixed with glistening sedge shoots on fresh mud.

"It's good you came," whispered April Coldsnow.

"I wanted them to know how sorry I was about Frankie's death."

"The younger ones shouldn't die," April uttered. "It's very hard."

"It's tragic," echoed Jennelle. "It never should've happened."

Tightlipped, they stayed to the trail's middle and avoided the ruts half-filled with effluent seeping from under the homes. In winter, septic pools froze over on top of permafrost and, with spring's thaw, formed mini-sewage swamps.

When they arrived at the Dlam, Jennelle sought an understanding. "April, did you believe me when I told the Nowells the vaccine had nothing to do with Frankie's death?"

"Yes, of course."

"Will you please contact me right away if they come to you with more questions so I may help?"

"I will. That's very kind, Jennelle."

"April, perhaps you may know … ah …"

"What, Jennelle?"

"It's a little awkward."

April straightened defensive.

Jennelle reassured, "Before I arrived here, I stopped in Glennallen to look at Frankie's clinical records. The info we had on him was incomplete, so I looked at the clinic's—"

"To help with questions Theo might ask?" offered April.

"Yes, and help me understand too," confirmed Jennelle. "But I'm still missing quite a bit about him."

Wary, April stared at the Nowell lodge and said quietly, "Go sit in my kitchen. I'll fix tea."

April condensed the gaps in Frankie's medical history. When twelve years old, his peer group had smoked meth-laden cigarettes before they advanced to popping it outright. Twice he'd enrolled in the First Peoples' detox program, but treatments ended once he'd suffered a seizure a year ago. Within six months, the convulsions had progressed from rare to daily events. Frankie quit school, walked strange, and ate like a whale yet still lost weight. Exhorting that meth caused the sickness, Theo and the counselors pleaded with Frankie to stop abusing.

Theo suspected other illicit drugs had laced some or all of Frankie's meth. He tried everything to keep it away from his son.

But what April then revealed shocked Jennelle numb. Theo allowed the Glennallen doctors to track only Frankie's seizures in the medical records and tough-muscled them never to enter a word about Frankie's meth problems and therapies.

"How can he do that?" boiled Jennelle.

"Oh, it's so bad," said April, eyes dropping. "Theo heads trading meth here. He's powerful and doesn't want a thing written to link him to it, even his family's health records."

"My God, April, his son died from his dealing!"

"You must never tell anyone," pleaded April, examining Jennelle's eyes for lionhearted trust. "Theo's group are killers," she muffled, scared. "It'll be bad for May and me if he found out I told you."

Biting her lip, Jennelle pledged, "I promise I'll never make it worse for you."

April stared the floor, and mumbled, "It's worse."

"How?"

"My first husband, Johnny Toofish, showed him."

Jennelle bolted from the table to pace away the anxiety surge. Dozens of questions assembled in her mind while marching from the kitchen to the cavernous meeting room's fire pit and back. She picked one line to pursue. "Did Johnny recruit Theo into the drug cartel?" she asked, calm, offering a hand to April.

"Yeah," replied April, clasping Jennelle's. "They were partners."

"How did you and May cope with it?"

"Meth stole our way worse than alcohol," admitted April in forced, even tones. "Neither was here to hurt us 'til the whites came."

"Addiction took over control of the village and disconnected its life," rephrased Jennelle.

"My sister and I are shamed. A family is who you are. We got thrown to Johnny's meth problems in marrying him … We searched for hope … We worked to find it." April's fist shielded her mouth.

"I'm so sorry," said Jennelle softly.

"I kept May away when he made it in galvanized cans," floated April's fragile voice. She rubbed forehead and eyes to further catharsis. "He'd feel the wham in straight meth or heroin and add tobacco and weed to get a different rush and then want it more."

"He'd mixed drugs together?" asked Jennelle.

"Yes."

"How'd he get them?"

"A syndicate in Burma and Indonesia controlled Johnny's group. They dumped meth drums along Knik Arm to Ketchikan, and Johnny got 'em to the lower states bribing crabbers and fishermen to haul 'em. Coming back from Seattle, he'd bring heroin and weed. He was so proud of all the easy money made."

April's story reminded Jennelle of the melamine contamination in Chinese food exports to the United States—the toxic industrial chemical had caused kidney failure in humans, dogs, and cats after it had breezed past FDA inspectors.

"The Sinaloa cartel came and recruited Johnny away from Burma with Mexican meth and cocaine," said April.

"So Johnny started as a meth supplier," said Jennelle, "and added other drugs to boost him out of poverty—"

"And aimlessness and welfare," inserted April. Psychic pain gripped her body steel hard. "Suckering whites out of their money was another rush he wanted. He felt he could do things he never could before. He cut three grades of powder and hid it from the bosses. They killed him . . . Theo gave him away."

Jennelle keyed edited notes from Chitina into Nick's NIH data bank—the American counterpart to the WHO stockpile pertaining to the Senegalese mystery disease of seizures linked to progressive degeneration. She detailed two potential cases: Frankie Nowell and Robert Graywood. Both had developed seizures with elements of neurodegeneration, and both had exposure to the same remote Alaskan village. Frankie's probably was drug related, but Bobby's remained enigmatic.

To solve a rare conundrum, Jennelle believed it advantageous, yet time consuming, to trawl for truth with a wide surveillance net. Almost all initial associations, in time, were discarded as false-positives. But investigations had to start somewhere.

"Hello, Nick. Jen here."

"Well, Jen. Why am I so honored today?"

"Cut the brouhaha. I want you to know I reported two kinda iffy cases into your mystery disease data base.

"Really!"

"Yes, so now you know Alaska's a contributor."

"Wow, Jen, I don't know what to think. It's getting way bigger."

"Come again?"

"Well, it's gotten more complicated since we last talked."

"How so?"

"WHO and the Pasteur Institute are reporting potential cases from Algeria and France."

"Well shoot, Nick, this is starting to mushroom."

"And there's more, Jen. NIH now agrees with WHO's tentative recommendation that if anyone finds a case of undiagnosed neurodegenerative disease with seizures, then get brain tissue biopsy samples upon death. We're crosschecking everything, even mad cow disease and scrapie with USDA and state veterinarians."

"Nick, you have specifics for the recommended way to do the biopsy?"

"Hope to get it up on the website tonight."

"Then I'll check it out. Bye."

"Bye, Jen."

What had happened to Graywood's kinetic Bobby boy? The crisp timing and sharp moves skating hockey at school—why'd they disappear? Balancing on a boogie board with daring in the Hanalei surf. Arm strength to pull bowstrings taut or caress Campsite's lake for hours in the ky-canoe. Where did they all go?

By spring 2016, Bobby had atrophied like salmon in their natal streams after spawning.

From Bearhead and web searches, Graywood had learned Alaskan salmon survived the last two years of a five-year life cycle eating prodigious Pacific Ocean shrimp, large plankton, small squid, and fish before they embarked on the terminal journey to their home streams. Over the final three months, dormant connections in the salmon's brain reactivated to program the quest to spawn. Once they entered fresh water, they never fed again, and their digestive systems shrunk to nonfunctioning tubes.

Graywood wondered what activated the neural cells to trigger anorexia, controlled acts of redd-making and milting, and locked in the eventual wasting within this species. Were the salmon's age and size a double impetus to start the final clock to drive it to spawn? How much was it augmented by the permanent change from sea salinity to fresh water? Or was it an intricate combination of feedback loops spliced to age, size, and decreased salinity, coupled to hormonal changes inherent with spawning, that led to ultimate atrophy?

Bobby's mysterious epilepsy had begun at age eleven but mutated into horrifying clashes where Graywood feared the child might never regain consciousness. Frightful images plagued Graywood's dreams ... and kept his nights. One out of twelve repetitive seizure victims died from a convulsion.

With puberty at age thirteen, the unbalanced muscle wasting in Bobby's left arm and shoulder had become grossly apparent. His fits exhibited more chaotic eye-rolling, less tonic-clonic shaking. Mentation plunged ... and there was less of him. Chronic fatigue commenced months later with the physical need for a wheelchair. Plasmaphoresis to correct hyperviscosity syndrome capped the final eight months.

Cardiac involvement manifested in many patients who suffered neuromuscular diseases, but not so with Bobby's enigmatic affliction. Brave heart pulsing strong, he never required a pacemaker or implantable defibrillator.

On the Tuesday night shift at the nursing facility, a tenacious spasm gripped Bobby's shallow frame, and copious vomit aspirated into the lungs. Struggling for air, he convulsed again and inhaled more acidic puke. This time, he needed no medical-induced coma to stop follow-on seizures. They ended on their own from damaged lungs without sufficient viable membranes to exchange the necessary air. Without oxygen, his heart stopped until nurses and paramedics resuscitated him.

At Providence Medical Center, two sea lions hold up stop signs on the doors to the pediatric ICU.

The reasoning part in Graywood's mind now allowed letting his child die. No higher cortical function equaled brain death. Let the mechanical rhythm by the life-prolonging respirator stand still …

No, wait a little while …

Father squeezed son's ten fingertips in succession. He retold the old bedtime story where Rum Tum found the courage to ride in the belly of Uncle Oo-otek's seaplane. Graywood had to do something with his hands … Bobby couldn't die if they both stayed flesh-pressed together. He massaged the boy's arms and motioned the legs to coax blood circulation.

Exhausted.

Let the respirator bellows cease …

He did.

The life beats fought, flickered, last to go.

My boy's tough little heart.

Let the rhythm stop …

HE did.

To the void, Graywood spoke, "My only son begins his painless journey home," and left the room.

Two preternatural pairs of feelings descended and congealed within him: grief-stricken hurt of mortal separation cleaved to the certain knowing Bobby had overtaken the sun in heaven; and the twin phantoms—sorrow and sublime—cloaked him as only they may, and have always, for the parent who's lost a child.

But they dislodged.

"Gary, it is possible Bobby died from the same syndrome as young people in Senegal?" soft-pedaled Jennelle. Awkward, her frame stiffened to pursue NIH's request for a piece of Bobby's brain tissue.

Motionless, Graywood zeroed on the cityscape beyond the house deck. In the long fight for his child, he'd lost everything. Embittered, he believed they'd become unwelcomed immigrants from the twentieth century searching in vain for twenty-first identities. Unmet millennial expectations had left him and Bobby behind and overwhelmed. Absent his son,

Graywood lacked meaning. Feeling desperate and decayed, he wished to cross back in time.

Jennelle justified, "DNA sequences from the African brain samples suggest a common abnormality in neural tissues of those deceased that's not found in aged-matched controls in the same communities who died from something else."

Grieving, Graywood's eyes closed. Lungs inflated drawn-out volumes. Her talk meant nothing.

A brain sample meant a modified autopsy. In life, Bobby had suffered so much. Did it have to continue? He wanted her to go, yet his tongue remained limp.

"If Bobby has that anomaly," she finished, "we're dealing with something very bizarre."

He remained mute.

She wished to tell how NIH, CDC, and French colleagues approached the families for tissue samples from recently deceased victims suspected for this unknown illness. They needed to ascertain any ties to Senegal's genetic picture and, if they existed, by what biogenetic pathway that connected these cases from such diverse continents. Was it a natural or man-made worldwide agent? Mystified, scientists contended that neural genetic blueprints from the victims would best elucidate the ultimate cause.

Timing was also critical. A biopsy within forty-eight hours of death provided optimal DNA to sequence genetic code with minimal chromosome decay. Pending Graywood's consent, Jennelle had prearranged the medical examiner to extract samples before Bobby was embalmed.

Tortured, she wanted to wed to his agony. Stepping beside him, she rubbed his neck and stroked her palm down his right arm. She remembered the willful Bobby of six and seven years, how he'd molded compromises to the worldly wonders each day, bestowed and aided unconditionally by his loving father. They were so fortunate then.

Tragedy had engulfed two people Jennelle loved so dear. She forced back tears and sobbed in secrecy to a blurred horizon.

How might this man be helped? She regretted the sample request. Execrable … it wasn't the time. Should she have even dared ask it?

Four northern shovelers, led by a green-headed male, soared overhead and disappeared to western breeding grounds.

Clueless, Graywood clasped Jennelle's hand. A dimmed sun arched above mountains as an austere arm wrapped around her shoulders.

Human DNA is packaged into twenty-three pairs of chromosomes for every cell. There are four chemical letters in the DNA language code—A, T, C, and G—each representing a sugar acid. Every chromosome braids 100 million coded acids, plus or minus, into its double helix.

Before the twenty-first century, DNA blueprint researchers had to start from scratch and employ the ancient Sanger sequencing methods developed in the 1970s: chromosomes were chopped into overlapping pieces and painstakingly fitted back together using marginal software hardly robust enough to process the task.

To devolve the entire human sequence at the end of the millennium, the Human Genome Project wisely split off parts of DNA, seven hundred letters long, and computer match-searched the pieces for unique overlaps. Through thousands of researchers coordinated across the globe, the project completed the first human genetic layout by 2003 at a cost of three billion dollars.

Thereafter, decoding technology matured exponentially. By 2016, upgraded computers and improved chemical scalpels spliced various DNA portions from prepared cell samples and paired them to deciphered, archived genetic blueprints at a cost less than eight thousand dollars per full genome. Within one week, a person's twenty-eight thousand functional genes could be DNA-sequenced.

A light storm illuminated the scudding clouds pillowed over Mount Susitna. Graywood wished that stretch in heaven held nature's wealth. And his blessed son.

If Bobby's tragedy missed inclusion with the Senegal outbreak, it did appear ideal for genetic coding. Applying the cutting edge technology might determine cause of death.

Graywood consented.

CHAPTER TWENTY-ONE

Transformations

Finished.

The red planet had pinned low and baleful in the short night sky. In autopilot mode, Graywood had buried his child and gone to the wake.

Brandy Belle approached when he entered the house. "You must be hungry, little one."

He forked a quarter can of cat tuna on a saucer and filled the water bowl. Exhausted, he parked next to the kitchen table.

Panic compressed reality into tortured fear … life had stopped having meaning. The months Bobby suffered had forced Graywood to search out ways to vanquish the torment, usurp depression, absolve rage, and negate the abandonment hurled on him by death's advance.

He's gone … So what matters?

Winning a skirmish against Emrick and the bureau? That might recharge one hundredth of the joy compared to seeing Bobby's blue eyes alight with delight whenever Graywood entered the nursing facility.

He pinched the president's unopened condolence card and rotated it counterclockwise. He agonized for the ten thousandth time if all had been done for his son.

A Saint Jude's advertisement crept into mind: "Saint Jude Children's Research Hospital—We have science on the fast track."

Graywood never trekked Bobby to Memphis, Tennessee, although he'd consulted their physician referral team at length. They were extremely good at treating children's cancer with pioneering research. Many cases were curable. Not so with neurodegenerative diseases.

Fiddling the official presidential envelope, Graywood flipped it toward the table's edge, and it fell to the floor.

From the cabinet above the refrigerator, he opened a fresh liter of Siberian vodka and poured a tumbler. Kamchatka had introduced drinking it like water. It aided selective forgetfulness for any sane parent cast anguished and adrift on relentless seas mourning the loss of a gravely ill child.

Yet some memories he'd cherish forever:

How Bobby's tiny lower lip quivered cherubic when he'd entered the world from Maren's womb—turning red from dusky blue, aided by nasal-blown oxygen …

The August night when the boy and Roe had pounded the drums under the lunar eclipse, told stories, and drunk hot chocolate …

The Campsite episode when Bobby perched precariously in the canoe and released Bearhead's bowstring to almost pierce Roe between the eyes instead of the alder tree's target …

And the day Brandy Belle came home as part of their family, and little Bobby twinkling whenever he heard a Rum Tum bedtime story. If Graywood developed Alzheimer's the last endearing remembrance ever lost, when all others had unhinged away, would be tucking the sweet child in bed with Rum Tum.

He watched Brandy Belle finish her meal. Supposedly the life sentence of being a parent ended once a child died, but Graywood denied it utmost. Bobby had been, was, always would be his son …

He gulped vodka and picked fingernails in succession. Brain snippets rebooted from Bearhead's wake:

"What am I to do, Roe?"

"Try letting yourself off the hook, Gary. Find one thing that puts your heart to rest."

"I prayed so terribly hard for God's help. I worked damn hard to save him. I really did."

Bearhead embraced Graywood as Bearhead's uncle had done after he'd lost darling Sophia. Attempting to explain or speculate God's dynamism from humanity's perspective would have waxed prideful, incomplete, and absolutely foolish.

But the unanswerable had empowered rage. Slurping tumbler number two, Graywood circled about the kitchen and smashed his moral compass with God. He and God must have it out … and on Graywood's territory. Nostrils flaring, he ground a heel on the president's condolence card without pity and resolved to battle God at Campsite.

He shot emails to his staff outlining work priorities and called Rachel and Cub to look after Brandy Belle.

The landline rang as he packed a rucksack. "Gary, I've just finished up at Bearhead's," said Jennelle. "I'll be over in twenty minutes."

"Ah … thanks, but no need to come tonight."

"What? What's the matter, Gary?"

"I'm going to the airport. I'll spend what's left of tonight getting *Seneca* refitted and take off for Campsite."

"Oh! Ah … how long will you be gone?"

"A week, maybe more. I need some explaining done."

"Explaining? Gary, who? I'm worried for you."

He itched to say he'd taken on the Almighty not knowing the outcome but, nonetheless, confident. But he replied, "Thanks, Jen. I'll call when I'm back."

Jennelle approached several at the wake's bereavement circles after she'd volunteered Rachel to take Graywood home. Most important, she wished to know from April Coldsnow how Theo Nowell and his family had coped the past three months since Frankie's death.

"It's still very bad," said April. "Theo doesn't believe meth destroyed his son."

Theo's denial, no doubt, stemmed from his illegal network that provided the means for Frankie's death. Instead of broaching thick psychology, Jennelle opted to listen and asked, "Did he say why he didn't think it killed him?"

"No. He doesn't understand why Frankie got seizures on meth when others he'd hung with didn't," said April, shrugging shoulders.

Overhearing, Bearhead asked, "You don't think it's the hep C vaccine, do you, Jen?"

What he spoke grabbed and shook Jennelle's heart and mind hard. Could there have been a seizure outbreak within her field trial?

"I really doubt it," said Jennelle with a resolved tone. "You can bet I'll look into it."

Something bad happened after an inoculation—a temporal relationship for sure. And the dependent connection shined so obvious between injecting someone and the following poor outcome, regardless of the subsequent time frame of days, months, or years. It appeared the easiest correlation for passing blame, suspicion, and guilt.

After detailed investigations, however, nearly all the temporal adverse associations were proven coincidental. Circumstantial or not, the cause and adverse-effect mentality remained the bane to all immunizations seeking or maintaining approval for general use.

The federal government acknowledged the public's angst and passed the National Childhood Injury Act in 1986. Within two years, the NCIA created the Vaccine Injury Compensation Program to recompense individuals possibly harmed by an immunization the CDC had recommended for common use. Also derived from the NCIA was the Vaccine Adverse Events Reporting System—VAERS—which collected and analyzed reports of harmful events that followed any dose.

The week Graywood and God holed up in Campsite, Jennelle and the CDC broke the double-blind code designated for Chitina which pertained to Theo's son. Frankie had received the control inoculation, hepatitis B, in the field trial, not the hepatitis C candidate.

Jennelle reverified Frankie's complete immunization record. All in compliance with accepted standards, except one minor glitch: by age six years, he'd still not received the routine hepatitis B series recommended for infants. A sequence of three hep B injections at the Glennallen clinic had then caught him up without complications. Upon enrollment in

Jennelle's field trial, in essence, Frankie had received an extra dose of a previous inoculation.

She reported to VAERS Frankie's temporal circumstance of developing seizures with degeneration after a hep B booster, but she already had deemed it coincidence. Frankie had episodes like Bobby, and meth abuse caused convulsions in many. That appeared to be the leading culprit.

Yet something else perplexed Jennelle in Frankie's medical record: for another preventable childhood infection, chickenpox, the nurse had not recorded the product's manufacturer and lot number, although Frankie had received it on September 2, 2006.

Peculiar, it must have been a documentation error.

Graywood anchored *Seneca* and pitched camp. Sounds of the ax cracking on fallen wood bounced off the Seven Sisters.

Puffy clouds spilled over the sky to obscure the solar roadway. Graywood rested by the shore and clipped into all the times Bobby and he had conjured the blank cumulus masses into creatures, trees, and manmade things.

And seeking the familiar in night's mysteries too, they'd made shapes from the stars flung across the firmament. Adventurous sagas sprung from fixed stellar formations—Bobby's favorite, Orion defending against charging Taurus, the bull—mixed with the campfire stories of mythical Arcturus, Capella, Canis Major and Minor.

Yet the fond remembrances faded. Bobby's tree, the mature alder that had held the archery target, summoned Graywood. From its bark still protruded the arrow point's rear metal rim to mark Bobby's overshoot from the ky-canoe. The tempered steel fragment confirmed Graywood's shattered life. A cold heartache coated him scalp to sole.

I'm so terribly alone. God, my boy made me, made us, special. The pain's so polarizing. How do I go on?

Out of the tree's canopy, a swirling resin-scented reply whiffed brusque ... "As we all do ... We may live mundane lives of second choices ... We find a way ... tolerate and avoid devolving to pessimism. Follow not those who make the most of blandness, or it shall be Earth's only privilege ... and we'll never see hope ..."

Searing orange painted the cloudscape anew. Placid waters nudged the lake's edge. Driftwood littered the beach. A kingfisher alighted on *Seneca*'s tether and flipped a fresh-caught meal with its beak to swallow.

Watching the opportunistic bird recreated the final time Bobby and Graywood had cast in the pure water. Bobby had dipped an aluminum can for a quick drink but spilled it over his face when a rainbow trout hooked the line and well-nigh jerked the rod out of his grip. In the explosive yelling and reeling melee, the container hurled overboard and sank. Thereafter, Bobby called the tarn "Tin Cup Lake."

Graywood dragged the ky-canoe from its wood-hewn shelter and paddled to the modest river milking the Seven Sisters' northern watersheds. On the drumlin set above the merging waters, he kindled a fire in the coiled stones Bobby had laid to roast morning-caught fish and marshmallows for lunch.

Graywood had shared the wonder and the terror of many things. It felt softer to sit and troll for sadness rather than beauty. For hours, flames popped and whistled. He yearned to empty bitterness.

To the shortest Sister, he cursed, "Maren, you never came. Damn, I'm so angry."

He could not close the book on her while Bobby lived. By the circle of flames overlooking Tin Cup Lake, he locked and threw it away.

"Maren, I'll never know what killed our boy. Life's not fair. I understand that. You're the perfect teacher. I'll figure out someday why you didn't want him. You didn't abort him. For that alone, I forgive you everything."

She'd been expelled. Logs burned to cinders. He added more.

"God, the struggle's too great. You lost a son. How'd you recover?" Fresh eye-tearing smoke drifted divine. It cohered above Graywood's skull in imperfect clumps not making sense at first.

More bush branches burned. And more. And from the tormented years of defeat, Graywood's unflagging hope to heal Bobby matured into an ethereal cure for the rift in Prisontown's schizophrenic health program.

What would Abraham Lincoln have done, Gary?

"With malice toward none and charity for all," Graywood answered. Bearhead was right to appeal to Graywood's better angel to find a medical way to treat all banished felons as equal human beings, regardless confinement level.

How could he bring top-notch facilities like the Providence Medical Center in Anchorage to the prisoners instead of denying them the equivalent access dictated by the bureau's interpretation of the Grand Compromise?

What would Lincoln do? Albert Schweitzer? Sir Thomas More?

"They'd say no to limited health care and yes to equal access to heroic measures."

By revelation or self-enlightenment, Graywood commenced to link Prisontown and Alaska on one firm path to broaden inmate care, regardless of circle. He included the surrounding areas of Kamchatka too. Summoning operating principles and procedures employed by the Peace Corps and third world non-governmental organizations, Graywood expanded the concept that had already brought Jennelle's hep C vaccine trial to Prisontown. Multiplied a hundredfold in ten directions, his mind sculpted a thousand pocket-sized ways to extend health support across the Bering Sea and end the double standard forever.

Beneficent atonement shrouded Graywood with grace on the hallowed rock of at-one-ment. Airstreams pulsed off the greatest Sister, akin to a Bearhead voice, "If you don't do this, who shall?"

Genesis renewed meaning and value.

The fire simmered to embers.

Before, Graywood had gone part way into Circle Three. Now by equal deeds, he'd care for all circles. He'd champion the special meaning of life for all without prejudice. Prisontown had become his extended family. Out of the flawed struggle committed to Bobby's terrible disease and death, he'd become an inured leader who'd sever the bureau's shackles with a new Kamchatka-Alaska medical alliance. From pernicious grief, he'd forge the Kamchatka-Alaska medical initiative ... and call it KAMI.

Only ashes remained within the blanched stones. He stirred for sparks and uncovered none. Skyward, he spoke, "Lord, you fight in mysterious ways to have me turn my will."

Stroking the ky-canoe to Campsite, he passed the granite scarp where Bobby and Bearhead once had witnessed a marbled murrelet surface from the underworld with a fingerling in its beak. Few humans ever saw the secretive bird: it nested high in coastal trees of old-growth forests and dove from secluded lofts to pursue underwater prey. Bobby and Bearhead had eagerly recounted its rise from the deep. A blessing.

Graywood observed no sign of the resident sow and cubs.

On the morning he returned to Anchorage, he found tufts of fur and fresh marks clawed on the dominant tree behind the nylon tent. The ursine overlord had watched over Graywood. He still allowed him to come and go in peace.

"Jen, the probable cases we've uncovered in the continental US have this in common," said Nick at the webcam's start. "They've all spent time living in Alaska."

"What? How's that?"

"Here's how they're similar," repeated Nick. "Hard to control seizures over time, chronic neurologic losses, and having lived in Alaska several years."

"What exactly were their connections to Alaska?" she asked.

"Seventeen-year-old male now living in Oklahoma City whose parents work in the oil industry had transferred from Anchorage five years ago; a fifteen-year-old girl whose military father rotated out of Elmendorf to Travis Air Force base, honorably discharged, now living in Charlotte."

"Nick, okay," interrupted Jennelle, "send me everything your people have turned up."

"Of course. Jen, you're one of the best to rule in or out associations. From now on, consider being part of my team."

"I'll clear it with Atlanta," she said, showing a pencil thin smile. "How many probable cases?"

"Got thirteen, working on twenty-one. Next is an eighteen-year-old man born in Juneau, relocated to Sacramento in 2007. His old man lost a state job in Palin's shakeup after she got elected governor."

"I'm convinced, Nick. I'll start a search for more cases still in Alaska."

"Great Jen, I'll get our particulars to you today ASAP."

Based on the three Alaskan locations Nick specified, Jennelle downloaded hospital admissions at Anchorage, Juneau, and each Alaskan military installation. The Anchorage and military data did not match the NIH case definition, but she struck gold in Juneau: four potential patients—two within city limits, coded eighteen months apart, a third from West Juneau, and one out of Auke Bay.

Juneau also was a primary participant in the hep C field trial. She cross-referenced the four candidates against the recruited volunteers and instructed her secretary, Miss Taylor, to arrange an immediate flight with Piper.

Pratt Emrick agreed to Graywood's KAMI concept so long as it remained within DOJ budget parameters. KAMI needed free transportation to bring elements of Providence Medical Center, or its equivalent, to Kamchatka. That came courtesy of the United States Air Force.

The Elmendorf medical center's executive officer, Colonel Sulmasy, approved all medical operational flights. The twice-per-week support missions to Petropavlovsk-Prisontown were high level responsibilities he coordinated with Elmendorf's flight line from the second-floor Command Suite in the 2D Moose Zone.

To direct foot traffic, the air force had divided the extensive medical center into three "ranges"—Wolf, Bear, and Moose. Graywood's offices were on the main floor, spliced into 1A Moose with the occupational and public health sections. From Moose 1A to 2D required a ninety-second march and a flight of stairs if one shunned the elevator as Graywood often did.

He briefed his KAMI brainstorm to Colonel Sulmasy off a laptop and broached tapping the semiweekly Boeing 767 flights to meet KAMI's transportation requirements. A forward-thinking careerist, Sulmasy wanted a general's star. Graywood's bold presentation seemed innovative and doable to risk hitching onto.

"What's the payload?" asked the colonel.

"Mostly people, some added supplies and equipment," replied Graywood.

"How many personnel?"

"A handful … sometimes a team or two, say six to twelve at a time," estimated Graywood.

"Well, Gary, we've got plenty lift for that. We hardly use half as is. You'll handle the DOJ entry procedures with passports and Petro's customs so your people can off-board once we land."

"Yes, sir."

"I'll alert flight ops and assign one of my majors to handle details."

"Thank you, sir."

"One more thing, Gary, if you've got a minute."

"Yes, sir, of course."

"The air force has supported Prisontown five years in all kinds of weather relocating staff and prisoners, delivering routine and emergency supplies and equipment while heeding Russian air corridor restrictions without incident. You know the story."

"Yes, sir. You're our lifeline. There're no outside roads to Petropavlovsk or Prisontown. Only way in is by air or sea."

"Think on this, Gary," encouraged Sulmasy. "I'm heading up a documentary mission to film what the air force has done in Kamchatka. I want to devote a good chunk of it to your medical support mission tied to flight line ops and Russian diplomacy."

"Yes, sir. I'm glad to help out," volunteered Graywood.

"And if this KAMI project of yours works, Gary, we might put its piece in too."

"Plan on it, sir; I'll make it work."

Well-nigh one thousand miles of Kamchatka presented as primeval wilderness, landscaped by snow-covered volcanoes sloping to exquisite black-sand beaches. Geysers, mineral springs, boiling lakes, and hot mud vents speckled the peninsula. In excess of 160 mountainous craters had sprouted over geologic time, and twenty-nine plumed gas, ash, and rare spurts of lava. Klyuchevskaya, at 4,750 meters, emerged the greatest.

Brown bears, ten feet tall and identical to North American grizzlies, roamed the untouched tundra meadows and birch forests. A quarter of the Pacific's wild salmon spawned in Kamchatka's frigid rivers and streams.

A strategic Soviet military region, the jutting landmass remained closed to outsiders for most of the twentieth century. As a recluse defense outpost, it had state farms and a robust fish-processing industry that produced milk, vegetables, and meat for Russian markets.

Yet the unforeseen economic transition and martial drawdown after the post-Soviet collapse closed most cultivation and the salmon packaging plants. After a decade, entire villages lacked jobs; the regional government announced bankruptcy. To survive, poaching became a billion-dollar economic engine.

Children in the post-Soviet generation were raised with indifference toward the region's resources. The lucky ones witnessed the sole employment their parents had: illegal fishing from the terrain's waterways and the Okhotsch Sea. In summer and fall, villagers taught youngsters to strip the eggs from hundreds of salmon to sell as red caviar, casting aside the rest to rot on riverbanks.

For the few who operated helicopters, unlawful brown bear hunts became lucrative for sport or taking ursine gall bladders—valued by Asian folk medicine. American and European sportsmen, out-of-shape yet compelled to slay a trophy, paid ten thousand dollars for a guided flight to shoot a big male. Once located by the pilot and driven into a killing zone, the animal had no chance, gunned down without effort from above. Worse were the reapers who killed every bear within a region to harvest gall bladders. Males, sows, and cubs were slaughtered by rifle blasts to the backs of heads. The indiscriminate poachers sliced their bellies open for the small organ, leaving the remains for scavengers.

Tri-P and Prisontown had become local boons to Kamchatka's Avacha Bay. Both enterprises supplied good paying jobs that mitigated the persistent rape of the region's wildlife.

Geothermal energy potential had influenced the location of Tri-P's prefabrication factory. Anticipating business production to double or triple to meet worldwide demand for its products, Tri-P took advantage of the intrinsic thermal hot springs to augment driving its turbines.

The technology to tap heat-mined sources to power facilities or warm tracts of homes had been employed for two decades in Iceland. Not intermittent like wind or solar, geothermal energy remained steady and renewable. Tri-P estimated the higher costs from start-up drilling would decrease to a fraction needed to maintain the system. With zero fuel expense thereafter, recapture of the initial outlays would occur within five to seven years.

But once oil prices had spiked beyond $140 per barrel, the near-term uncertainty of higher fossil fuel prices favored heat pump technology. Tri-P consulted a Finnish company that operated a ninety-megawatt plant on heat released from wastewater. Also, a system of compressors and condensers in Oslo, Norway, produced eighteen megawatts from raw wastes—enough to heat nine thousand apartments or save burning six thousand tons of oil. Through Scandinavian contractors, Tri-P moved forward with a series of heat-extraction pumps for its factory and the sewage plant in Petropvolitin, its company town.

Tri-P excavated a three-hundred-meter tunnel in a hillside midway between Petropvolitin and Prisontown's future site. Sewage ducts from both locations joined the wastewater from Tri-P's factory and brought the combined effluents to the machines that sucked out and transferred heat into a water-pipe network feeding thousands of radiators and hot water taps down-line in the buildings and homes.

Animal fecal droppings from the dairy and chicken farms, in excess for compost needed in the prison's vegetable hot houses, were funneled into the system via a portal at the end of the wastewater conduit. Street rainwater and snowmelt also entered after filtering had excluded gravel and debris.

The mixed refuse flowed in 48°F and out at 40 as the refrigerant extracted thermal energy. In turn, that resource warmed the parallel water grids to 131°F for usage within the two communities and the factory.

The cooled contents settled into septic tanks, each holding two million gallons, and from there into connecting drainage fields. As the solid waste condensed, anaerobic bacteria fed into the tanks knocked down organic odors. When blended with leftover lignin from Tri-P's pulp mill, it produced a specialty fertilizer for export to China.

The Norwegian heat pumps ran on any reliable source of flowing water. At peak operation, Tri-P's factory provided adequate wastewater amounts for efficient thermal extraction. Any marginal shortfall got made up by the sewage streaming out of Prisontown and Petropvolitin; yet those inputs varied and predictably diminished in the early mornings of workdays. At the other extreme, on weekends in Petropvolitin, enough consumed vodka and beer—filtered first through the kidneys of factory workers and prison guards before urinated—insured an abundant supply. In essence, the hot water in a worker's flat was heated every time the toilet flushed.

In 2011, Tri-P and its Alaskan allies had entered the bidding contest offered by the US Senate's site selection committee to win the overseas penal institution contract. They touted the novel use of green technology in factory operations and the willingness to aid Prisontown to meet its own financial bottom line by "greening up" the prison. Those tactics shifted eight senate votes away from Saudi Arabia's proposal and sealed the deal.

The combined effluents generated from Prisontown and Petropvolitin made the heat extraction process economically feasible once the prison inmate level reached 63-percent capacity. The Federal Bureau of Prisons projected that occupancy within seven years.

As reported in the 2016 Congressional Record, this form of power produced significantly less pollution than burning fossil fuels: over two-thirds the combined energy expended at Prisontown, Petropvolitin, and Tri-P came from heat-extracted wastewater and sewage. The remaining fraction was generated by the factory's natural gas and oil turbines. City and regional leaders throughout eastern Siberia demonstrated keen interest to exploit their own sewer power potential and consulted Tri-P.

Energy extraction from waste flows had worked from Norway to Kamchatka. With modifications, the technology was advocated even for seawater and, therefore, championed by international organizations as a feasible solution for many cities worldwide.

The minivan rambled on bumpy Prisontown Prospekt with its snowfall of summer trash from Petropavlovsk to Petropvolitin and Birch Acres—the housing subdivision for contracted Americans and other non-Russians employed at the prison. The road terminated at Circle Three's main checkpoint. After receiving clearance, the vehicle proceeded on paved avenues to the prison's headquarters in Circle Two.

Graywood had a loaded agenda for this assistance visit. Besides supporting the medical staff and verifying prison-wide progress on the hep C vaccine trial, he planned to set in motion several KAMI initiatives he'd briefed the warden two days earlier via Skype from Anchorage.

For Kamchatka's time zone, that had happened yesterday because the five-hour flight west from Elmendorf to Petropavlovsk crossed the International Dateline. A lost day and an adjustment that Graywood's body never mastered.

He met with prison section chiefs for feedback on the current care dispensed by the onsite medical department to staff, guards, and prisoners. After noting every raised strength and weakness, he presented an overview with timetables regarding the equipment installation and training that added palliative radiation to treat terminal cancer pain for those admitted into hospice. He closed with a three-month summary review on the electronic Intensive Care Unit link with Harborview Medical Center in Seattle.

He found Doctor Pawar in her office.

"The eICU you set up with Seattle for our backup is, how you say in your country, a godsend," Pawar chortled.

"Any problems communicating with Harborview?" Graywood asked.

"None at all," she replied with an expansive smile. "We access the critical specialist for each worker, family member, or inmate patient we admit to our ICU. Harborview graciously reviews our procedures and makes recommendations. Those we cannot fix right away, I have written down for you." She handed him a page and a half of requests for equipment, supplies, and advanced staff training.

"We'll see how much we can implement in the coming six months," Graywood sighed, turning pensive upon reading it—demands exceeding funds yet again. "So do Harborview docs have any qualms about helping you manage the prisoners?"

"None at all, Doctor Graywood," she said, drawing closer to clarify. "When the specialist recommends transfer to Anchorage, then we say this patient is not allowed to go. That is when they know they have consulted on a prisoner. They say they do it all the time for walk-ins from Pioneer Square, wherever that is."

Graywood held back explaining the derelict haven in downtown Seattle. "Let's go walk about and see your good work, Doctor Pawar."

Anxious to fly anytime to Juneau, Piper shoehorned Jennelle's urgent request into his air-taxi schedule. With *Sky Woman* and decent weather, it took less than six hours.

He disembarked Jennelle at a Gastineau Channel pier and returned once she completed her investigation. Unfortunate for Jennelle, Piper vented Juneau politics the entire roundtrip.

"They're worse than scum who shoot wolves from planes," Piper repeated with bitterness to Jennelle over the com system. He vowed to fight the next damnable governmental "taking" or send Juneau all to hell.

Piper's great middle-age quest centered on moving the capital from Juneau to Willow, a hamlet twenty-three miles northwest of Wasilla. Juneau stood inaccessible to over 90 percent of Alaskans—isolated in the southeast panhandle without a land link and only reachable by air or water transportation. Piper believed all should have easier avenues to petition state officials in person and not get shut out by distance and the means to travel there.

And Piper agonized over politicians not leaving the permanent fund alone. It had been created by law out of Alaskan North Slope oil royalties. Those, in turn, were reinvested to generate revenues sufficient to disperse annual checks to each Alaska resident often in excess of one thousand dollars. But salivating Juneau bureaucrats persisted in eroding its sanctity. Piper believed they'd dare not risk their electoral livelihoods if forced to legislate from Willow and suffer the encounters from droves of angry citizens in the flesh.

The Juneau government had attached strings to the permanent fund checks after the US Congress had approved the Alpha-Omega Health Care Act and financed it with the nationwide 2.4-percent VAT. Bold Juneau amended its state law such that new residents arriving after 2015—newborns in Alaskan hospitals and out-of-state transfers moving in—would have 2.4 percent deducted from their annual permanent fund remittances to help bankroll the state's Basic Health Care Plan.

Like a gillnetter pulling salmon with abandon, Juneau's arbitrary division of the people into taxed and non-taxed groups appeared to Piper as a clever ploy toward even grander schemes to snip away everyone's permanent fund payments. Piper reasoned the majority of non-taxed residents would not object to newcomers getting plucked and many might even support it. But once the unlucky ones had been assessed a few years, the mandatory deduction would then be levied, out of fairness, against all Alaskans. Juneau's charade piqued Piper's anger further when the state encouraged the current non-taxed citizens to voluntarily donate 2.4 percent of their checks to the Alaskan Basic Health Care Plan as well.

Juneau's repeated attempts to tie the permanent fund checks to Alpha-Omega's federal weight standard had galled Piper the most. For each tax year an Alaskan was classified overweight, Juneau proposed he or she receive just half the annual payment, and those identified obese on their 1040WTs received nothing. The forfeitures would also support the state's Basic Health Care Program.

On the return flight to Anchorage, Jennelle directed Piper to dogleg to Chitina. He'd set down *Sky Woman* on Two Mile Lake north of the village, and they'd flag a ride to Bearhead's longhouse. Dreading Theo Nowell picking them up, she tuned out Piper's political rants and pretended sleep.

Jennelle had uncovered three of the four Juneau cases, like Frankie, had been meth abusers. The desire for mind-altering substances appeared wired into Juneau's psyche, and many sought to lose control drinking worb water—the leftover, laced liquid in a water pipe after smoking methamphetamines. Other illicit drugs, such as Ecstasy and LSD, were often suffused into Juneau's worb.

At the AIDs outbreak in the early 1980s, downing "poppers" had been associated with its spread. Jennelle suspected a similar tie between Alaska's illegal drug trade and the current unknown illness distribution. Tracking meth supply routes through Alaska might lead to more hidden cases … and more clues. She needed to glean from April Coldsnow more information on the geography of Toofish's and Theo's covert drug networks.

Once at Grace Hall, Jennelle matched chart maps constructed from April's memory to the annual admissions from hospitals across the Forty-ninth State. From the towns and villages scattered within the southeastern panhandle, she found several potential patients: two each at Skagway and Haines, and single cases in Sitka, Wrangall, Petersburg, and Yakutat. The

Sitka facility also had entered into the state's electronic medical records a potential second victim from Hoonah on remote Chichagof Island. Farther south, Wrangell's health center had logged two latent individuals from isolated Klawock and Craig on Prince of Wales Island.

Playing a hunch, Jennelle contacted Nick and pleaded for NIH to re-evaluate everyone for illegal drug exposure who had been entered into its disease index, with emphasis on methamphetamine abuse. Astonished by her summarization of events, Nick requested she verify the suspected linkages in Alaska and forward copies of the possible cases. He'd present the findings to WHO and the Pasteur Institute.

"Professor Bearhead, wherever there's a case of Bobby's disease, there's a Public Health clinic," observed Masi, scrolling on a computer in the Consortium Library. "So I might get to follow one after all." The fourth year medical student searched WWAMI clinical sites for locations to take his clerkship in family practice.

"How'd you come by that?" queried Bearhead from the terminal to Masi's left. The Raven had taken a break from his web-chat with village elders.

"It's a special credit project Doctor Daniels assigned me. I survey the cases and crosscheck their medical homes. Each one with Bobby's disease has a PHS clinic for its medical home."

"Why do you call them Bobby's disease?"

"'Cause Doctor Daniels calls them that," shrugged Masi.

With Masi's help, Bearhead outlined Bobby's disease to the web-net of elders and requested they forward information on First Peoples suffering from it at their villages. In quick succession, two chat mates indicated knowledge of a victim and worried it may have come from the hep C vaccine trial Bearhead had persuaded them to undertake.

"Masi, when do you see Doctor Daniels about this?"

Sheepish, he replied, "I was supposed to last week, but she's gone the whole time. She's back now and wants it like yesterday."

"Well, Masi, let's get my truck and go see her," directed Bearhead.

"I was checking on PHS affiliated clinics for where I'd like my family practice rotation, and over half I'm interested in had a patient with the unknown disease, but every new case was linked to a PHS clinic except one," explained Masi to Jennelle and Bearhead at her office.

"Where was the outlier?"

"Elmendorf's medical center."

"All government clinics," she concluded. Obvious to her, the scenario resembled the Nigerian polio outbreak in Africa she had connected to the oral polio immunizations dispensed in 2006-07. She made a mental note to check every inoculation given over the past decade at the Alaskan clinics.

"Some village elders in my chat group worry your trial is causing the disease in their villages," said Bearhead in red-flag tones. "They're talking, Jen. Do you think there's anything?"

"No, Roe, I don't." Realizing the grave threat this rumor would have on the hep C field investigation, she formulated the format and data collection necessary to combat it. "Masi, do you remember how John Snow in 1854 discovered that the Broad Street water pump in London had caused a cholera outbreak there?"

"Ah … he made a spot map of London to visualize the epidemic's distribution."

"Did that prove it?"

"No, but it helped him focus his investigation toward the pump."

"Very good, Masi. Doctor Graywood has taught you well," she complimented. "The power of a spot map is how it excludes assumptions about what's causing something," she amplified, looking straight at Bearhead. Shifting to Masi, she said, "I want you to make a bigger spot map of all of Alaska. Put on it all the Alaskan PHS clinics, all the federal government clinics, and the clinics we've recruited into the hep C field trial. Mark the ones in red that are the medical homes for every case of Bobby's disease."

"Jen, what will that prove?" asked Bearhead.

"I bet it'll show a visible discordance, a poor match, if you will, of cases of Bobby's disease separate from the clinics involved in the hep C study," she replied. "There will be many more cases associated with medical homes that are not the least bit involved with my field trial."

"I understand now," said Bearhead. "You're sorting out if there's truly a signal in all the noise but already thinking this can only be noise pertaining to the hep C vaccine. May I suggest marking the hep C clinics in blue to emphasize the mismatch?"

"Agreed. And one more thing, Masi," said Jennelle, "expand your net to see if the cases of Bobby's disease we know about in the Lower Forty-eight are linked to any PHS clinics down there or up here in Alaska, or both."

"An inkling of yours?" asked Bearhead.

"Sometimes random events occur in clusters, sometimes not," she noted, making her way for the door. "I've got to catch a plane, gentlemen. Sorry to leave you."

"So how did John Snow confirm the pump was the cause of London's epidemic?" yelled Bearhead.

Jennelle spun around, saying, "Snow took the handle off the pump, and the epidemic stopped. People had to find water from the competing company that piped it from an uncontaminated source."

CHAPTER TWENTY-TWO

Documentary

"While waiting for Jen on the dock by *Sky Woman*," began Piper, "I was reviewin' my flight plan, and a raven landed on the beach within spittin' distance."

Graywood, Bearhead, and Piper had cornered a table near the bar at the Glacier Brewhouse. Out of character, Piper hadn't fumed about Juneau hatching another nefarious Alpha-Omega plot to take away everyone's permanent fund checks. The other two were grateful and ordered drinks. It was the first time they'd come together since Bobby's death.

"So what did Raven do so close to you?" asked Bearhead.

"He went pickin' through rocks, turnin' some over, lookin' for a meal of hermit crab or whatever." Piper raised an index finger to the bartender to signal the customary martini. "Someone must've tossed a wadded gum wrapper earlier 'cause he found the foil and pecked at it to inspect every silver crease."

Bearhead eyed Graywood and asked Piper, "How close were you to him again?"

"Ah, not more than six feet. He was right by the dock."

Bearhead twinkled. "Ravens are smart. They never get that close unless to impart a lesson or warning." Twisting in his chair, Bearhead faced Piper head-on. "So what happened next?"

Hesitating, Piper wanted to know what Bearhead had meant by a bird's warning but went on with the story. "Like I said, 'stead of huntin' crabs, that raven beaked away at the shiny foil like a woman primpin' diamond rings. Then another raven landed 'bout a yard away."

Graywood and Bearhead glanced at each other as the little drama unfolded.

"The second one wanted the wrapper but faked not wantin' it while the first teased by tossin' it all about. Both started a lot of caw-jawin' and head bobbin' back and forth like they were haggling over its price at a second-hand store. That's when a third raven came in and tried to steal the wrapper, but the other two had none of it, so all three made circles makin' a helluva racket. Then out of nowhere, in a wink of an eye, a fourth one swooped in and grabbed the wrapper and took off. None the other three could stop him."

On the peeled log surface before the storyteller, the bartender placed a martini with three olives. Piper took a couple of slurps.

Perplexed, the other two wanted to hear more. Bearhead asked, "So after the fourth raven left, what'd the others do?"

Piper tabled the glass and said, "Oh, well … since there was nothing to fight over, them other two ravens flew off leaving the first alone. He went back to scavenging, snatched a crab 'bout a minute later." Piper plopped an olive in his mouth and chewed slowly to savor it.

"Roe, you think it's significant the ravens and Piper crossed paths?" asked Graywood.

"Don't know," responded Bearhead with a distant face. "Raven is both trickster and hero in many of our legends."

"Piper had no trouble flying back here with Jen, so if there's a warning in it for him, I can't make sense of it either," agreed Graywood.

"You two are plain crazy jawin' about birds acting like us," interrupted Piper, amazed. He thumped a hand once to his chest. "They're just creatures like us tryin' to survive."

"You know how Roe likes to argue Raven is an extension of God," said Graywood, stroking fingers up and down the side of his head.

"Ah … yeah … ah sure," discounted Piper. He rotated his drink to admire the clear contents surrounding the two remaining olives. "For him I'll respect that notion, but really don't believe it."

"Do you think dogs are smarter than ravens?" queried Bearhead.

"Ah … yeah … ah, for sure. Cub swears by how smart all dogs are," returned Piper.

"He still planning to race the Iditarod?"

"Yep."

"Can you ask him a question I've been thinking about?"

"Sure, Roe"

"If dyslexic, can a dog be closer to God than man?"

Piper straightened up. "What the hell you mean?"

"When dyslexic, a dog is closer to God than man, right?"

"Well I'm goddamn dyslexic, and I'm closer to God 'cause I'm a bush pilot. That much I know," snorted Piper. He drained the last of his drink and nodded at the bartender to bring a second. "I'll admit after landing I'm not so close to God like you two."

"No, that's not the point, Piper," howled Graywood in gulps. "Roe's … just being … a smart ass." He hadn't laughed so hard since Bobby's death and couldn't choke out the old joke's meaning for dog spelled backwards.

Amused, Bearhead was glad Graywood's humor had resurfaced.

Piper didn't ask for an explanation yet retook center stage. "Come to think of it, Roe, something more did happen with that raven struttin' in front of me and *Sky Woman*."

"I had a hunch there was," chimed Bearhead.

"I'd just finished recheckin' the bolts on the floats when the fourth raven came back to the first and laid the silver wrapper down between them. The first one dropped his crab next to the wrapper and both stood really still."

"So what happened?" asked Graywood.

"They just stared at each other. Not movin'. It must've been over a minute. Then they looked straight at me."

"Really?" muffled Bearhead.

"I swear it."

"Did you feel anything when they looked your way?"

"Hell no, Roe. The first raven picked up the wrapper and tossed it in the air again, and the thief took the crab and flew off."

"That's interesting," said Bearhead. "Maybe they'd acted out the reason you flew to Juneau."

"What! Come on, Roe. I flew there 'cause of Jen's work and to fight the damn takeover of the permanent fund," retorted Piper.

"They're taking the permanent fund?" asked Bearhead.

"Shit, there's a big battle to tap the permanent fund for the damn Alpha-Omega mandate that the state's gotta pay to meet all the crap rollin' out of Washington," snorted Piper.

"There'll never be enough dough to fund all the health care everybody thinks he's entitled to," added Graywood.

"Well they goddamn better NOT skewer away our checks for some goddamn federal mandate!" blustered Piper. "That's our money. It's the sacred promise." He slammed his right fist into the other. "If they steal any part of our royalty or pay for some shit ass piece of health care by being caught overweight, we'll goddamn move the capitol to Willow. You bet your balls we will."

"Perhaps consider this," offered Bearhead, unruffled, "You and your movement to protect the permanent fund from Juneau politicians diverting it into health care payments might be like the three ravens haggling over the silver wrapper. While you jabber your heads off, a fourth sneaks in from someplace else, like Washington, and steals it all away."

"That bastard bird or anyone like him taking our money will be toast," declared Piper.

Bearhead ceased the analogy. Another round of liquor shifted the trio's talk to other concerns.

Leaving for home, each managed nightfall in his own manner. Piper came to Mary by way of Cub's kennel to stoke a father's pride. Cub had turned out fine and readied his dogsled team for the winter's races.

If Bobby had been alive, Graywood would have parked bedside at the nursing facility for three or four hours, grateful for any speck of alertness out of his semi-comatose son. Then he'd have shuffled toward the empty house and grasped at sleep. But tonight he stared cold at the Big Dipper.

Bearhead approached from behind. "Gary, I'd like to do a remembrance for Bobby."

Startled, Graywood spun and said, "I'm sorry, Roe; what'd you say?"

"You search the stars and think of him," sympathized Bearhead. He'd done the same for Ume and Sophia.

"God, I sure miss him, Roe," said Graywood. "Not the years when he got really sick. I just miss when he played hockey without fear and the times we flew off to Campsite to fish and shoot arrows.

"Yeah, he really loved that and got pretty good with the bow," added Bearhead.

"You're a good teacher."

"I miss him too, Gary." Bearhead cupped a hand to Graywood's shoulder and gazed skyward.

"Thanks, Roe."

In silence, they beheld majestic constellations brighten into night's advance.

Bearhead expanded his request. "Gary, I'd like to carve something to remember Bobby, maybe a mortuary totem."

"Oh God, Roe, I'm not ready for that," uttered Graywood, tilting down his chin.

"I understand. Goodnight, Gary." Bearhead pressed no further and walked away. In the spring, he'd ask again.

"Where would you stand it up?" Graywood shouted, striding to catch up.

Not surprised that fickle eddies coursed upon grief's river, Bearhead turned and said, "At the grave or your house or maybe Campsite."

"I don't visit the grave."

Confused whether this might be denial, confession, or declaration, Bearhead shrugged, "Yeah, Gary, it's really a tough time. Goodnight."

On the road home, Bearhead wished his friend's grief cycle would end within a year. Each season held indestructible memories that needed work to heal. Graywood's intent to shepherd KAMI along might make living his coming years less onerous.

Bearhead elected to carve four mahogany pieces based on Piper's bar story: four conniving ravens manipulating the worth of silver wadding and hermit crab. Value appeared as relative to them as it did to humans—all bargaining, like the permanent fund money rerouted by governmental fiat to pay for health care if one got caught overweight.

He imagined what Cashel Goodlette might opine in a North Slope message if told Piper's raven story: "Our collective girth is increasing, so we tax it to make it less. Governments develop cap and trade policies on abdominal girth in the righteous belief the best environmental legislation combines diminished fossil fuel use with one's shrinking belly ... the bastards!"

How would Alaskans accept an outside entity swiping the wonderful permanent fund? If they gave up its royalties, would they get back improved medical services in return?

Bearhead grinned his yellow teeth when he imagined the fourth raven bringing back the foil to the first. It might have been a repeat of when the First Peoples' Raven had brought the moon to man.

"Sorry I'm late," Graywood gasped. "My webcams with Emrick back east take extra turns these days." He entered Colonel Sulmasy's office out of breath from two-stepping the stairs.

"No problem, Gary. Let me introduce you to Evans Harl," said Sulmasy. "He's one of Hollywood's masterful directors. We're going ahead with the documentary on air force support to Prisontown."

"Colonel Sulmasy has told me much about you, Doctor Graywood," said Harl, extending a hand. "May I call you Gary?"

"Yes, of course."

A pleasant-faced Asian-American, Evans R. Harl presented the visionary filmmaker in the rough. Taut, intelligent eyes searched for beauty glued to pity, and they balanced the completely shaved head. With a northern European name, Graywood suspected Harl had been adopted.

"Before you came, Gary, I'd summarized for Evans our logistical support mission to Prisontown," recapped Sulmasy. "I'd just begun on how we were, at one time, a backwater DOD and Veterans Administration joint venture hospital until Washington added DOJ's banishment mission, and how—"

"With the Prisontown documentary," interrupted Harl, zeroing in on Graywood, "we'll tamper with the mystery of existence, warts and all. We'll go deep inside the organism that makes up Prisontown and try to discover where it's thriving, where it's having growing pains, and how it reflects back on us."

Burying his chin in his palm, Graywood listened to Harl spin more. "So much goes into making a credible documentary, Gary. Trust, most of all. It illuminates us as a country. It's an American window for the rest of the world to see us. We in this room must believe our documentary is a team effort. I hope to make it inspiring, and I need your help."

"Well, how do I fit in?" acquiesced Graywood to Harl's recruitment.

"I'm a connoisseur for detail, Gary. I probe for twists, detours, and devils."

"Okay, so what details and twisted devils would you like out of me?"

"The fabric of Prisontown as you see it, Gary. Its health, the very essence in its culture."

Graywood's stony expression pleaded for less airiness, more substance.

Harl expanded, "I need you to help me capture insights that stand out from the daily struggles and dramas in Prisontown's life and offer your understandings on the human strife it creates and moderates while attempting to deal with its diverse personalities, politics, and economics. I hope to share your lens on all its culture and technology."

"Gary, I told Evans about your KAMI innovations," clarified Sulmasy.

At last something said that doesn't blow over my head. Graywood's hand dropped from his jaw.

"KAMI is such a prime piece for the film, Gary," said Harl, recapturing center stage. "Prisontown may hold a key, perhaps THE KEY to understanding the meaning of twenty-first century humanity," Harl emphasized. "I wish to display the grand puzzlement we all have with our modern natures and emotions, how often we're wrong about them, and how we've misread the emotions in others."

Christ, he's all over the place. "So ... um ... which emotions do you want to get at?" asked Graywood in a polite way to focus the film director, whom he and the Kamchatkan personnel would have to assist.

"The great emotions," Harl said, ticking off six, "fear, joy, grief, love, pride, and shame." Sensing Graywood's rising exasperation, he expounded, "Emotions have intelligence. They are the vital, personal strategies in our everyday lives, our health. They're sophisticated survival strategies, and today what better place is there to document them than at Prisontown."

Graywood grimaced and studied the air-force-blue carpet for a scrap of sense in Harl's Hollywood mind. For sure, Prisontown had its share of emotions, but so did he and every other scud alive. Should he light up Harl's goggles on life and reveal the stories of Bobby and Maren and

Jen—his own desperate trials of injury and survival? Should he dwell on Bobby's loss upon loss, every week a little less of him that God returned alive, capped off with Jen asking for a piece of brain the day he died? And Maren … damn her to Hell … she'd been life's carnal and mental flesh he'd negotiated, fought, and lost to. Maren … she didn't even come to the funeral. At least she didn't fake excuses about storms delaying flights. Christ, she'd never booked one.

Graywood's pensive eyes rolled up to gather the sunrays streaming through Sulmasy's window …

"You're a caretaker," they beamed, *"same as Jen … Change the wallpaper on your mind, Gary. As it always does, the world goes on when something mysterious or precious or magical as your son is lost or denied. Harl's a caretaker too, so are Sulmasy and the prisoners who've raised their spirits out of Ground Zero."*

"These are our weekly teleconference recordings since standing up Prisontown's medical department six years ago," said Graywood, tapping two shelves of stacked DVDs. "The binders below contain the meeting agendas, and at the first page's bottom, you'll find stamped the referenced DVD by date."

"Thank you, Gary. So every meeting's recorded?"

"Correct. Each scheduled one is on DVD, and there're written minutes too.

"Why both?"

"Government documentation requirement. Substituting banishment for the death penalty is a huge change for the country," deadpanned Graywood. "Guess one day these'll end up in the Library of Congress for historians to ponder over."

"They'll help magnificently with background," bubbled Harl.

"Here's the playing remote," said Graywood, handing it off. "Let my secretary know when you're finished so she can lock up."

Alone, Harl leafed binders and selected a half dozen DVDs. Tomorrow, he'd arrange the screenwriters to camp here. He loaded 14Nov2011 and fast forwarded to a younger Graywood speaking while standing in front of a whiteboard that displayed three bullets:

- Agency for Healthcare Research and Quality—annual budget $300 million
- Pharmaceutical companies spend $34 billion/year on drug development
- Prison Health Care Budget—To Be Determined

“Each incremental advance in medical therapy is tempered because many prisoner patients will not receive recommended treatments and therefore not benefit by them,” spoke Graywood, machine-like.

“Efforts to improve fidelity, defined as the extent to which our system provides prisoner patients the precise interventions they need, properly and precisely delivered when they need them, is greatly diminished by the generic treatment protocols put in place by the Bureau of Prisons and Department of Justice.”

“Pretty interesting shit made dull,” mused Harl out loud. He jumped to a different section, Graywood still speaking:

“A daily aspirin reduced the rate of recurrent stroke by 23 percent. If we have a population of one hundred prisoners who have survived their initial stroke, and if all of them are placed on daily aspirin, twenty-three recurrent strokes would be prevented. To prevent the same number of strokes as aspirin, this newer, heavily advertised medication would need to prevent forty recurrent strokes to justify its higher cost. That’s the financial break-even point. But longitudinal studies show it will only prevent twenty-five recurrent strokes. That’s why it’s not on our formulary.”

Harl observed Graywood’s stolid body language and inferred the half-hearted attempt to present reasons for dispensing generic drugs, rather than cutting-edge ones, to the prisoners for cost control. Indeed, Graywood sounded like a blunt Alpha-Omega bureaucrat. Harl zapped further and listened.

“Symptoms of intermittent claudication, also called chronic peripheral arterial disease, can resolve spontaneously, remain stable over many years, or progress rapidly to critical ischemia, which endangers the limb’s viability. We can expect the annual incidence of critical limb ischemia to be one per three thousand prisoners, or one to two episodes per year once the prison is full and aging. Coronary artery disease is the major cause of death in persons with peripheral arterial disease of the legs. In five years after diagnosis, overall mortality is 30 percent, and 70 percent after fifteen years.

"Treatments approved for claudication in the bureau's manual are aspirin, regular walking exercises three times per week, and smoking cessation."

Bored, Harl ejected that DVD and loaded 23March2013. Once he saw the dark-skinned woman wearing a white doctor's smock, he stopped, fast-forwarding to hear her speak.

"Each prisoner harbors a self-inflicted chaos that corkscrews into blackmail and deception that in the past culminated in homicide. That is how he or she was sent here. Therefore, in the beginning, each prisoner must reside in Ground Zero and rediscover his or her margin of sympathy for self and for others. We try to help the prisoners find that sympathy within themselves. When they find enough, we move them up to Circle One and even further as they progress over time. If people are given a chance to make healthy choices, they usually do.

"To achieve any degree of atonement, it must be watered with forgiveness. Progressing into Circles One, Two, and Three are signs of acceptance by all parties involved."

Impressed, Harl rifled the binder for her identification—Doctor Nayna Pawar, onsite medical director. She emitted a knowing smile over a tempered-steel core. She'd provide balance to Gary in the documentary.

Harl switched to the DVD entitled "Graywood's 2013 Guidelines on Discussing Terminal Illness with a Prisoner" and opened a laptop for note taking as he listened.

"Our challenge is that we are pretty much limited in our ability to treat the chronic illnesses present in our prisoners. Our mandate from the Justice Department is NOT to intervene in the progression of diseases normally treated under Alpha-Omega to extend someone's life. Instead, the political reality is very stark: the prisoners were spared execution in order to die a natural death WITHOUT any medical interventions to prolong their lives. The current political consensus is that the social mercy granted by ending their death-row status is much more gracious than what they had rendered without mercy upon their murdered victims. So when banished, that's all they get medical-wise."

Wide-eyed, Harl paused the DVD to key impressions. First, Gary of 2013 had a harder edge than the Gary of 2017 he'd just met. *What's changed in him?*

Second, the political will advocated behind the mandate to forego chronic disease treatments for the Kamchatkan prisoners spilled out, in a way, from the same dark well as the restrictions attempted against illegal immigration starting back in 2007. Secure borders and amnesty were the code words of that time, and amnesty was not granted to illegals living and working in the United States. Not allowed to have access to American fruits of a better life, the illegals had to return to their country of origin—go to the back of the line. That was the pecking order. If ever sick while in the United States, they received only urgent care hardly better than first aid in overcrowded hospital emergency rooms. Rarely had they received chronic disease screening and treatment. An illegal alien with kidney failure in 2007 had an ice ball's chance in hell of snaring a renal transplant—same as the felon sent to Siberia in 2013. Both groups were booted to the back of the line or completely off.

Harl resumed the recording.

"How do we implement this?" said Graywood, skewing a robotic face. "Let's gave two examples:

"A prisoner survives a heart attack but afterwards develops congestive heart failure. We are to stand by and let his condition progress to its terminal stage. There will be no administration of agents to increase heart function, no consideration of heart transplantation, no mechanical augmentation of cardiac function or placement of pacemakers to improve heart rhythm. For congestive heart failure in any prisoner, we are to practice medicine as it was done in the 1950s. And that basically amounts to easing pain and discomfort.

"My second example is HIV infection. There shall be no anti-HIV treatment cocktail other than two pills distributed per day that only cost a few dimes in the third world. Likewise in third world fashion, there shall be no antibiotic prophylaxis. However, everyone will follow blood-borne and body-secretion precautions to protect the staff and other prisoners. There will be prisoner isolation if active tuberculosis develops. For HIV infection in a prisoner, we are to practice medicine as it was done in 1981 before any anti-HIV drugs were developed. Again, that amounts to easing pain and discomfort, most likely with elements of isolation to protect others from contagious infections.

"I can describe a similar scenario when a banished prisoner develops Alzheimer's disease or has a stroke or cancer or develops any form of organ failure. Our role will be limited to easing pain and discomfort. Bottom line, they are to die a natural death as our grandparents did in the mid-twentieth century."

Harl skipped the end-of-life communication guidance given face-to-face to prisoners and listened to Graywood discuss pain management.

"When the patient's pain fails to respond to acetaminophen and other generic anti-inflammatory drugs, or otherwise becomes intractable, opioids are recommended, although the studies that compare opioid agents for effectiveness are lacking. Consensus by those who manage cancer pain is to start with short-acting opioids. When the pain persists throughout the day, switch to longer-acting opioids two to three times daily to provide twenty-four-hour relief.

"If methadone is prescribed, be aware it's metabolized very slowly and can build to dangerous levels. During the first three weeks after starting methadone, patients must be monitored closely because they will vary greatly in their response to it, and so they'll need to be inched up from lower starting doses.

"If pain continues to worsen, this may be a sign of worsening disease, opioid tolerance, or constipation, or abdominal pain induced by the opioids. Reevaluation for underlying causes is warranted. Bear in mind that the effective dose for pain relief can vary from patient to patient. Patient treatment variation in a disease as complicated as terminal cancer is the true challenge in the art of medical practice."

Harl ejected the DVD and summarized inputs on his hand-held device: Gary had started out calling them prisoners but switched to saying patient by the end, and Sulmasy's briefing about KAMI revealed the opposite of what had been recorded in 2013. The earlier Gary appeared disgusted by the way he had to practice some treatment components—that may have fueled his creation of KAMI.

"What's their common plight?" thought Harl. "The prisoners, Doctor Pawar and Gary, KAMI and Kamchatka—and the future of Alpha-Omega within the United States? What linkages and contrasts should the documentary present?"

Plenty of material, perhaps too much.

Rubbing excited hands, Harl patted the DVDs like a pet dog and returned to the Sheraton to sequence the production mechanics with the film crew.

To discover additional Alaskan victims, Jennelle aligned the illegal drug networks gleaned from April Coldsnow to Masi's expanded data sets and obtained a remarkable association: close to half the cases had either confirmed or probable drug exposures that included methamphetamines, and another 20 percent had possible abuse histories.

Masi's work also verified Nick's NIH observation that all US cases had once resided in Alaska, and the overlay spot maps revealed an uncanny concordance: every case when living in Alaska had a medical home either at a PHS clinic or an affiliation to one. No private medical care organization had been identified, except for Bobby's episode. Since 100-percent linkages never happened in epidemiology, Bobby's case being the sole outlier astonished Jennelle.

"Doctor Severstal on line one, Doctor Daniels."

"Thanks, Taylor." Jennelle skipped toward the desk and grasped the landline.

"Hey, Nick, any news?"

"You bet, Jen! I wanted to tell you first. Your idea to follow illegal drug distribution is spot on. WHO and the Pasteur Institute think they're on to something with meth and the cases in Senegal and maybe in Algeria too."

"Wow!"

"And there's a possible case in France," added Nick. "The French are now calling it a public health emergency.

"Just from one case in France?"

"Well … that's how they are. You know the French, hundreds of victims in Senegal aren't a problem, but if there's one in their backyard, then it's a disaster."

"Did the French case ever live in Senegal?"

"No, she's thirteen years old, never left the country."

"Hmmmm. Nick, what if it's the other way?"

"The other way? I don't follow."

"What if their thinking's backwards?

"Huh?"

"Look Nick, Alaska seems to be the potential source for all the cases of Bobby's disease in the US. It's like the annual flu epidemics every autumn crossing from Asia into the States first through Alaska. And I'm thinking contaminated meth from Alaska shipped down to the Lower Forty-eight might explain it all."

"So you're speculating that France is the source for the cases in Africa instead of the other way around," reasoned Nick.

"That's right. Everyone's thinking Senegal to France, but what if it's the wrong way? What if it's France to Senegal, like Alaska to the rest of the US for Asian flu?"

"Well, Jen, the case number size and earlier outbreak in Senegal make that pretty far-fetched."

"Yeah, on the surface, it'd seem so." For a moment she detoured back to Cashel Goodlette and his ranting against scientists who had often placed cause and effect backwards. She missed Cash's unannounced visits, laced with sarcasm for his peers. He'd moved to larger offices in Glenn Olds Hall after his climate change grants had received federal approval and enabled hiring assistants.

"Nick," asked Jennelle, "can you send me what they have on the French girl?"

"It'll take some time. You know with the French it's all take and very little give."

"Yes, but I know you can do it if anyone can."

"I'll buzz you as soon as I come by it. Bye."

Jennelle studied Masi's overlay on the office wall. The map beside it pinpointed continental US cases, dated and color coded to their medical homes when they had resided in Alaska. Jennelle's brain replayed the multiple potential connections: Alaska to the States, Senegal to France, France to Senegal, Alaska to Senegal, Senegal to Alaska, Alaska to France, France to Alaska. Was the disease an infectious agent and yet not anything like the flu, an unknown chemical contaminant shipped through a meth cartel, or something else?

"Doctor Daniels," interrupted Taylor, "the Juneau clinic just called and wants to know where to send expired hep C vaccines."

"It's in the protocol I've explained over and over to them," she snapped. Once composed, she reiterated, "They ship them here first so I log out unused vials before I forward them to Atlanta."

"Thank you, Doctor."

Where was I before Juneau's expired vaccine question ... Oh, yeah, France and Alaska ... What possible connection is there between France and Alaska for all this? Not Asian flu. Maybe an international meth cartel... France and Alaska ... Oh, My good God! That expired French vaccine!

Jennelle raced to the basement's cold storage locker and found the pristine vial retrieved from the Glennallen clinic.

"I'd forgotten all about you," she whispered, reading the label: Cannes Pharmaceutical Internationale, Anti-Varicella. "How did you and your companions ever come here?" she thought. "A French product sent to Alaska. You should've been tossed a decade ago."

Jennelle contacted colleagues in Europe, WHO, CDC, FDA, and the pharmaceutical industry. She accessed the retired public and secure electronic files on Cannes Pharmaceutical Internationale. Its chicken pox vaccine, VaroCell, had been manufactured from cloned human embryonic cells—one of the early biotech inventions brought to market employing that premiere business model. The biopharmaceutical company, listed CPI from 2002 to 2008 on the French stock exchange, was disassembled in 2009 and sold to other industry giants.

Before she resurrected Cashel Goodlette's time-tested harangue to follow money trails that exploited profit through science, Jennelle detoured into the cloning techniques utilized between 2000 and 2010. It shocked her how nigh shotgun approaches were employed by reputable institutions in the United States, Europe, and Asia to tout discoveries and cures derived from cloned stem cells. In aggregate, they resembled the puffed-up promises made by the cosmetics industries when they advertised their plethora of concocted stews for eternal, youthful skin if only forever slathered on.

At that same time, ethical controversy surrounded research protocols that employed human stem cells. The most sought experimental substrates meant for biomedical manipulation appeared to have been the extracted stem cells from discarded days-old embryos or from the eggs donated by healthy women. Those derived from newborn umbilical cord blood, amniotic fluid, or adult skin or bone marrow stem cells were regarded inferior. This dichotomy perplexed Jennelle since a stem cell remained a stem cell, regardless of its derivation, and in theory, it possessed the ability to develop into any of over two hundred tissue types.

If Cashel Goodlette had been looking over her shoulder, he'd have inferred leftover embryo usage from fertility clinics had a crass financial motivation—cheaper and more plentiful, compared to creating stem cell lines from scratch.

Jennelle doubted the widespread speculations made in that decade's newspaper editorials and Internet blogs. Many had implied a sinister plot to ghoulishly harvest fetal tissues to pursue a spectrum of cures for each old-age illness as the immortal boomer generation approached Social Security. Yet she also perceived a purer investigative relevance to exploring this novel frontier.

Stem-cell research money became sparse in 2001 when President Bush limited its federal funds. He personified the social conservative view that embryo destruction for harvesting stem cells was unethical. Opponents countered the strict policy hampered critical science.

To bypass federal restrictions, California organized its own stem-cell agency in 2004 with a voter-approved, three-billion-dollar bond. Sixteen research grants were awarded totaling forty million dollars by September 2005, but lawsuits challenged the agency's legality and prevented further dispensing of bond money. Only private loans and donations advanced the bulk of embryo stem cell research, and the United States lost ground to other nations in the biotechnology race.

Jennelle matched the grant proposals in that time period to those approved. Cashel Goodlette's basic critique against science proved correct—research had bowed down truth to power politics. She found whoever controlled the purse, government or private, had been biased towards funding research proposals that involved stem cells derived directly from human embryos. Those who obtained stem cells harvested from adults or other tissues, such as newborn umbilical cord blood often got chucked. The winning grant applications had broadcasted their research would advance biotechnology and contribute to the universal foundations of regenerative medicine: stem cells, once cloned, could be matured into replacement parts for diseased and injured organs or repair severed spinal cords or cure diseases, such as juvenile diabetes and Parkinson's. And any moral objections to the proposals should be negated by the potential cures developed.

Jennelle discovered and downloaded the cloning competition at that time between South Korea and the United States. It amused her how much it had played like the space race between the United States and Soviet Union after Sputnik's launch.

South Korean scientists, led by a veterinary professor at Seoul National University, had cloned the world's initial human embryo and within a year had moved close to growing replacement tissues for eleven sick or injured patients from fresh, embryonic stem-cell lines genetically matched to each. Meanwhile, the Americans bewailed how the United States had become a second-class power in biotechnology.

The Korean team started with 185 eggs allegedly donated by unpaid women who each underwent a month long series of hormone shots to ripen a dozen or more ova for extraction. Upon removing each egg's DNA, it was fused into a single skin cell taken from one of the eleven individuals who had either diabetes, a spinal cord injury, or an inborn disease of poor immunity. Out of the 185 original ova spliced into skin cells, thirty-one grew into hybrid embryos. The Koreans then extracted stem cells from eleven hybrids and cloned subsequent cell colonies that genetically and immunologically matched the person who had supplied the skin cell. On average, it took seventeen eggs to produce one successful cloned cell line.

But the succeeding steps—worldwide verification of this brand of stem cell research—were torpedoed by the lack of ethics in the ova collection. Twenty Korean women who had donated eggs were paid, and two others had been members of the research team. Viewed as taboo outside Korea, these procedures demonstrated potential coercion. When globally known that the team leader had withheld the truth about the ova acquisitions, the other institutions canceled their collaborations, and the Korean government scrambled to salvage the nation's reputation by creating a state-run egg bank under stringent guidelines.

Jennelle searched further online into CPI's history and the concurrent European efforts in embryonic stem cell research. CPI had developed its cutting-edge varicella vaccine, VaroCell, with a biotech variation that cultivated human embryonic stem-cell lines on beds of mouse cells, modified to secrete a cocktail of hormones to support their finicky growth. Yet internal CPI memos voiced concerns about how potential embedded mouse viruses or other cell contaminants might risk the vaccine's effectiveness or cause something unexpected. And they messaged frequent refusals to adopt the Korean method for cultivating stem-cell lines in dishes without any animal cells. From there, the trail went cold.

To glean CPI's primary business philosophy, Jennelle backtracked to its origins. In the 1990s as a start-up with venture capital from an anonymous foundation, CPI had employed advanced bioengineering to augment the nutritional content in the East African highland banana. When compared to other bananas, the Ugandan species contained low amounts of iron, vitamin A, and iodine. Despite an average consumption of two pounds per day, half the Ugandan children under five years had iron deficiency.

Ugandan leaders preferred to retain this particular fruit for growing instead of importing a more nutritious one. Officials feared a foreign species, such as one from Australia, might damage their ecosystem. There would be less environmental disruption if CPI's scientists improved the current one cultivated. Implementing its maiden biofortification process, CPI complied with the Ugandan concerns and increased the genetic mineral, vitamin, and protein contents in the highland banana.

CPI went public in 2002 after the Ugandan success and retained the anonymous foundation as the major partner to head off hostile takeovers. Buoyed by international acclaim for its ecological prowess and the revenue from its tropical fruit patent, CPI focused on improving the varicella immunization.

They usurped a marketing strategy made famous by a competitor: "We don't make the injection; we make it better." CPI had a two-pronged goal. First, improve the inoculation's immunogenicity such that a single vaccination—compared to the two-dose standard—would provide life-long immunity to chicken pox. Second, arm the product's effectiveness to prevent shingles from erupting on the skin of elderly people who earlier had been infected with varicella as children or young adults.

Characterized as a painful, vesicular rash along the distribution of a sensory nerve on the skin, shingles occurred in older people who had contracted chicken pox decades earlier. The virus wedged itself into the nerves toward the end of the initial infection and remained dormant to avoid its outright destruction by the immune system. If immunity significantly weakened, the virus could restart multiplying in one of the infected nerves and produce an eruption. Each year, over one million people suffered an episode, and by age eighty-five, half the elderly had endured the malady.

In order to multiply the responsive vigor in an immunization meant to last a lifetime, CPI's scientists reasoned the viral substrate necessary for a one-shot product had to be grown in cloned, embryonic human stem cells, instead of conventional fetal chicken eggs. They hypothesized such modified cells for the substrate would better approximate the natural processes of wild chicken pox interacting within human neural tissues. Therefore immunity should be enhanced.

CPI also bolstered their logic from the discovery that the rabies vaccine more than doubly improved potency once its viral substrate had been propagated on diploid human cells instead of duck embryos. The switch decreased the number of shots needed for rabies immunity from over a dozen down to five.

CPI's marketing plan emphasized the duel life-long protections from both chicken pox and shingles. It would be the vaccine for all generations: a single immunization given at one year of age to replace the three current doses—the first two for childhood chicken pox prevention and the third to decrease shingles risk in the older adult. Simplified, one CPI inoculation reduced to zero the risk for chicken pox and shingles in all susceptible populations.

In a no-stone-left-unturned manner, Jennelle located the product's approval and licensing request records. Dated 10 January 2006, CPI had submitted them to the European Union's counterpart of the US Patent

Office. Like previous patent requests, CPI had stressed the unique qualifications. Three stood out:

- Their work emphasized the human imperative to develop treatments, even cures by harvesting the widespread promise and appeal of embryonic stem cell technology.
- Cloning techniques developed through stem cells insured an endless supply of reproducible, homogeneous substrates that exceeded the European Union's quality control standards for biotechnology.
- Bypassing United States restrictions, the human fetal stem cell lines were derived from aborted fetuses in France and Senegal during the vaccine's 1999 to 2005 development.

FRANCE and SENEGAL … the CPI vaccine had been developed in Senegal and France!

There was more, but Jennelle didn't need it. She deemed the commodity a potential common source for the neurodegenerative disease's outbreaks on three continents.

She notified Nick and shipped to NIH the vial discovered in Glennallen for analysis. She contacted colleagues at the American Immunization Registry Association and coordinated historical tracking of CPI's VaroCell within state and local web-based immunization registries.

"Gary, here's what we came up with," said Harl, handing him a screenplay draft for the Prisontown documentary. Harl had deserted the film crew in the aft of the aircraft to join Graywood once the Boeing 767 had left Elmendorf. "Look it over and tell me what you think."

Graywood lifted the manila cover.

"Gary, please start at page fifty-six. I want impressions on the segment about prisoner marriage by proxy."

"You're including that in the documentary?" Graywood asked and squinted to find the page.

"I'm inclined to. Films aren't really about life so much as imitation."

"I'm not following you."

"Sorry, Gary," said Harl, adjusting the seatbelt. "After years in the business, I've come to believe films are often mistaken for reality because they perpetuate so many illusions we have of life."

Graywood frowned a quizzical expression, so Harl added, "In the film industry, the documentary is closest to reality, so all those sweet, electronic wives the prisoners have are an illusion I want to include for contrast."

Digesting Harl's explanation, Graywood pulled out a pen and said, "I think I get it. If e-wives are an illusion, you're adding them in the documentary so viewers can assess the degrees of illusion throughout Prisontown and then compare them to themselves."

"Couldn't have expressed it better." Harl grinned, trading to the seat across the aisle for more legroom. "Besides, e-wives add a touch of pizzazz. Sex sells, Gary, even e-sex."

Graywood held back smiling in agreement and flipped to page fifty-six. He hand-covered Harl's scribbled notes for the film crew and concentrated on the printed voice-over: "Death penalty opponents argue how violent and vile prisoners deserve a dignified, human life. In time, they believe some bad people can change. We cannot identify who will find their inner goodness from those who will commit more outside evil, nor can we tell how long it may take them to discover so.

"The premise behind banishment in lieu of judicial execution is emblematic of our evolving humanity—banishment provides a chance, with enough time, for human beings to step into a larger heart. In the past, the death penalty symbolized society's knee-jerk embrace of reciprocal barbarism, yet today we have found within ourselves the audacious hope our American culture can do better."

Graywood turned to page fifty-seven: "Banishment to Siberia's Kamchatka is a dramatic change from the austere confinements allowed on past death rows.

"A decade ago, a condemned inmate sat alone in a stateside cell the size of a small, walk-in closet, perhaps permitted one hour each day for isolated exercise and a shower. He communicated with the outside world only by snail mail. Some lucky ones might have listened to a small radio.

"Prisontown's Ground Zero resembles those stark, death-row conditions but for one exception: it erased the foreboding anxieties of execution which had lurked in America before the Grand Compromise. Beyond Ground Zero is Circle One where the banished prisoner has earned a much improved living condition, even an opening to the rest of the world. It's an earned behavioral choice."

Page fifty-eight: "Circle One's Internet connections come from the prison library access telebooths, called PLATs. PLATs are the midwives to a similar phenomenon of proxy marriages seen on stateside death rows between the condemned prisoners and their female pen pals. Circle One inmates log on to multiple websites seeking contacts to fill their respective black books of willing correspondents. The pen-pal-like, email relationships mature into e-dates with or without sexual e-intimacy, which in Prisontown jargon is labeled PLAT-sex. Even e-engagements and e-marriages may follow. Many relationships are compromised by e-bigamy. Some prisoners sweet talk their numerous contacts into personal e-harems, often including six or more e-wives."

Graywood flipped to page fifty-nine: "The harems are graded into the four ranks of bronze, silver, gold, and platinum. A bronze harem sports a minimum of three e-wives with at least one photo-perfect blonde who must reside in California or Florida. Silver is the bronze requirement increased to six e-wives. If the six e-consorts hail from six different states and all show blonde perfection, then the inmate is crowned sheikh of a gold harem. Platinum status is reserved for any harem of six or more e-spouses consisting of two blondes, one each from California and Florida, and at least one e-wife from a country in Europe, Africa, Asia, or Latin America.

"PLAT time availability for each Circle One prisoner often cramps the creation of larger harems. Significant PLAT minutes are expended every week on precious harem maintenance. But the shrewd Circle One prisoner entrepreneurs reserve a few PLAT minutes to barter other favors or delve into flashes of e-cheating. Because no e-wife ever visits Prisontown in person, this Internet activity remains immune to social ridicule, modifications, or threats from any disadvantaged e-partner or partners."

Harl had underlined page sixty all in red: "Smarter prisoners strengthen their relationships by encouraging handwritten letters and photographs with selected e-wives. Lacking access to printers or fax machines, they request their e-partners mail provocative posed pictures. Nude and semi-nude prints are the most coveted. They are hung on the bunkroom walls, traded as baseball cards, or sold for extra PLAT minutes."

Graywood closed the script and contemplated the proxy marriages. Most harems were heterosexual and headed by a sheikh or a pre-sheikh, designated as a Potentate. And "Potate" was the shortened term often used. Yet other significant e-households existed such as clandestine homosexual "Pens" controlled by a "Peacock." Plus a handful of banished prisoners had bloomed to become "Shepherds" of bi-sexual "Herds." These other groups, Pens and Herds, Harl had edited out from the documentary.

Graywood reasoned the women involved in e-marriages by proxy had to have received something too. Both parties must have felt a net gain, or the relationship wouldn't exist. Because e-romance was physically never consummated, that alone promised a sizable element of safety. Plus it appeared exciting and wicked—to be ardently allied to a banished man, the worst of the bad boys, rather than a boring, stateside male gave the e-wife something to flaunt. Her clique, in turn, viewed her as interesting too.

Perhaps other impulses motivated these women. Were they trying to reason through past violence or sexual abuses? Or had their compassions to nurture been ignited by their e-husbands' pitiful confinements in a faraway land forever?

Possibly they had rationalized achieving, at last, society's relentless requirement to marry. Yet they expended scant physical and emotional resources on the token men, locked up like convenient shoes or dolls in closets to be taken out on effortless electronic whims to be worn or played with … a true expression of their power.

Maren crossed Graywood's mind. Leaning into the seat back, he stretched the comparison: it's a fashion statement to have a relationship with a banished prisoner … an accessory to die for in order to make oneself more exciting and unique.

Whatever motivated an e-wife had to make sense for her own good reasons.

Manipulation of women by men, and men by women, had always been in play for money, sexual stimulation, and sport. Once a Circle One prisoner established an e-harem, he remained loath to return to Ground Zero for any prison rule infractions.

The guards monitored the inmates' Internet keystrokes from the communications section on the headquarters top floor. These proxy e-relationships were tolerated, overall, as acceptable carrots that stabilized inmate behavior.

Still, a few convicts bounced back and forth between Ground Zero and Circle One. They sought exclusion from the higher-order social responsibilities layered into the latter. In their minds, at times, Ground Zero grew akin to a vacation refuge or monastery.

The 767 arched across the International Dateline.

For Graywood, there existed no science to explain the evil manipulations in murder. It seemed too gracious to say murderers simply chose not to appreciate the rules of right and wrong for their culture and century. No, there had to be more. Lethal aggression so far in excess of reciprocity suggested, at the minimum, wiring deficiencies within the felon's orbitofrontal and medial-frontal lobes.

Graywood recalled the three-dimensional MRI and magnetoencephalographic tests Bobby had undergone at the University of Washington. The multi-colored splotches and ribbons revealed cortical maps that processed information through complex neural networks that widely interacted between brain regions. When instructed to do exact arithmetic, Bobby's left side showed greater activity. When asked to approximate a calculation, bilateral distributions more equally occurred. Perhaps MRI-ing some prisoners in 3-D might light up an area map and identify the brain's homicidal center.

Graywood pondered how much plasticity still existed within a killer's head to foster the abilities to learn and adapt during banishment. Would any felon have the coping capacity like Bobby? And to what extent would society accept an individual's willpower being limited by the integrity and molding capability of his or her brain? All minds were not equal—morality, marriage, and murder were individualized.

From e-wives to homicide to Bobby, the screenplay had triggered another attempt by Graywood to make sense of the world. He pushed them all away to avoid a looming numbness. With tired eyes and aching neck, he set aside the manila binder and forced sleep.

The Kamchatka peninsula, part of the ring of fire, might suffer earthquakes or volcanic-induced disasters that could overwhelm the medical facilities at the prison and nearby Petropavlovsk.

In 2012 when Graywood had organized the triage and evacuation procedures with Russian counterparts, they cautioned how large parts of Petropavlovsk—similar to coastal Alaska—were threatened by tsunami. The potential casualty risk had forced authorities to broaden the local contingency responses into a regional Pacific strategy with linkages to Alaska and northern Japan. Developing those international commitments had excited Graywood as much as when Bobby had scored a hockey goal for O'Malley Elementary.

After the child's death, Graywood expanded the emergency care document to give birth to KAMI, the Kamchatka Alaska Medical Initiative. He bound together the Petropavlovsk and Anchorage medical communities once the diplomatic blessings had been obtained from the United States and Russia. He borrowed the University of Washington's business model for medical school support to Wyoming, Alaska, Montana, and Idaho, and he advanced overlapping partnerships between Prisontown's medical department, Anchorage's Providence Regional Medical Center, Elmendorf's Medical Group, Seattle's University of Washington medical school, and Petropavlovsk's Peoples' Hospitals Numbers One and Two.

Advancing beyond regional mass casualty management, Graywood championed the medical training opportunities available at Prisontown and Petropavlovsk. At times he felt like the secretary of health for a third world country who advocated unique, real-world experiences in rural and semi-rural health care.

In September 2017, he implemented the initial collaboration by the University of Washington with Kamchatka: UW placed seven donated pacemakers into patients with heart disease—three prisoners, one prison guard, and three Petropavlovsk residents. All procedures were performed at Peoples' Hospital Number One.

UW provided the placement team of one staff cardiac surgeon, two doctors in residency training, one anesthesiologist, and a recovery nurse. They flew to Avacha Bay, courtesy of Elmendorf's Boeing 767. To erase a technical shortfall identified in preparation for the mission, they brought and donated the missing equipment needed at Petropavlovsk's facility.

Prisontown sent its senior nurse and two operating-room technicians to provide liaison with the Russian hospital. It also provided lodging for the visitors and meals produced by its farms and bakery.

Besides the cost-free transportation, Elmendorf detailed a medical evaluator to compile a report for the Department of Defense for future planning. The assessment had rated the medical exercise successful. Highlights included:

- The University of Washington staff surgeon performed the inaugural pacemaker insertion; the two resident surgeons split the remaining six cases for first-rate training experiences.
- Seven patients had improved heart function.
- Prisontown nurses initiated a new training proficiency.
- Hospital Number One received serviceable equipment that would have been discarded in the United States.

The positive DOD evaluation was forwarded to the Departments of State and Justice. It confirmed Colonel Sulmasy's initiative for making the documentary.

In contrast to the droll report, within Graywood, the exquisite mission had verified his piggyback insertion of scarce resources onto existing medical structures and operations. In a greater sense, it had created a fresh, tangible strand to connect the northern Pacific medical communities from Kamchatka to Alaska to Washington. Most important to him—the right care had been given at the right place, at the right time, to patients, regardless of social standing. Ethics, science, and economics had combined to do the correct thing and embraced a bold future in the form of KAMI.

Graywood opened his eyes … less than an hour to Petropavlovsk by his wristwatch. He perused the health parts in the screenplay and fumbled past the rest.

Jotting at the top of Harl's scene-by-scene sequencing notes, Graywood suggested juxtaposing the 181 Circle Three convicts selected for full-time work at Tri-P's prefab factory against the sixty-three felons who'd volunteered to be caregiver aides in the prison's medical department. Tri-P paid the inmates wages; Graywood paid zero. The contrasts and similarities between remunerated and volunteer prison labor might help to humanize the murderers to the viewing public.

The screenplay had four pages dedicated to "Kamchatka, the Musical," a prison-wide morale and welfare activity, as well as a segment on "The Banished Wife Calendar." Graywood recommended both pared down or eliminated, especially the narcissistic pin-ups. In the script's margins he penned two replacement shoots: felons who donated to the international red-blood-cell transplant program and inmates who clamored to become patients for the visiting students from Washington and Oregon dental schools.

Tri-P had constructed a double-suite dental module, transportable in a C-130, the workhorse cargo plane for the third world. Before volunteer dentists repaired decayed teeth somewhere in the boondocks, Graywood had arranged to fly them to Prisontown and orientate on the unit's characteristics: they provided oral care to the guards and prisoners and gave feedback to Tri-P. Subsequently, he recruited several schools and community colleges to join up and contribute free dental care to the developing world and send their faculty, students, assistants, and hygienists to Kamchatka for familiarization. Elmendorf's 767 provided free transportation, and the lodging and meals came courtesy of Prisontown.

Graywood also initiated a voluntary program for prisoners to donate into the worldwide, allergenic hematopoietic cell transplant program. HCT served as the curative treatment for victims living with sickle-cell disease. In the prior decade, HCT protocols to treat sickle-cell patients had improved to reduce infection and the inherent toxicity of graft-versus-host disease. Yet the shortage of human leukocyte-antigen-identical donors remained the main barrier to HCT's widespread use.

Whenever found as suitable, the inmates accurately matched to patients helped to fill the treatment gap until biogenetic research discovered the means to correct the sickle-cell patient's actual genetic code and allow each to then make normal hemoglobin instead.

Otherwise, Graywood concurred with Harl's documentary film as written and the warts-and-all conclusion that wove together Prisontown, American culture, and Alpha-Omega's future: "Health care rendered today in Kamchatka foretells the future of health care administered under Alpha-Omega. All countries ration their good medical care, and sadly, some must ration all of it, both good and bad."

In the film's credits, the female narrator questioned her audience one final time: "When Alpha-Omega runs a deficit due to our demands for improved quality and access, will our government increase the VAT to cover the expanding costs or will people with ailments such as Down's syndrome or Alzheimer's be excluded, partially or wholly disguised or not, by caps on their care? The winnowed access to health care has profound implications on the future ways our country will treat its elderly, its infirmed, and its criminals … and how we Americans will ultimately think of ourselves. Should we fear our pragmatism if it slants us away from generosity? If so, perhaps our country needs what's found within KAMI."

"Jen, I'm sending the access codes from the French Ministry of Health so you can open files on their securities exchange investigation of CPI," Nick said over the phone.

"What's that all about?" she replied, setting a mug of tea on her office desk so to log on NIH's website.

"CPI wasn't above board in its business before getting dismembered and sold. I skimmed some of it but don't have time to pick apart every page."

"And you want me to get into your weeds."

"Jen, you're the best to find unethical behavior in research," soothed Nick.

"Does this earn me a trip to Paris?"

"Well, who knows? I guess they'd like to meet you."

"That might be good or bad, depending on what I find," she scoffed.

"Jen, you're so good for doing this for me."

"Maybe, I suppose," her voice softened as she closed the cellphone. She was doing it to solve the grotesque mystery.

She'd once saved her youngest brother from drowning in the Pacific. The summer before Jennelle entered college in San Francisco, the Daniels family had vacationed on California's Ventura Beach. A rogue wave had swallowed precocious little Kent. She'd fought the oblivious tide to reach him in time, beating the lifeguard by a minute.

Bobby was like Kent once. She was doing it for Bobby … and Gary.

Before Nick's call, Jennelle had uncovered that the bulk of CPI's immunization shipment to Alaska in 2006 had gone to Juneau's borough for distribution to outlying primary-care clinics. The rest had been stockpiled at Anchorage to cover vaccine gaps elsewhere within the state—sixty doses had been routed to erase a shortfall in Glennallen. It was strange that the cases of Bobby's disease traced to Alaska had received CPI's VaroCell at either a federal or state public health clinic. For now in the investigation, that connection only made a suspected, not actual, association.

Villages in Alaska also hid methamphetamine laboratories. Jennelle expected any day the Drug Enforcement Administration's report detailing the locations of meth labs uncovered and destroyed since 2005. If they overlapped with the clinics that received the CPI product, she'd have a second, plausible association.

Thankful not having to hack into the French Ministry of Health, Jennelle set to work with Nick's codes. Within an hour, she concluded CPI and the French-British conglomerate it was sold to had been corrupt—profound greed had biased their research. CPI's scientists had revealed confidential information to a select group of elite hedge fund investors who'd sought out results not yet published or announced.

International fund managers in 2005 had searched for secondary derivatives in the biotech market, primarily the companies headquartered in the United States and Western Europe. They correlated stock security risks and dollar fluctuations to the euro to create annual yields of 20 percent or more. They bankrolled the lead investigators and doctors of various corporations for inside information on drugs and vaccines under development and timed their market transactions to minimize risk.

Matching researchers who agreed to divulge critical knowledge to Wall Street and European stock-market professionals provided the cardinal means for insider success. Monetary compensation swayed willing scientists to leak whether a pharmaceutical's new product tested better than a competitor's or would receive FDA or EU approval. By paying four to five hundred euros, or the dollar equivalent, an hour, more than thirty thousand researchers had signed onto an intermediary matchmaker registry that brought scientists and investment professionals face to face.

Timing was critical. If the financial wizards knew in advance of a superior result compared to a competitor's drug or vaccine, they'd buy the company's stock at its current low price and sell it high once the product's apparent success was announced. Conversely, if studies revealed less benefit than a competing brand or a documented side effect which harmed consumers, then the biotech's shares were sold short to fatten portfolios before the general press release. A 40-percent return or more was possible within two or three weeks by the adroit executions of divulged secrets.

Livid, Jennelle simplified the financial victimization of the public as a sure-fire conduit to introduce bias into research. Forget the ordinary investors swindled by fund managers. Worse were the doctors talking for a fee when they knew better: They'd make off-the-cuff summaries based on incomplete data or on-going collections of results that lacked adequate statistical analysis. A researcher might even prematurely suggest a survival benefit for a cutting-edge drug or immunization when the opposite occurred later, such as with the 2007 HIV inoculation trial that increased the risk of illness rather than prevented it. And regrettably, the development pipeline for other competing products that truly were life-saving might be abandoned. Society dearly paid many times over.

Jennelle accessed the meeting minutes and documents from the European Medicines Agency to understand how CPI's cloned-cell vaccine had received permission for public use. She only found "Approval Pending" stamped in French and English on a letter addressed to CPI dated 11 November 2005. That married well with the hedge-fund practice to game the system: Buy 9 percent of the company, distribute the official "Approval Pending" letter, plus talk up the product to increase the company's potential commercial value … then unload the stock for a handsome return in less than six weeks.

She also uncovered a disconnect: In February 2007, CPI pulled its application request from the European agency. Why?

Jennelle tracked countless CPI files and uncovered the camouflaged sale orders that revealed the product lacked market competitiveness unless sold below cost. In 2006, a vaccine lot was distributed gratis to the French national health-care system, another twenty thousand doses sent to Senegal, and six thousand to Alaska. She found nothing more on deliveries. CPI had unloaded the product to give the appearance of building market share.

She discovered a company memorandum, dated 12 March 2006, that endorsed an advertisement brochure touting tentative immunization sales to Africa, the Americas, and Europe, soon to be followed by Asia. It smacked of hedge fund manipulation.

How the biotech product had gotten past FDA to enter Alaska rankled Jennelle the most. She logged out France and plowed through related, confidential FDA files. A four-hour search found the critical linkage. The same letter, dated 11 November 2005, had been translated into English with a cover memo marked March 31, 2006. CPI had expressed a willingness to sell at below cost to introduce the inoculation into the United States after its successful applications in France and Africa.

Where were the final permits from FDA and the European Medicines Agency? Who'd dropped the ball?

Jennelle never found them. She suspected the commodity had entered the United States without FDA approval. Likewise, it appeared it had been exported at a financial loss to Senegal without European Medicines Agency certification.

These procedural lapses smacked of a CPI setup to recoup money from a technologic sinkhole that had never been economically competitive. Jennelle inferred CPI's bigwigs were in bed with shady fund managers. Both parties had counted on the French government to act painstakingly deliberate with the approval process to allow sufficient time for them to manipulate the scam. She'd pass her suspicions to Nick and recommend adding legal authorities to their investigation.

Or had CPI been honorable? Perhaps the organization had denied bribing French officials to speed up the product's license, thus the bureaucrats had let it languish. From prior international experience, Jennelle knew the fastest way to retard anything in France was the refusal to wire a covert kickback.

Yet she could not dismiss the written exhortations of profit and pride contained in CPI's files. Their bioscientists wanted to show the world how immunizations created from cloned cells could be done. They proved their prowess for the same reason climbers conquered Mount Everest. No doubt it enhanced their future professional prospects as well: biotechnology trademarks this advanced placed them at the pinnacle for future benefits and prestige in the medical-industrial complex. Competing biotech companies would bid bundles for such skilled researchers and their hot technological insights.

At the same time, Jennelle detected within the correlated FDA records a quasi-political mission to encourage medical usage of embryonic stem cells. Increased stem cell applications discovered by foreign scientists might force the Bush administration to reverse course and expand federal funding to develop human embryonic stem cell lines in the United States. Could such an agenda have motivated someone within the FDA to allow an unlicensed French vaccine into the country in 2006?

And Jennelle speculated on how the cloned VaroCell presented a new type of microorganism. It had been released on humankind without knowing any of its unintended consequences. Most advanced drugs and vaccines, when marketed to the public, have unknowns not detected within the clinical trials leading to initial FDA approval. Only after three or more years of clinical exposure will the dangerous side effects become reported. If the agent does more harm than good, only then is it recalled.

If VaroCell lacked FDA approval, no recall could have happened.

"That does it for the Canadian system and how it compares to our Alpha-Omega for providing health care," concluded Graywood. He switched off PowerPoint and keyed reference notes on the questions asked for future use.

The discussion had compared the pros and cons of health care delivery in the United States, Great Britain, and Canada.

"Next week we'll cover intentional and unintentional biases in the medical literature. See you then."

Inconspicuous, Jennelle had entered the classroom as Graywood finished. The place where Bearhead often sat was empty. Once the last student had exited, she approached, pensive eyes averted back and forth toward the composite ceiling. In her brightest voice, she said, "You certainly cover a host of subjects with this course of yours, Gary."

"Jen! When did you sneak in?"

"Just the very end." Torn, she looked away. "Didn't see Monroe. Did he leave early?"

"He couldn't talk today; bad case of bronchitis. So the students get a free hour."

"I hope he's not too ill."

"He'll be okay. I wish he'd quit smoking," said Graywood. "So are you here to remind me to send updated hep C results from Prisontown?"

"You're only two weeks late," she kidded. *If only you knew why I'm here.* "Gary, I know you're extremely busy on the film the air force is putting together."

"I promise I'll head straight back to Elmendorf and zip everything over."

"That'll be fine," she uttered. Her courageous voice had failed to launch into Bobby's illness. "Gary, I have data back in my office I want to show you."

Impervious, he opened his cellphone to check appointments. "Shoot! I've gotta hustle back for a meeting with Sulmasy. Jen, if I come tomorrow afternoon at four, I'll have enough time to finish your hep C report and can bring it over myself. Maybe when we're done, we can head out for some dinner."

"I'd like that, Gary."

"Great. See you then." He rushed away.

Head bowed, she crumbled at a student's table.

How would she tell him her suspicions about Bobby's disease?

CHAPTER TWENTY-THREE

A Testament

Graywood perused the four Alaskan maps coded with bright red, blue, green, and yellow pins. An atlas of the Lower Forty-eight and one of Senegal covered the opposite walls in Jennelle's Grace Hall office.

She breezed through his hep C follow-up report on Kamchatka and pronounced it first-rate. Switching gears, she detailed the associations implied within the cartographic portraits regarding the mysterious outbreak of a neurodegenerative disease with seizures on three continents.

Graywood simply listened.

Jennelle wove in the work completed so far by WHO, NIH, and French investigators. She pointed to Masi's map and asked, "By chance, Gary, did you ever take Bobby to one of these clinics?"

"Which clinics?"

"The ones marked in red."

His eyes focused on the layout.

She waited the longest two minutes.

"No. How'd you come up with this?" he asked, emitting a vocal edge she'd never heard.

Jennelle recounted Masi's construction of the visual aid with Bearhead's careful help and how her investigation had stemmed from it. She summarized the working hypothesis that CPI's cloned product seemed the probable agent for the disease.

"You sure Bobby never went to any of these clinics and got this vaccine, Gary?"

"Jen," he curtly declared, "I never took him on my flights that checked the clinics."

All the red herrings he'd once pursued on Bobby resurfaced. All the years he'd desperately tilled and forgotten flooded back. All those illogical tests he'd ordered to discover a remote cause for his son's disease—so many—yet he'd never considered a rogue inoculation.

Even Bobby's biopsy that Jennelle had requested came back inconclusive: "generalized neuronal atrophy lacking significant inflammatory markers of massed T-cells, activated microglial cells, or reactive astrogliosis." It had ruled out chronic occult encephalitis, even an unknown variant of Rasmussen syndrome and other rare maladies.

But an unregulated vaccine?

With God's help, Graywood had locked up frustrated grief at Campsite with the Seven Sisters and moved forward to live with a bit of purpose. Now the dreaded ghosts of anguish clamored to escape. He grappled for control.

"You know what this sounds like, Jen?" cracked Graywood's voice.

Staying silent, she looked expectant.

He cleared his throat. "This reminds me of that old Nigerian polio outbreak from an overripe oral vaccine you solved a decade ago," he said, with harshness. "You're overreaching."

Rolling her eyes, Jennelle held back escalating into argument. "I don't know for sure, Gary," she intoned neutrally. "All our investigations are still incomplete but appear to point this way."

"One basically could say you want to relive your past success," he brusquely added, thinking out loud.

Despite the deflation jumbled with ripples of anger, Jennelle kept composed. Any other colleague who'd chided this way would not have escaped without a blistering counterattack. She and Graywood were friends … once they'd been lovers. She wisely let him vent.

"And what does the connection to meth have to do with it?" he snidely asked. "Is it a cause too, or a cofactor, or nothing but coincidence?"

She stomped to the map with meth lab locations circled in school-bus orange that the Drug Enforcement Administration and Alaskan police had destroyed since 2004. In steady controlled tones, she replied, "Earlier, I'd suspected an unknown contaminate cut into the meth might have caused the outbreak." Methodically shaking her head side to side, she elaborated, "When we followed up the abuse, it helped us capture more potential cases in the US and Senegal. Still, that didn't come close to explaining everyone affected."

"So how close did it come?"

"Near 30 percent initially. NIH and the French investigators went back through each patient's history and got 54 percent of the victims or their families admitting to some form of illegal drug.

"Not much better than flipping a coin," Graywood said, distracted. "I bet there was some coercion, too." He wheeled to dissect Masi's prodigious work, but air ceased to move from his lungs.

Gritting teeth, Jennelle went to her desk, thumbed Graywood's hep C report for overlooked errors, and waited for him to normalize.

Eyes glued to Masi's chart work, he back-stepped to the doorway.

"Lost my appetite, Jen. I'm sorry I'm not good company tonight." The man's blue eyes brooded in a much paler face, like two trout trapped in eddies. "Can I offer a rain check for later?"

"Yes, of course, Gary. I hope it won't be a long drought," she encouraged.

Looking down, he left.

She'd miscalculated his response to her collaboration with NIH. Something revealed or inferred had twisted deep to the core.

Graywood had remembered bringing to Snowline Drive a vial of an advanced varicella immunization to inoculate Bobby before he'd turned six years old. Doctor Timm's practice had suspended administrating vaccines that year due to Alaska deferring certain prevention subsidies to private clinics in order to pare budgetary costs as promised during the run up to the state election at that time. Yet O'Malley Elementary School had mandated that its first-graders attain all required injections for admittance.

Graywood also had recalled recruiting Cub to take the same shot to force Bobby to tolerate the needle-stick without a tantrum in front of his best friend. Because Cub exhibited strapping good health, Graywood discounted a cause-and-effect connection between this chicken pox product Jennelle suspected and the lethal illness Bobby had suffered.

Yet her reasoning made him anxious, and the hunger to uncover and condemn whatever had killed his son returned in pernicious full force.

To quell suspicions, Graywood accessed Nick Severstal's NIH website. Masi's map with the affected villages circled in red pointed the way.

"What are you going to carve with this?" Graywood strained, hoisting the end of a twenty foot beam toward Bearhead's back porch.

"It's my practice pole," grunted the artist.

"What? How's that?"

"My pole to practice on." Bearhead set the timber's opposite edge on a support block below the awning. Graywood did likewise. "That'll help air keep her dry," observed the sculptor. He placed both hands on the shaft and rendered an inaudible blessing.

The hewn wood from majestic western red cedar held natural antifungal properties that prevented rot—ideal for canoes, houses, and totems. For Bearhead and the First Peoples, it possessed great spiritual importance.

Completing the tree-of-life prayer, Bearhead looked skyward. He nodded twice to affirm an occult message and then said, "Let's go in and eat."

"What do you want to practice on?" asked Graywood, puzzled.

They crossed the carving room. The mastodon-elephant remained paired with the nameless, still incomplete, winged creature.

"This summer we're raising a totem at the potlatch. My skills need work."

The oolong-tea-scented kitchen beckoned.

Graywood detoured to wash hands. An elongated, brass ashtray stood on patrol by the toilet. Menthol tanged the bathroom's air. Roe had switched cigarette brands again.

Tobacco was a funny thing—a pleasure and evil to Bearhead—which parched the throat whenever indulged too much. Everybody growing up in Chitina had smoked.

Bearhead had made one serious attempt to quit while in Tokyo as an assistant chef dicing overlapping jobs along *Shibuya Crossing*. The other cooks and scullery crews had exhaled enough second-hand smoke to where he didn't need to add to it first-hand. Despite nicotine being his strongest craving, there was something else in the fumes discharged by these kitchen co-workers that tempered him from lighting up. The peculiar qualities inhaled from Tokyo's culinary hazes, however, were lost once he migrated to Bangkok. He restarted the habit and never tried to stop thereafter.

Graywood towel-dried his hands and recalled how his mother had smoked to death. Roe would do the same. Why couldn't they stop? What cemented them to nefarious addiction? It caused her death and would shorten Roe's life too.

Looking in the mirror, Graywood reengaged reflected eyes with the haunting questions left over from Bobby's funeral. Why did his boy have to die? What caused it?

As a teenager Graywood had accepted his father's untimely death. As a young man, he'd willed to move on after scattering his mother's ashes in Oregon. Yet grave be damned, he could not let Bobby go. Jennelle's working hypothesis derived from the NIH investigation had made that even more impossible. He washed hands a second time.

"Still smoking, Roe?" Graywood half-asked, half declared when entering the kitchen.

"Only when I shit."

Bearhead brought to the table two tureens of curry soup floating chunks of celery, fennel, and sweet potatoes. A platter of smoked mozzarella wedges on brittle flatbread squares completed the meal.

"Believe it or not, Gary, I learned this recipe exploring Cairo. It's one of my favorites."

"In heaven's name, Roe," shifted Graywood, "I don't believe you need practice cutting on wood."

Bearhead spoon-dribbled curry broth on a cheese square and bit off half. "I must skill up, Gary, to shape a big cedar into what's needed for the totem." He chewed the rest and poured tea into two porcelain goblets. "For Chitina, it'll top sixty feet. I'll craft the one here at one-third scale."

Impressed with the sizes, Graywood asked, "So when you're done, what'll happen to the twenty-footer?"

"Give it away."

"Come on, Roe, your models are one-of-a-kind and worth a whole lot."

Bearhead smiled and dipped a second wedge in his bowl. "It'll have many errors to mask its merit. Gary, it's humanlike … cannot be priced. So I give it away, a daughter in marriage to whoever will have and care for her." He popped the saturated bread into his mouth.

The two Ravens supped and gossiped about Chitina village, the Coldsnow sisters, Cub, and Piper and his fourth wife. Graywood avoided Jennelle's investigation.

Bearhead retrieved a dessert hidden in the oven and announced, "Warm lemon tart. Hope you want some."

"Please."

Bearhead pulled lemon sorbet and a plate of lemon slices from the refrigerator. He scooped a frozen sphere on Graywood's turnover and garnished it with three citrus pieces. "I get high on curry and lemon," he said, eyes sparkling. "Wish I could smoke 'em."

A nameless fifth taste abided on the tongue. It searched for the subtle existence in any food being prepared, and it refined and rounded out the other four—sweet, salty, sour, and bitter. It remained the chef's duty to bring that essence out with reverence and respect. A dash of self-humor helped too.

Partway into dessert, Graywood tackled the reason for coming. "Jen told me about the NIH investigation and asked for help," he said, face tilted down. He'd embraced the art of diplomatic mendacity from Emrick where a falsehood was blended into a truth. Jennelle had never asked for assistance.

"I'm amazed you're getting involved," returned Bearhead. "Won't it concern a sickness like what could've affected Bobby?"

"Maybe. I think all the time about him and that," answered Graywood, downcast. "I gotta find out anything and everything that would've killed him."

"So what are you going to do?" Bearhead wished Graywood went on with life but knew he'd stay stuck until he'd found the answers on his child's death. The investigation might give clarity.

"Jen and I figured I'd start double-checking the information Masi mapped out."

"I know it well, Gary. I helped him put it together."

"Yeah, and Jen told me about your web of village elders. I think it's time to contact them for updates and compare them with the stuff Nick Severstal has found out at NIH."

"The elders talk at noon on Tuesdays and Fridays. I'll introduce you."

"Good. Your office?"

"Nah, I use an account in the Consortium Library."

"Why there?"

"It keeps the library staff employed when we use their equipment."

"Well that doesn't make much sense, but whatever. Guess it's the university mindset."

"I don't mind," declared Bearhead.

"Before I go, Roe, you've got to tell me what the totem is really for." Another tactic Graywood learned from Emrick in delivering believable falsehoods was swiftly derailing the person one spoke to.

"Ah, Gary, what do you mean?"

"You've never carved a totem for your potlatch, and your artistic skills are still damn fine. You invited me to lunch for a reason. I think you're up to something."

"I need a smoke."

"Don't do that, you old fart."

Exasperated, Bearhead came clean. "It's a mortuary pole for Bobby."

"Damn it, Roe!" Angered and surprised at how his own ruse had actually hit true, Graywood regrouped and pressed. "I've told you before not to do that."

"I know, I know, Gary, but he's my godson. It's my custom. It'll help me mourn him."

"I'm not ready for that, Roe. Please listen to me! That's my custom."

"Okay, okay, okay … I'll wait."

"Thanks."

Stone-like, they sat a long time inhaling lemon-scented kitchen air and then cleared the table in silence.

Graywood exited the front door to the old Subaru.

"See you Friday noon, Gary. I'm in the second computer row."

Graywood postponed scanning Prisontown's electronic chatter or Elmendorf's flight manifest. He reported a sink faucet needing repair in the staff men's room nearest his office before he accessed Jennelle and Nick's CPI files.

A CPI offshoot had entered the cloned livestock market. The whole point of cloning was creation of animals with desirable qualities, such as champion milkers, excellent fat marbling, or desired body distribution of meat. By cloning the original, farmers and ranchers could produce more offspring possessing those preferred traits for human consumption. The public would not eat the clones; they'd eat the children of clones.

But cloning remained an imperfect science in the decade after CPI was cleaved and sold. It took several attempts to birth a healthy animal, and the entire process often overstressed the clones as much as the animals they'd been cloned from.

Graywood believed to intrude this way into the animal realm played God. Even more absurd were CPI's attempts to produce a human vaccine from cloned tissue substrates. The state of cloning knowledge at CPI's time could not safely support the intended mission. They had tried to force bioscience to run before it could walk.

Overall, science lacked the higher levels of intelligence necessary to understand fully the human genome's biopsychology. Graywood feared that probing around it for profit would spawn a number of mistakes.

His cellphone jingled …

"Say Gary, I need help getting *Sky Woman* switched over to floats," declared Piper.

"When do you want me at the hangar?"

"Well, right now, if you can."

Not in the mood for Kamchatka or the sway through CPI, Graywood replied, "I'll be there pronto. You're buying drinks when we're done."

"Damn straight!"

"How many years we come to GB's?" asked Piper, signaling for the customary martini.

"Right when I started flight lessons," answered Graywood with a pencil-thin grin. He scouted the bar's liquor display for his favorite vodka to chase down Moose Drool beer … a mundane combo to confine the anguish creeping within his saner borders.

Both pilots remained mute. They mellowed the initial round more out of reflex than fatigue. As long as they'd known each other, Piper had inclined toward the less talkative. Since Bobby's death, Graywood had devolved to soundless introspection as well. But today Piper discerned Graywood's tied tongue was permanent. After ordering the second hit, he proclaimed, "Gary, I want to give you something special."

Graywood hesitated to respond, not wanting whatever it was.

"This year at freeze-up, I'll be sixty-six."

"Piper never mentions his age," thought Graywood. "Something big's coming. Hope it's not bad like cancer."

Piper belched from the half-gone cocktail and dropped the surprise. "I'm gonna shut down the flyin' business and put the Beaver up for sale."

Motionless, they spied each other.

Graywood's disbelief shrugged to confusion. In the past, he'd pepper questions about such a life-changing event, as he'd done when stupid Piper had divorced sweet Rachel to marry the serpentine bitch. Now everything swirled in uneasy flux. Adding his partner's announcement only cycled more turbulence and gnawed him nervous.

"Why? You're one of the best," said Graywood, attempting to condense the uneasiness.

"I'm an old bush pilot who's lived long enough to collect Social Security, whatever it's worth."

"Phhhth! It's worth only whatever the government cuts payouts to match the taxes grabbed away from the younger workforce."

Piper sparred back, "Then one day that'll be worth less than co-pilot's snot blown on your instrument panel."

Graywood was half-inclined to dismember Piper's caustic reply, but he'd lost the mental surge to pry into the real reasons for Piper giving up his wings. And retirement had to happen sometime. Both aviators had to adapt.

Graywood envied Piper's cool ability to handle life's great changes. In flying and artistry, Piper's courageous, independent spirit had dazzled.

He'd explored the wilderness to capture brilliant places on canvas and had survived shit-clearing encounters with landslides, moose, and bears, plus the most tenacious weather Alaska had ever stewed. With four marriages added in, time had ripened the bush pilot into the witty, grouchy, and generous man he now appeared, despite the advance of years.

Graywood feared never getting beyond the colorless numbness of Bobby's death … an excruciating cross far heavier to shoulder than all those that burdened his longtime friend. Why should he probe Piper on quitting the air-taxi business when he couldn't understand himself or God for what had happened to his son?

Piper squared up and uttered, "I'm losin' my balance to where I'm afraid to fly."

"What?" Graywood saw defeat in Piper's eyes.

"I'm losin' my ways with the Beaver and *Sky Woman* … I can't sense wing air like I used to." He stroked tired hands over a broken face.

Astonished, Graywood felt Piper's stunning hurt. "I'm sorry your reflexes are going."

"Hell, man, they're shot to nothing!" Piper cut swift to his trump card. "Gary, I want you to have my share of *Sky Woman*."

Guided by Masi's map and the scribbled notes from Bearhead's tribal elders' Skype, Graywood reworked each known Alaskan case of neurodegenerative disease with seizures.

From Jennelle and Nick's websites, he verified the chicken-pox product he'd procured from the Anchorage Community Clinic in August 2006 had indeed been CPI manufactured. The records at that time indicated no other varicella vaccine had been stored in the facility, so it was the biotech product injected into Bobby's and Cub's arms.

If Jennelle suspected CPI's vaccine as the potential agent, what protection had Cub possessed then that Bobby lacked? What spared him from the inoculum's unintended, devastating effects? Was it Cub's older age at the time of immunization? Possibly was it the protective effects from swelling pubertal hormones in the half-dozen or so years afterwards? Or anything else? Did Bobby have exposure to something Cub didn't that made him vulnerable?

Graywood compared both boys … They differed in four ways: parents, age, medical history, and prescribed drugs … none for Cub, yet for Bobby numerous anti-seizure drugs and, before all those, the sustained-release Ritalin … Ritalin!

Prescribed to treat ADHD, the active ingredient in all forms of Ritalin was methylphenidate hydrochloride. Earlier in Jennelle's office, the methamphetamine association she had cautiously connected to the international epidemic had made Graywood uneasy. Now he understood the ensuing rancor toward her and the cancelled dinner date—derivatives of meth, such as amphetamine and dextroamphetamine, had been prescribed in the past to treat ADHD. Could brain pathways exposed to ADHD medications such as Ritalin and meth derivatives, or even meth itself, be crucial to causing the lethal effects Jennelle had connected to CPI's product?

Graywood pursued the association for CPI vaccine exposure and ADHD treatments. Did it have the legs to explain the other Alaskan cases similar to what Bobby had suffered?

He started with Juneau's four victims. Jennelle had uncovered that three presented histories of meth abuse. She'd followed that correlation throughout the state yet had investigated the fourth no further. Graywood contacted the Juneau school district's Special Ed program and verified the remaining individual had been a middle school student who had an integrated education plan with ADHD therapies. Graywood searched the student's electronic medical record for clinical confirmation but found none. He fired off requests for summaries of diagnoses and treatments to every clinic in Juneau that might have had a hard copy of her medical file.

Then Graywood contacted the tribal elders of each village in Bearhead's clique where at least one member had the disease: On Prince of Wales Island lived a boy in Klawock and a girl in Craig who'd received the CPI vaccine and had meth exposure; on Admiralty Island, one student in Angoon had Ritalin prescribed with the CPI inoculum codes in his health files; at Katkwaahitu by the Chilkat River northwest of Haines resided a student with CPI recorded, along with a newer ADHD med similar to Ritalin; on Chichagof Island, a deceased boy from Hoonah village had an apparent CPI immunization and episodes of meth abuse; and so it went. Graywood combined the village data with updated sources from Skagway,

Haines, Sitka, Wrangell, and Petersburg—a third of the cases in Alaska had ADHD as a co-diagnosis.

Afraid to enter the uncanny findings into the office computer for statistical analysis, Graywood shaped the robust data set on paper instead. He constructed frequency tables and derived joint, marginal, and conditional probability grids. Utilizing a series of statistical tests that correlated the outcomes of neurodegenerative disease plus seizures, he found the dual events—receiving the CPI vaccine and having subsequent exposure to either methylphenidate or methamphetamine—to be strongly co-dependent variables.

Simplified, Cub and Bobby both got CPI's vaccine. Cub remained healthy, but Bobby died. Cub had no exposure to meth or Ritalin. Bobby did …

Shattered! The breath of blackness blew on Graywood's soul.

No way to whitewash the conclusions. In Graywood's mind, the analyzed facts turned as daggers. Worse, he'd injected his son with a cloned vaccine and had treated the boy's modest ADHD with the drug. Was Graywood destined to make two calamitous choices?

Embittered, he scourged his methods and analyses—data set insufficient, methods faulty, reasoning biased. He ripped the charts and graphs to ribbons. There had to be mistakes.

He departed Elmendorf and sought vodka stashed at home.

A sober Graywood emailed everything to Jennelle and Nick two days later. They'd find the errors he'd overlooked.

With French assistance, NIH had the unencumbered access to the Senegalese data and its superior vantage to determine what had happened worldwide. Graywood prayed their final analysis of Senegal's outbreak would contradict what he'd uncovered for Alaska.

Prior to the morning Skype with Nick, Jennelle munched Wheat Thins and read a translated Interpol summary from Lyon, France, forwarded by the Drug Enforcement Agency.

"Subject: 2000 to 2010 Illegal Drug Traffic between Asia, Africa, and Europe, Section IVc.

"A longstanding insurgency in Myanmar between the government and ethnic groups on the Thailand border had devolved into cauldrons of drug trafficking, cross-border criminality, and massive refugee flight. After the scorched-earth offensive in 1990 by the Myanmar army had failed to gain control in mountainous eastern and northern frontiers, the government switched to inducements. It negotiated with ethnic leaders, cut deals to clear-cut teak forests, and cultivated opium for export. Once a cease-fire was signed, soldiers were deployed to each village in rural northeastern Myanmar and ordered the population to grow opium for tax collection and shipment to aligned drug cartels.

"Disrupting the traditional farming culture, opium production and heroin addiction had become part of village life. Men imbibed drugs instead of working farms and relied on wives and daughters for income or sold family possessions to purchase more drugs.

"Ensuing power struggles between several district leaders and the government over monetary kickbacks from opium exports and tax collections led to crackdowns on poppy cultivation in areas of eastern Myanmar. As opium declined, criminal gangs in league with local leaders opted to manufacture methamphetamine and smuggle it through Thailand. With assistance or threats by terrorist groups demanding a cut in the trade, the methamphetamine was sold or resold to Indian Ocean countries and routed around the Horn of Africa to Western Sahara for shipment into major West African cities or trafficked to Europe.

"For decades the vast desert stretching from southwestern Algeria, Mauritania, and Western Sahara had remained a primary base for contraband traffickers. The area also provided havens for drug runners and terrorist sleeper cells.

"Midnight dashes across frontiers to elude detection by Customs agents or patrols, however, were rare feats whenever shipping methamphetamine into African counties. Sophisticated schemes to outwit authorities, instead, had become the norm. Deft ruses rigged piggyback methods to hide methamphetamine in foodstuffs arriving in ports from countries such as Australia and the United States that donated surpluses through the United Nations. When compared to manufactured goods crossing borders, access to these commodities remained effortless due to the lax chains of custody applied to bulky grain shipments.

"Agricultural products locally grown also were recruited as covers for methamphetamine transport. For example, a reliable secure route into and out of Dakar, Senegal, employed peanuts. Because peanut agriculture appeared an innocuous front for illegal drug shipments throughout Dakar and western Africa, it was harnessed by international drug traffickers for cocaine, opium tar, hashish, and Ecstasy. Wealth in Senegal appeared easy to come by with peanuts."

Jennelle chuckled at Interpol's conclusion and returned to deciphering the wall maps. She scrutinized the cross-border smuggling and methamphetamine labs in the Alaskan villages April Coldsnow had indicated. The North Pacific meth circuit passed from Myanmar through Java, Indonesia to Canada before doubling back on Alaska to enter Washington State by leaping around potential Canadian-US border interdictions.

Mexican cartel meth also routed along western Canadian ports, fought for sole control of the vital Alaska to Washington conduit, and bumped out the Myanmar supply chain. Near the turf war's end, Theo Nowell betrayed and drowned his smuggling partner, Johnny Toofish, in the Tasnuna River where it joined the Copper.

Jennelle had protected April for two years. Not disclosing Chitina's criminal activity to authorities had made her complicit. Tolerating illegal limbo was not her strength. Bewildered and emotionally paralyzed, if ever found out, she'd lose her federal job and serve time too. Somehow she'd have to ferret out the means to safeguard April yet stick DEA on Theo's tail.

The Wheat Thins had exhausted to crumbs, so she stretched and window dreamed. Cones of sunlight darted past broken clouds—spring in Anchorage. As done eleven years ago, the kelly-green trees leafed out brisk and full. She marveled how nature here transformed in such a few days, not the weeks Georgia needed.

Computer chimes interrupted the reverie: Nick had signed on Skype. Bittersweet, she returned to the work station.

"NIH worships looking at weird illnesses," crowed Nick, "and Jen, this is a beaut! From this disease outbreak, we've discovered whole new thought circles on cellular development."

"What are you talking about?" she asked.

"Redundant DNA in the nucleus of a neural cell, or junk DNA as some call it, communicates with mitochondrial DNA. We never suspected that."

"What? You're saying there's a connection between junk DNA and mitochondrial DNA?"

"Yeah, Jen, and it had to persist all the way back in primitive times up to today. It's like squaring a fresh, gigantic circle in our thinking about genetics and cellular development."

"Nick, dear," she said, holding a palm up to the screen to slow him down, "you want to explain how you and NIH got to such a shocker?"

"Recall you sent that frozen CPI vial from the Glennallen clinic," reviewed Nick, "along with your preliminary mapping of the cases and clinics where the other vaccine vials got sent." He drew a series of circles on a legal pad and framed it to the monitor for her to see. "Without that old CPI material, we wouldn't have solved so many abnormal biocellular processes so fast on what you call Bobby's disease."

He added line appendages to the circles and talked rapidly. "First we propagated the vaccine material and verified it was varicella DNA by polymerase chain reaction. Then we tagged some of it with green fluorescent protein and added its chemically colored cousins in orange, red, magenta, yellow, and violet." He labeled the central circle GFP.

"GFP stands for green fluorescent protein, right?" interrupted Jennelle.

"Yep." He penciled another group of six smaller circles and pressed on. "We injected them into discarded, living human embryos and employed DNA microarrays to study the genes and their manufactured proteins and where they went into action elsewhere inside and outside the nuclei. Our GFP techniques enabled us to simultaneously follow multiple cell lines and the proteins made by those cells."

"Nick," intruded Jennelle, "the microarrays should link particular genes to diseases that are quite complex, right?

"You bet. And we carefully set up GFP and its colored cousins to tag out the proto-brain embryonic cells and got a 'brainbow' of colors," he said proudly, gesturing with two extended fingers from each hand like quotation marks.

Nick drew a box at the pad's bottom with arrows directed to the cell groupings. "We digitalized the genetic codes in the brainbow and fed the data petabytes into our decamag-petaflop operating systems for analysis and theory testing."

While Nick delved in further with NIH's world-leading expertise in cellular biology and the workloads accomplished in-house or farmed out, Jennelle's mind disengaged and rolled through the developments in computers.

Intel, Microsoft, and Cray had worldwide involvement in the data-intensive human genome project undertaken in the year 2000 by scientists and bioengineers. In the eighteen years thereafter, computing power had accelerated within innovation cycles to create teragigaflop, petaflop, and mag-petaflop operating systems. The data petabytes and zetabytes mined, assembled, and processed from bioscientific research had led to unexpected, cutting-edge, microbiological insights. Similar endeavors had also hastened advancements in weather-system modeling, structural engineering, and national defense capabilities.

The state-of-the-art supercomputer at NIH operated at five orders of magnitude beyond the once highly touted Roadrunner supercomputer—a technologic gem from a decade earlier, jointly managed by IBM and the Los Alamos National Laboratory.

Tuning back in, Jennelle asked, "Nick, what did all your theories come up with?"

"We believe we've discovered an area on the embryo junk-DNA domain that got reactivated by CPI's vaccine. Once turned on, the junk DNA made RNA snips, called micro-RNA."

Nick repositioned the legal pad crammed with the interconnected, colored circles and lines for Jennelle to see clearer.

"Now, for a long time, we've known micro-RNA regulates a host of activities in the cells of animals and plants, but what really surprised us was the junk DNA got reactivated by CPI's product, and it played either a controlling or a damaging role in the cellular ontogeny of the embryos," explained Nick, voice swelling enthusiastically.

"Nick … ontogeny?" Jennelle questioned, overwhelmed. "Are you saying the vaccine interfered with natural development in embryos by turning on some junk DNA?"

"Yeah."

"You better talk me through this."

"Sure, Jen. Our genes are made of DNA, and they collaborate with thousands of other strands of DNA genes, which ultimately program the developmental processes that make all the tissues, organs, and eventually a complete body.

"It takes a huge, culminated cartel of orderly genetic programs, which, by design, turn on and shut off in an ordained sequence to make an embryo out of a fertilized egg, then develop a fetus out of that embryo, and then finally create a baby from the fetus. The genetic programming codes are like integrated sets of cellular scaffolding that are erected in an orderly stepwise series where each set supports and manages a few days, or even just a few hours, of embryonic or fetal development. Then it gets shut down, disassembled, and replaced by the next designated set of codes."

"So what's junk DNA got to do with it?" asked Jennelle.

"Jen, that's the point," emphasized Nick. "A lot of those sets of cellular scaffolding and their genetic operating programs are derived out of what we've been calling junk DNA for years. We now believe this is why the human genome has always kept so much of it around."

"Nick, as you talked, I imagined all the successive layers of scaffolding needed to build the Duomo in Florence, Italy."

"Oooh, that's a good one, Jen. I'll have to remember that. Anyway, I now like to think of junk DNA is the biocellular equivalent to physics' quantum mechanics and its probability equations. In fact, a few of us here say junk DNA has become to our genome what dark matter and dark energy are to our universe. Junk DNA serves an essential purpose, or it wouldn't be there in the genome in such great quantities, just like dark matter and dark energy make up most of the cosmos."

Rolling eyes to the heavens, Nick pressed both hands to his jaw and added, "Think of it, Jen. Darwinian natural selection wouldn't have allowed the expenditure of so much energy to constantly reproduce junk DNA unless it served a critical purpose to survival, unless of course Darwin's theories are wrong."

"So you're saying junk DNA isn't junk in the least," interpreted Jennelle.

"You bet! Don't know how much of this goes on after birth or in an adult, but for darn sure, it's essential for embryonic and fetal development."

"How do you propose these scaffolding transitions basically work?" she queried.

"What we've discovered blew our minds," he crowed. "There's a communication system between different parts of junk DNA in the cell's nucleus and with its mitochondrial DNA, and there's a different piece of junk for each cell type among the different cells and tissues. Junk DNA's gene expression produces a micro-RNA that turns on or turns off the DNA in the mitochondria, directly or indirectly, by the unique amino acid chains it produces."

"Okay, so you've got amino acids joined into mini-proteins acting like little turnkeys. So how does CPI's vaccine fit into all this?" asked Jennelle.

"There I have to give credit to the French arm of our investigation team. They unlocked CPI's old trade secrets and found CPI's product was made out of cells cloned five times over. With each cloning cycle, we believe there was a partial loss of the overrides that kept the junk DNA dormant, so some of the junk in those cells got turned on after the fourth or fifth cloning, just as the junk had done in the ontogenetic state."

"So how did the activated parts of junk DNA cause Bobby's disease?" she pursued.

"CPI used cloning technologies, now considered primitive, to get their chicken pox immunization vigorous enough to protect a child against that disease and shingles decades later as an adult," said Nick. "Unfortunately, the junk DNA that was reactivated from their cloned vaccine was the shutdown program for the child's neural cells—"

"Oh my God!" blurted Jennelle, comprehending Nick's explanation. "The cloned virus was made into an injection that got encrypted into the victim's nerve cells in such a way as to reactivate a piece of the nerve's dormant junk DNA. That encoded a junk protein which turned off the metabolic workings of the DNA in the nerve cells' mitochondria."

"Yeah, that's about it, Jen," said Nick, impressed by her clairvoyance. "Eventually the vaccine simply shut down the neuron's mitochondria."

"So each cell's little energy factory ceased to operate," rephrased Jennelle.

"Yep. Without energy, there's no cellular respiration, and the poor little thing sputters and dies," finalized Nick.

Jennelle heaved a grim sigh, pushed back her chair, and replayed in her head what he'd presented.

Nick knew from Jennelle's position to stay quiet until she restarted the conversation.

Rubbing her forehead after a couple of minutes, she leaned forward, filled the monitor with her face, and declared, "Nick, you're not smart enough to concoct all this about junk DNA and how it talks to and turns off mitochondrial DNA."

Nick almost fell from his chair. "Well, Jen, we had some help," he confessed.

"Nick, you start over and tell me how your team came up with this."

"Okay." He unconsciously raised his right hand to swear to give the whole truth. "When Doctor Graywood forwarded his data and analysis about how Ritalin might add to the picture along with methamphetamine as separate but equally potential cofactors for Bobby's disease, we relooked at the pharmacodynamic interactions where two drugs act on the same or related target sites in the brain cells. Of course, that suggested additive or synergistic or even antagonistic effects."

Then he raised his left hand. "We tested a leftover part of Bobby's brain from the biopsy you sent a couple of years ago and confirmed CPI's vaccine footprint all over the neural cells."

Nick clasped both hands together. "We hypothesized that a physiologic signaling mechanism existed that somehow got oddly magnified by repeated doses of either the meth or the Ritalin, but that became an impediment."

"What … how so?" asked Jennelle.

"It seemed very likely that the disease, as a whole, was greater than the sum of its parts, and that meant we were dealing with a nonlinear, dose-response relationship."

"So you got stumped."

"Yep, we definitely were," confirmed Nick. "The erratic, unpredictable side of nature had us hard by the balls, so to speak. In order to solve it, we had to get away from thinking like reductionists and forego the logical sides of bioscience."

"So, Nick, what did you do?"

"Without yielding up all our beliefs on how cellular biology remains a system governed by deterministic laws, we nevertheless acknowledged that it still could behave unpredictably and that chaos might have crept into the cells' clockwork and disrupted it."

"Good God, Nick, please stop hedging! What'd you do?"

"We did computer-thought experiments."

"What? … Really?" replied Jennelle, amazed, yet in tones laced by sarcasm.

"It's a great way to amplify the mind, Jen," defended Nick.

"So you used that mega-whatever-computer at NIH to find some form of order out of all your disorderly chaos," she smirked.

"Jen, I've gotta make two points to you. First, chaos is not the absence of order. It's a subtle state poised between order and randomness," he said, wounded. "There's a shape, a structure to chaos and, over time, an exquisite order within it."

"And point number two?" she pushed.

"We brought in computer scientists from MIT to help us use what you call our mega-computer."

"Okay, okay, Nick, I apologize. So what did your hired geek guns do?"

Nick swallowed hard. "You never give an inch, do you, Jen?"

"All right, I'm sorry. I'll stop tweaking you."

From time to time, Nick enjoyed how Jennelle toyed with him, but today he wanted to barrel forward. Over a long-nose smile, he replied, "Thank you."

"You're welcome. Now tell me, Nick, how did MIT help out?"

"Instead of puddling through the millions of possible variables of DNA coding sequences, MIT recommended we concentrate on the clusters where we'd picked up the inoculation's footprint in the cell's nucleus and mitochondria. From there, we used their chaos-theory testing expertise since we were probably dealing with a nonlinear, dose-response relationship between CPI's product and methamphetamine or the Ritalin. We wanted to find out how each one of the vaccine-stimulant duos had wrecked its havoc on the neural cells."

"Nick, I got the part about the genetic footprints, but you gotta hit me again on the chaos stuff," returned Jennelle, confused.

"We believed the interaction between the vaccine and the stimulants was non-linear. Examples of nonlinearity are all around us … such as the life-saving power of combination therapies for cancer treatments, the multi-drug cocktails prescribed for treating AIDS, or the dangers of a toxic interaction whenever someone drinks grapefruit juice and swallows one of the newer antipsychotic meds. Jen, chaos theory helped us take our focus off the accepted laws of genetics and cellular biology and shifted us to its holistic consequences."

"You mean shifted you to the erratic, unpredictable side of nature," interpreted Jennelle.

"You could say that," confirmed Nick. "Chaos took us away from the reductionism inherent within the stringent walls of science. When the MIT geeks matched up our data using chaos theory, it all came to life."

"Well, my dear Nick, that's quite a story," said Jennelle, sitting back engulfed.

"It's complicated, but it's marvelously simple too, and that's where I need your help."

"My help? You've got MIT and all your French contacts in the Pasteur Institute."

"Jen, I've been tasked to prepare the brief for the Federal Claims Court hearing on CPI's immunization and all its unintended, disastrous effects. This morning, we discussed our theories and findings with Health and Human Services and Department of Justice. They're hot to trot to have everything specified before they crank up the Vaccine Injury Compensation Program to mitigate CPI's monster. They expect a hellish number of petitions for compensation once we go public."

"So what can I do that I'm not already doing?" she probed.

"Come here for a month and help me prepare the hearing."

Jennelle's management of the hep C field trial had rolled into its fifth year and was now proceeding on autopilot for routine surveillance and data collection. She could spare the time. More so, she savored the challenge of presenting CPI's adverse creation before the Court of Federal Claims.

If Graywood had been around, she'd have turned the hep C monitoring over to him, but he'd left Alaska four weeks earlier. On the chance he'd checked messages, she emailed about assisting in Maryland and expected to return near June's end.

The raw wind rustled off Knik Arm the day before Graywood departed. After muddling through the WWAMI lecture and seeking out Bearhead, he'd driven the dirt-streaked Subaru—interior littered in fast-food wrappers, Coke cans, and paper coffee cups—back to Elmendorf Air Force Base.

But prior to teaching the medical students, he'd crossed to Jennelle's office. Grace Hall's curbside sign had been corrected—RESEARCH was no longer misspelled. Arsenic-grey clouds billowed in the morning sky.

"Hello, Jen," Graywood said, having entered her open doorway without stopping by the secretary's desk in the foyer.

"Gary ... ah, come in," she said, taken aback.

Creased clothes and a disheveled face amplified the groaning from his heart.

"Please, sit down." She joined him on the leather couch.

Ice pellets stormed against the windows. She reached and squeezed his hand. Not letting go, she waited.

Rain followed. Hail melted.

"I don't read Nick's emails anymore," he uttered.

"He sends way too many on what they're doing," she said, nudging him to keep talking.

"They made any progress?"

"Nick and NIH are working round the clock, Gary. We'll hear about any breakthroughs before anyone else."

"So you haven't heard something yet?" He let go of her hand.

She leaned to him. "Nothing significant. Nick will definitely let us know first."

He stood and watched the splashes on the panes form tiny rivulets. "I've sent both you my take on what must have happened to Bobby and Cub."

Catching her breath, Jennelle rose, heartsick, and rubbed his shoulders. "You did the bravest thing, Gary, telling us what might have happened and how things could interact terribly between CPI's vaccine and Ritalin."

Exhaling through pursed lips, he plodded to the color-coded, geographical maps, tacked like a psychopath's photograph wall in an FBI homicide room. Staring at Southeast Alaska, his finger inched along the Copper River to Chitina.

"I remember when Theo Nowell, Wayne Secorr, and I rescued Bobby and Frankie off that sinking sandbar. The two little guys were the same age. We were so damn thankful we didn't lose them."

Graywood's flashing eyes darted to Jennelle. "Rescuing them then was brave, not me now" he groaned, "not by a long shot for all this bullshit." He wanted to shred the maps to dust. Head shaking, he gasped, "Saving them didn't count a damn, did it?"

"Gary, come here." She ached to hold him through the misery.

"To perish how I think they did … God," he crescendoed, "they weren't supposed to die that way!"

"Oh, Gary …"

"Ritalin and CPI killed my son; CPI with meth doomed Frankie," he mechanically fired and laughed manically. "Isn't the world damn straight crazy?"

"Gary …"

"Theo and I … damn," he spattered harshly, "we did every right thing for our kids!"

"Gary, please," she blurted, "you did all the right things for Bobby; Theo didn't for Frankie."

"What?" He scoured Jennelle as if she were an outer-space alien. "I don't understand." Seeping rage morphed to bewilderment.

"Oh, Lord Jesus, please forgive me," whispered Jennelle, looking skyward. Outside rain had wisped into mist.

"Was there something wrong between Theo and Frankie?" Graywood demanded.

She escaped to the protection her desk offered between them. Teeth clenched, she jumbled loose papers into random piles.

"Jen, you tell me what happened with them."

Clutching the mahogany edge for support, she confided the horrid circumstances surrounding Theo's drug smuggling network and the threats of lethal harm to those who divulged his crimes, April Coldsnow and her sister, May, included.

"Roe's never told me this," said Graywood, shocked.

"Monroe doesn't acknowledge or deny what Theo ever does," confessed Jennelle, mimicking April's excuses for her husband's inaction.

Like family, Graywood cherished Bearhead, April, and May. And Jennelle. All were in peril. Bearhead had to stay wary of Theo, yet he'd hold to dignity as Sir Thomas More had done until England's Henry the Eighth had axed off his head.

Graywood's crushing grief alone would have made it excusable not to help save them. Depression's trappings easily cloaked one to avoid the far greater dangers awaiting others. But now Theo appeared akin to the Satan who'd diced the brains and licked the bodies of the people Graywood dearly loved. Their frantic shadows had been captured and made afraid within Jennelle's dark secret … and his as well.

He cleaved to the window.

Who am I? Is there some way to protect them, make it right, and bring them to safety?

Without Bobby, why even try? I'm not Maren on the run. She didn't care. She fled all this for her own way. So why do anything?

It doesn't matter.

"Gary, you must never say a word to anyone what April said," warned Jennelle. "Theo is relentless. He'll kill her if he finds out she spilled what I've told."

Without a blink, that shit-faced dealer will kill you too, Jen.

Christ, how do I prepare? Jesus Christ, what would you …

Jennelle stepped sideways attempting to see Graywood's profile rather than the back of his head. Out of her reflection, dulled on the drenched glass, Graywood's mind's eye opened to crude truth. He'd make certain she and Bearhead and the Coldsnows remained unharmed … and the meth got stopped.

"Jen, I want to say something to you." Turning to her, he declared, "I'm going away."

Her chest tightened from instant loss. She discarded the desk shield and embraced him. Into his shirt, she muffled, "Where are you going?"

"Alone, to a place I love," he said enigmatically. "Listen, Jen, whatever happens to me, you make sure Cub never takes any stimulate, and you damn well better find a way to finger Nowell to the police but only blame me for it."

"But, oh, what're you going to do?"

"Don't ask, Jen."

They uncoupled.

Mouth dry, she swallowed three times to speak. "When are you coming back?"

"Weeks, months, longer, I don't know … maybe never." He kissed her forehead as he'd done with Bobby.

The jagged scar that trenched his soul had healed a mite. Rain had cleansed the outside. Like the hail that had hit the window, he'd been washed pure.

A preparedness mission on Elmendorf's flight line had set the four F-35s on the runway in diamond formation. The sweeping, metallic takeoff boasted a raw prowess.

Oblique sunlight bounced off the tactical drill and collected to the triple-layered panes shielding Graywood's office. And a reflected teal-blue shirt hung loose over a thin, human frame. Gauntness cried out to hoist the antidepressant dosage.

The wisdom Bearhead revealed after the morning WWAMI lectures did not provide relief.

"If what you say is true, Gary, your mistakes were honest." Bearhead sought to repackage Graywood's guilt for causing Bobby's death.

"I gave him … tainted … vaccine!" Graywood spat out. "I made him … take Ritalin … I really didn't want him to."

"You believed you did what was best. You always have for him."

"Damn! God, Roe, my insides are ruined."

"Please, Gary, just think," Bearhead negotiated. "You said your data was incomplete, likely full of errors. Your fears could prove wrong from what NIH knows in Senegal."

"I pray you're right, but what if I'm the one right … I'll never feel joy."

"I'm … ah." Bearhead bit his tongue, aggrieved. And he so wanted a cigarette. "I'm sorry, Gary."

"If I'd never forced him to take stupid, stupid, STUPID Ritalin!" Skin without color, Graywood's voided eyes zeroed on Bearhead's. "God, Roe, I've murdered my child." He'd committed the world's most heinous crime.

"No, Gary, you didn't."

Staring at the floor, Graywood whispered, "You know what I should've done?"

"What?"

"Forged records to show Bobby had gotten the two damn varicella shots required to start school. The injection Doctor Timm had given when he was only one would've been enough protection. But no … no, no, noooo … I made sure he had two because that's how it's done."

All sides of grief lingered fresh and heavy in the air. Bearhead held silent.

Withered, Graywood bargained out loud with himself. "I put off getting the booster. Shots anytime were a battle with him. It's so damn hard being a single parent, balancing it all … getting him ready to start first grade. All the running around … a nightmare … him, me, everything. I got him to Doctor Timm for the preschool physical at the last minute. Her clinic had none of the usual vaccines, so I took that damn CPI stuff from the community clinic … gave it to him and Cub so he could start O'Malley on time."

"Gary, you're a very good man," consoled Bearhead. "I understand blaming yourself, but be fair to yourself too." Bearhead tried to lift him from total self-recrimination. "Put more blame on the vaccine makers." It was futile.

"Agonizing pain, Roe," choked Graywood. "My little boy writhing in those fits … God, seizure after seizure after seizure … horrific!"

Graywood's linkage to reality bordered mirage-like. "I raised and loved him so hard, and I betrayed him. I didn't protect him." Spent, he slumped to the chair abutting the bookcase, crammed with philosophy texts.

"It's so tragic, Gary, what happened." Bearhead strived to reset Graywood's moral compass. "It doesn't make a wit of sense. Your world got shattered, but it's not all your fault."

"Then whose? God's?"

"I beg you, Gary, please. Mistakes were made. One can't ever fully understand God's plan for this world or this universe, but you can understand your place in it."

"Phhtt! I've lived a lie … science and Maren, the two biggest, goddamn lies. My mistakes, Roe, were to trust medicine and love a narcissist." Thumb and index pinched the ring finger like a vise. "You agree?"

He didn't wait for Bearhead's response. "You know what? I don't believe in God, and I don't believe in science. Where were they when Bobby died, eh? I followed them, and they killed my boy."

"Gary, you're not right to your nature."

"Cash doesn't believe in God. Why should I?"

"He's got reasons."

Anger narrowed Graywood's eyes. "Tell me damn straight what they are."

Neutral and steady, Bearhead divulged how Cashel Goodlette's grandfather had been recruited from Ireland to hunt down Tasmanian aborigines. He reiterated Cash's core reasoning behind the world's suffering being caused by mankind or nature, nothing else. To Cash, if a god existed, the deity would've never allowed such misery, especially race extermination by his grandfather. So he'd blanked out God's existence. He solely believed in nature and the sciences to which he sought better understanding.

If Bearhead had been in a classroom, he'd have broadened Cash's boxed-in reasoning to argue how mere slices of culture, science, and nature had become the finite gods of current atheists and agnostics, despite abundant manifestations of so much more in the infinite universe than science could ever explain. But not now with Graywood.

"A belief system of disbelief is a belief system, nonetheless, Gary. Disbelief doesn't work for me, but it works for Cash," finished Bearhead. He wasn't sure if Graywood understood, but the interlude had drained the room's tenseness.

To pry Graywood back, Bearhead added another tilt on life. "What happens in the world every day to each of us can be viewed as an exercise between choice, chance, and fate. Often they're lumped together, and sometimes we're smart enough to split them apart by our own desperate attempts to make sense of the world. Gary, in the past, you and I have done this so many times."

"I can't make sense of it, Roe," mumbled Graywood, face dropped in anguish. "I'll never make sense out of our world again."

Bearhead had never heard such somber tones from his friend. They marked an eroded will and how far Graywood's compassion had evaporated.

Shriveled, the haunted figure compressed like frozen tundra exposed to incessant polar winds. Barren and broken, he'd lost all self-respect.

Derailed when Maren left him, devastated when Bobby died, he was doomed once he'd discovered his cardinal role in his son's demise. He'd known rejection, suffering, and excruciating wounds to such degrees he'd never find peace.

Bearhead had learned as an itinerant chef that possession of sympathy for others and for one's self first required self-respect. An individual without it would not cherish life. Both self-esteem and compassion were crucial for the nascent trances of forgiveness to ascend out of one's grief filled from guilt. Somehow, Graywood must start the long trek to healing and find his self-respect. Then he could grab hold of a shred of peace … and grace.

"Gary, let's do some time at Campsite," Bearhead spoke in the belief the endeavor might inch the tortured soul before him out of the abyss.

Graywood's head lifted. He'd reveled in the back country. Campsite had never failed to recharge.

"We haven't flown there for a long, long time," Bearhead encouraged. He skipped over recollections of Bobby shooting arrows and fishing from the hybrid canoe. "I wonder how the great bears have managed."

Wordless, Graywood scanned the ceiling.

"Tell me old friend, when should we fly out?" Abrupt coughing forced Bearhead to clear the sludge twinging his windpipe. Not spitting, he swallowed the pollution and sat with pursed lips to steady the airflow. "It would be good to go there, Gary," he half-croaked, leaning back, determined not to move until he heard a confirmation.

Graywood hunched over, face buried in hands.

The office landline buzzed unanswered.

Neither man budged until Graywood's spine straightened. He observed the round-faced clock atop the doorway. "It's late, Roe. I've gotta head back to Elmendorf. I'll let you know when."

"Gary, I'll be ready."

The four F-35s had boomed skyward and returned. Sometimes glass-paned portals, resembling mirrors, have an eerie penchant to reveal …

Single parenthood had felt at times like contests where mothers or fathers kept score. Before Bobby entered school, Graywood cared less about the tallies. He believed he'd raised the child well … until halfway through first grade when a teacher said Bobby lacked concentration, constantly rocked in his chair, and had fallen behind in reading. The final score ended in death.

"I don't dream in pictures anymore," he told the window. "Can I ever be the person I liked?"

Too late to raise Emrick on webcam, Graywood emailed he'd take thirty days' leave. He sent short messages to Jennelle and Bearhead.

He deposited Brandy Belle with Rachel on the way to the airport and flew commercial to Kauai.

Later, he searched for the old family house by Coos Bay.

CHAPTER TWENTY-FOUR

Untitled Prophet

"Nick, I'm here."

Jennelle had recovered from the shock of June's mugginess in DC after the overnight flight from Anchorage had landed at Dulles International Airport.

Nick Severstal worked in Bethesda, Maryland, at one of the National Institutes of Health's twenty-seven entities—the National Institute of Allergy and Infectious Diseases. The lead investigator for the Bobby-disease epidemic, he directed the NIH team members selected out of his organization, the National Institute of Biomedical Imaging and Bioengineering, and the National Human Genome Research Institute.

Through the half-opened entry, Jennelle surveyed two jumbled, computer work stations, surrounded by stacks of journals, reports, and spreadsheets—all extending the over-cluttered mind of a valiant man. Absorbed, he collated piles into fresh mounds and added more from the endless, disgorged splatterings of two office printers. She marveled how he orchestrated the daunting mess.

"Hey, Nick, I'm here," she said louder.

"Oh wow, Jen, you look great." He prevented a mountain of papers from tipping over when they hugged and exchanged pleasantries. After family updates, he switched to the Court of Claims task ahead.

"It is biological plausibility that makes the most points with the special masters when I present our findings in Washington," said Nick, dry and precise.

"Special masters, aren't they the ones someone else would call judges?" asked Jennelle.

"Yep," confirmed Nick. "They've been sitting on the Court of Claims since established over thirty years ago under the National Vaccine Injury Compensation Program. They'll want facts, reasoned out and tenable, before they approve a compensation payout for injuries caused by an immunization."

"Have you ever presented to them?"

"Nope. I'm giving NIH's two bits of expert testimony plus the medical record summaries gleaned from your work and the conclusions formulated in Alaska," answered Nick with shell-thin confidence. "So I need you there to help field questions."

"Fine by me," Jennelle replied, sensing his nervousness. "Nick, I see one huge problem right off the bat in a question they'll probably ask."

"What?"

"On the flight down, I reviewed my notes, and I didn't understand how FDA let CPI's vaccine come into the country from France."

"So far, we've found no paperwork trail approving it for use here," said Nick, shrugging shoulders. "It just may have snuck in. Jen, I need you to dredge that sinkhole as your primary domain while I prepare my side."

"Okay. Does that mean I go to Paris?"

"Sorry, no. Paris is coming to you, Jen, in the form of five gentlemen from France's Ministry of Health.

"*Mon Dieu!*" She smiled on the odds in her favor.

"Here are their names." Nick fumbled the documents strewn across the larger desk, unhitched an itinerary and summary sheet, and passed them to her. "They arrive at BWI tomorrow afternoon at two o'clock."

"Jean-Leon Dutertre, Georges Marsal, Augustin Fortuny, Emmanuel Devilliers, Gaspard Jollots," she recited with passable accent. "Do I pick them up?"

"A good idea," quipped Nick. "They're on the team you're leading."

"Holy Mother! You got any more surprises for me, dear Nick?"

"No. So how much sleep did you get on the jet?"

"I'm good."

"Then let's go around and get you settled in your work area. Before we start, how much do you know about the human genome project?"

"Completed in 2003 ahead of schedule," she replied. "Since then it's been a potential source for cures and profit, depending on one's motive. Otherwise, not a whole lot." She knew reams more but wished to hear about it from Nick.

"Well then … I'm gonna tell you about what I call Pandora's box that's hidden in the junk DNA of the human genome."

"Pandora's box? Sounds interesting, Nick." She sat on the only empty chair tucked behind the smaller desk. "Shoot away."

"There are forty-six chromosomes in each of the ten trillion cells that make up a human body. Out of those chromosomes, there are around twenty-four thousand active genes that express themselves to manufacture the enzymes and proteins and all the other cellular constituents necessary for our existence day-to-day. Now, Jen, estimate how much of the human genome does it take to account for those twenty-four thousand genes."

"I don't know, say about half."

"Would you believe just 3 percent?"

"Three? That's it?"

"That's all. The Human Genome Project discovered the genes that keep us alive represent only 3 percent of our DNA."

"So what d' you suppose the rest does?"

"Don't really know yet." Nick shook his head sideways. "Out of ignorance or wild speculation, some pretentious wags have called it junk DNA. But it doesn't make a lot of sense from the perspective of human evolution. Why would nature take the time and energy to replicate a whole lot of junk DNA? Some or most had to have a purpose. We just haven't figured it out yet."

"Maybe it had a purpose at an earlier time and became redundant through natural selection," offered Jennelle.

"A lot of us at NIH kind of agree with that, Jen. But let's think this through … The DNA we call junk could be a repository for all the evolutionary history of the human genome. Parts of it weren't junk when our proto-Homo sapiens walked the earth. But over the next million years or so, our evolution turned a bunch of it into today's so-called garbage."

"So it's leftover, redundant DNA," summed up Jennelle. She stood and moved three cardboard boxes filled with outdated journals off what appeared a more comfortable chair.

"Maybe so, Jen, but evolving organisms should have shed the redundant vestiges. From the point of view of energy conservation, it's not efficient for evolution to replicate a whole heap of so-called junk. So you've got to think maybe it's naturally advantageous to keep a gargantuan amount of ancient DNA around as a hard-wire backup or something like that."

"Ninety-seven percent, Nick, is a mountain of backup. You know how natural selection punishes the wastage of energy and time."

"Yeah, but we're humans. We've got to believe we're vastly more complicated," he sarcastically alleged. "We're so superior that we need obsolete, multilayered, genetic code to stop straying back into the evolutionary pit."

"Nick, you're implying, instead of being the pinnacle of evolution, we're kind of like an ultimate government bureaucracy," analyzed Jennelle. "We got redundant and overloaded with outdated layers of genetic regulation, in spite of natural selection."

"I was only joking, Jen. I actually disagree on that. All that extra DNA code must have had a positive effect on survival and reproduction because natural selection favored those who retained it."

"Or perhaps God had a hand in it."

"Oh yeah, Jen, sure that's it," laughed Nick. "God and his biological bureaucracy. So how much should we credit celestial unknowns whenever we don't have a clue what's lurking in our human genome?"

Rolling her eyes, Jennelle said, "Better to say we simply don't know—"

"Instead of dressing it up with spirituality," interrupted Nick, "or some mysterious biological rule."

"Well, it's the way we make sense of things we don't understand," declared Jennelle. "We either blame or credit it to some form of natural theory or God."

"But Jen, try this on ... A few here at NIH believe there's no such thing as junk DNA. As we learn more and more from the genome project, it's obvious we've haven't yet assigned a good purpose to all the pieces. Right now, we're just pretty much plain stupid."

"That's awfully refreshing coming from you, Nick. So tell me again how you came up with this idea that junk DNA isn't junk and that it could derail the DNA in the mitochondria, which you crowed all about to me last week?"

Nick opened a computer folder on the monitor at the smaller desk and booted up histological files showing fetal brain tissues indexed to genetic code sequences. "With the newest generation of DNA-sequencing machines coupled to our computer's magflop-drive, we did genetic maps on fetal brain cells for the effects of the CPI vaccine you sent us." He motioned her to view the screen. "Then we compared them with Bobby's biopsy. We examined the DNA equivalent of fifty thousand genes to determine which switched off or on."

"That's twice the adult number of genes expressing themselves, around 6 percent of the genome," said Jennelle, peering at the color-coded images as Nick methodically scrolled.

"Close enough," agreed Nick. "There was too much degeneration, too many cells turned off. But the brain maps helped reveal the genetic glitches responsible for the neural cell shutdowns."

Nick advanced to slides of malignant tumor pathology matched to mapped fetal biopsies. "In cellular activity, these are completely opposite to each other and show each cancer with runaway growth. Fundamentally, for me, cancer is an imbalance within the affected cells that prevents cell death, or it's a disequilibrium leading to uncontrolled cell growth. But we found this third imbalance that led to speeding up cellular degeneration. That, Jen, was the insight we needed to understand the processes going on in Bobby's disease."

Sorrow murmured within Jennelle's heart. Faintly she asked, "How'd you find that out?"

"Oh, that's a long story," Nick said with a slight jaw wiggle. He advanced to a split-screen picture on the monitor: left labeled, LOT3478QS-Kuru; right, AK06/2016-Bobby. Both appeared identical. He inhaled long and full to charge his lungs enough to explain. "Suffice it to say the chaos-theory geeks at MIT, plus our imaging and bioengineering folks, did an exhaustive search using a rigorous scientific approach. They discovered that CPI's vaccine had erroneously reactivated some dormant junk DNA in the fired up neural cells stimulated by Ritalin or methamphetamine. In turn, decoded junk messenger RNA got sent out, which untwisted the mitochondrial DNA like a reverse corkscrew. The mitochondria failed to produce enough cellular energy, so the neuron died."

Jennelle stepped to the doorway to refocus a woeful head. "Come on, Nick," she said, disconsolate. "Let's go admire your mag-flopping computer and probe the geeks some more."

Nick led the NIH-MIT group, and Jennelle directed the nineteen-member international team of experts from the French Health Ministry, WHO, CDC, FDA, SEC, and the US State and Justice Departments. For three weeks, subcommittees sifted through CPI's papers and research data from startup to being broken apart and sold. Recovered computer folders and hard copy documents were aligned to original correspondences catalogued and transacted with the European Medicine Agency and other international trade organizations. The specialists burrowed through crates of scribbled meeting notes, office memorandums, files, records, and confidential letters, all hidden for over a decade from public view. More than one thousand unfortunate individuals had received CPI's cloned product and had concurrent lethal exposures to stimulant co-factors, such as methamphetamine or Ritalin.

A flawed testament to hubris and greed underpinned CPI's deformed inoculation. In the beginning, CPI had a successful history in hybrid plant breeding—called biofortification. Yet in time, CPI's bioscientists likened themselves to modern-day biological watchmakers. As they adjusted a living cellular timepiece, they dared to believe they could manipulate the DNA and other internal mechanisms within any organism. These modern entrepreneurs boldly leaped beyond Galileo and Isaac Newton to control their versions of the clockwork universe. They presented DNA double helixes as ready-made for commercial exploitations. The clock masters from the Enlightenment would have stood drool-worthy envious.

The financial subcommittee analyzed CPI's balance sheets and unearthed a hedge fund network with contorted avenues to the Bank of France and Société Générale. SEC and French officials uncovered documents CPI had used to mislead investors with bogus claims on biomedical product lines under development. To influence New York trading, a stock-touting campaign on glossy newsletters and spammed faxes had inflated CPI's share value at the Paris and Frankfurt exchanges.

CPI's equity manipulations on both sides of the Atlantic were maligned by insider trading. Whenever Jennelle listened to the interim summations, she conjured Cashel Goodlette flinging wild arms and bellowing to follow the dollar and Euro trails and ending the diatribe thundering: "Whenever money becomes the primary motivator in scientific research, true science is corrupted. There's no escape."

Other internal CPI memos revealed an inability to pull off legitimate marketing campaigns like the other immunization manufacturers had done, such as the advertised push to prevent most cervical cancers in pre-teen girls. Instead, CPI's business model relied on outsourcing and field testing the culprit chicken pox vaccine in Senegal prior to selling it to France. They planned to accumulate third world results that demonstrated the inoculation's success and safety before broadcasting to the developed world, particularly American biomedical outlets.

Outright, a foreign product could not enter the United States without federal approval. The authorities on Jennelle's team deduced CPI had not sneaked the varicella injection under FDA's nose but, instead, had deployed a clever ruse: CPI had petitioned FDA to allow a field test within the country of its new immunization in an "effectiveness comparison" against the then-current standard chicken pox series to determine the reasonable payment should the cloned commodity become purchased by the United States.

CPI had extolled the "pending approval" status obtained by the European Medicine Agency as equivalent to governmental clearance for widespread distribution. Duped, the FDA had granted a limited-use waiver in February 2006 for entry and punted it to Alaska. The Forty-ninth State, at the time, had scuttled into cost-cutting mode prior to its next governor's election. Consensus on who should manage the protocol proved nonexistent between Alaskan state health officials and the FDA. By default, oversight descended to the borough level: Juneau city bureaucrats, in fact, had advocated for CPI's inoculum and aided its Alaskan distribution throughout the southeastern panhandle. No medical personnel, not even Juneau's coroner, had been tasked to follow the comparison study for potential effectiveness and side effects.

The entire routing and implementation was bureaucracy at its worst—no one in charge, no one responsible. Thereafter, the document trail dried up.

NIH verified all American cases of Bobby's disease had occurred in Alaska or were connected to it: each victim had received CPI's varicella creation from a federal, state, or local government clinic; the vaccine's cloned DNA sequence codes were found in each submitted biopsy. The investigative parameters for the exposed United States children and young adults matched tightly to those in Senegal and France.

In a rare break from work, Jennelle remembered the prime reason she had gone to Alaska in the summer of 2006: detect potential microbial threats—bird flu or SARS—that might enter the country from overseas. She never suspected the devastating Trojan horse concealed in a poorly researched French immunization.

"Our time slot at the Court of Claims has been advanced to tomorrow afternoon. Please look this over and tell me if it's on target," requested Nick. He handed Jennelle a fresh printing of the presentation.

Ignoring his pensive look, she nimbly thumbed the eighteen pages. "This could take some time," she sighed, uncapping a red pen. "I'll get right on it."

"Mark what you think needs fixing," winced Nick, "and be gentle."

"Don't worry, dear." Her careful advance through the document didn't miss a detail on the reasoning and conclusions the international team had elucidated for the pathology of Bobby's disease.

The two members from WHO advocated naming the lethal condition Viral Neural Atrophy Syndrome (VNAS) or Viral Atrophy and Seizure Disorder (VASD). Wherever these terms appeared, Jennelle overprinted in bold letters BOBBY'S DISEASE. In the margin by the first correction, she wrote: "Nick, give a human name to tragedy—viscerally better than fancy title."

After three-and-a-half hours, Jennelle entered Nick's office with the crimson-pocked draft plus four sheets of proposed changes.

"Nick, this is really good," she said and handed them off. "But there's a recommendation I'd really push that will make it easier to visualize the culpability behind CPI's vaccine."

Nick flinched yet said, "Go ahead." He beheld a manuscript flushed by raspberry-colored edits on every paragraph.

She grabbed it out of his fist. "Take these eight pages in the middle and shift them to an appendix. The special masters can read them there if they like. In place of them, substitute this double set of two by two charts."

	CPI Vaccine	**No Vaccine**
Meth/Ritalin	+/ + Disease	- /+ No Disease
No Meth/Ritalin	+/- No Disease	-/- Healthy

Nick circled the + + in blue ink. "As I interpret this, Jen, starting at the upper left, if a person is positive for the vaccine and positive for meth or Ritalin, then it equals Bobby's disease, and any of the other three combinations means no disease or a healthy condition."

"Yes. It's a plain double set of two-by-two squares making it easy to see how the vaccine was the necessary but insufficient cause behind Bobby's disease," she explained. "To actually have caused the illness required some social exposure to one of the critical cofactors, either meth or Ritalin."

Nick's finger moved up and down each column. "I like it," he said, "and it implies if you ever got injected with CPI's vaccine, for certain sure never take meth or Ritalin or anything like them."

Jennelle scribbled a note to contact Rachel in Anchorage and warn how Cub must never ingest or inject any stimulant for the rest of his life. As far as she knew, he hadn't.

"So Jen, what should I title my appendix?" asked Nick, scanning the earmarked piece.

"Oh something graphic to get them to read it," said Jennelle. "How about 'Pandora's Box Lurks in Junk DNA' or something devilish like that?"

Snorting laughter in bursts, Nick dropped the papers on the floor.

Jennelle's face twisted bittersweet. Pensively, she thought about poor Bobby and Gary.

"I'm tempted in court tomorrow to explain some other parts of Bobby's disease that we've got theories on," mentioned Nick once he regained composure.

"You should try them on me for practice," she half-suggested, half-dared.

"Sure." He located a mortality graph in the presentation binder and slid it to her. "It looks as if those exposed to meth developed the illness and died faster than those exposed to Ritalin."

"Why?"

"Perhaps because meth activated the shutdown processes in the junk DNA more efficiently than Ritalin. We think we'll have the data and analysis from Senegal in time to publish next year or early 2020."

"That could make sense," said Jennelle. She recalled how Chitina's Frankie Nowell had abused meth and manifested the disease swifter than Bobby. Her thumb flicked up positive for that inclusion. "What else, dear?"

"Unfortunately, the junk messenger protein is an extremely hardy compound. In an odd way it's secreted out of the neural cells into the blood much more readily than remaining inside to foul up the mitochondria." Nick flipped to the binder's back and unfolded a spreadsheet loaded with serum concentrations categorized into three-month time intervals.

"So far, Jen, our bioengineers can't locate an active part in the adult genome that makes an enzyme to degrade it. So the protein slowly builds up in the serum over time. Eventually the victim needs plasmaphoresis to reduce its concentration to avoid clogging up the circulatory system and kidneys."

"I'd mention that too, Nick," she said, voice sick with sadness. That had happened to Bobby only months before he died. Wheeling around, she wanted to leave.

"Wonderful," said Nick. "Let me speculate a little bit now. Junk DNA is a Pandora's box, right?"

"For now it is," Jennelle confirmed, yet faked interest. She'd reached the saturation point after having worked on this investigation for weeks.

"So floating around the institute right now," said Nick, "is an idea that Creutzfeldt-Jakob disease might actually be a shutdown prion-protein that's either intrinsically reactivated out of our junk DNA or innocently ingested as it is in mad cow disease. Some of us suspect that either type of prion infiltrates a neural cell and specifically attacks its mitochondria in an attempt to take over and replicate there, as the prions must have done for the past two billion years. So the prion-like protein infects the mitochondria, similar to CPI's vaccine. Our working hypothesis is prions initiate a physiologic signaling mechanism that shuts down the neuron's mitochondria, starving the cell to death."

Hiding irritation, Jennelle replied, "Nick, conjecturing on mad cow disease right now is way too theoretical for the court. They'll want facts for that, and you don't have 'em. Better leave it out."

"Yeah, guess you're right. It's too presumptive."

"Any more academic ideas?" she asked, hoping not.

"No."

"Nick, go home and say hello to your lovely wife and daughters for me and get some sleep. It's a huge day tomorrow." She left to phone Rachel in Anchorage.

Gratified, yet uneasy, Jennelle packed her suitcase and replayed the cell phone recording of Nick's summation to the special masters at the US Court of Claims:

"CPI's haphazard cloning technology had unintended consequences on both the junk DNA and the mitochondrial DNA. We knew very little about how these two areas interacted within the human genome, yet because of Bobby's disease, we now accept that junk DNA is essential to human development in the womb. Once the misnamed sections of junk DNA have done their timely, sequential portions of cellular programming and tissue development for the embryo and the fetus, they normally turn themselves off, and henceforth remain dormant.

"We also now know that repeated iterations of the cloning process will remove some of the overrides that keep junk DNA dormant and offline in the mature cell's nucleus. If reactivated after we're born, however, the effects of junk DNA activity in a child or an adult may prove grave or fatal. Let me say this as forthright as possible: cellular microbiologists must not negate the controls that nature has placed on junk DNA ... If ever done, as CPI did with its cloned product, Pandora's box is unlocked.

"The biosciences in the twenty-first century must decipher how these extensive DNA locales in the nucleus fully interact with mitochondrial DNA before further technological advancements in cloning may be safely derived and applied. If this research effort remains incomplete and lacks sufficient clarity, it will unleash potentially boundless dangers whenever and wherever applied. Discovering all the knowledge locked up in the human genome will require decades of stringent, prudent, and coordinated efforts with total attention to detail. Otherwise, there will be unanticipated mortal consequences.

"CPI's cloned varicella immunization has become one of those grave consequences: it created Frankenstein-like cells within its victims. These new Franken-cells killed critical brain tissues by reactivating a programming segment in dormant junk DNA—this unlocked portion of genetic code copied and pasted together hardened messenger proteins, and they, in turn, relentlessly shut down the metabolism in the brain. CPI's product horrifically diminished victims' minds and bodies before these innocent souls succumbed.

"The human race will not be destroyed from tragic thermonuclear war nor pulverized by gigantic, fatal asteroids striking earth. No, indeed! I submit it will be annihilated by crass mismanagement of our human genome and the genomes of other animals and plants that inhabit our world.

"In our futile race to become gods, we will overreach and lose it all. CPI's stem cell research and cloned vaccine development were reckless endeavors, wholly based on incompetent science. The ego trip to become the first to develop a commercial, human-cloned product curved into catastrophic mortality for those poor, unfortunate children and young adults who had received CPI's inoculation. Nature's warning to us is simple: Incomplete science, when commercially applied, kills.

"I request the court find in favor to compensate the families of those who have so grievously suffered from Bobby's disease."

Unknowingly, Bobby had been lethally bioengineered.

And lawyers smelled blood.

Listening to Nick's words, Jennelle remembered the boy running pell-mell to her when they'd met by the moose statue … and the love they both had for Gary.

She had to see him.

Graywood had not answered or returned phone calls or emails. From Coos Bay, Oregon, he'd contacted Pratt Emrick online and extended the absence from work.

Graywood returned to Anchorage unnoticed two days before the anniversary of Bobby's death. Entering the Snowline Drive house erased every sane part in his mind he'd excavated out of Kauai and Oregon. He'd accepted he lived in the wrong century. Could he continue?

He checked two months' worth of emails starting with Jen's:

Gary,
Gone to DC to help Nick prepare CPI debacle for US
Court of Claims.
Expect return by end of June.
Love, Jen

Skipping dozens, he opened two of Bearhead's:

Welcome Home Traveler!
Let's get together ASAP. Took over teaching your class.
Must say glad I heard your talking stick enough for that.
Believe I did well. Hope you agree.
Gave students last year's final exam.
Monroe

Gary,
Jen called from DC asking if you're home. I checked Elmendorf.
Told her you'd extended leave and were coping.
She has news on the claims court outcome.
Call Me When You Read This!
Monroe

He didn't.

Once he'd seen Masi's map in Jennelle's office, he'd forsaken the tattered peace blessed upon him at Campsite after the funeral and annihilated Bearhead's warning not to pursue Bobby's exact cause of death.

He emailed Emrick he'd returned early and requested the authorized access codes to the transcribed Court of Claims testimony. Come morning, he'd read the official proceedings at the Elmendorf office.

Foregoing vodka, he parked on the deck to view the twilight hues painted over the Chugach Range. By midnight, the sky had shaded dim.

He dreaded studying the court's documents, yet felt compelled. Not sleeping, he passed a mind-truncheoned night … and vanquished all hope.

At five a.m., Elmendorf's parking lot appeared flat, ordered, and empty—unlike his insides where disorder ruled.

Alienated and bone-weary, he was an absurdity in this world. Dankish, fungal, silent, sinking—condensed cold … abandoned … posthumous …

From the secure com-link, he uploaded the access codes for the recorded testimony at the US Court of Claims. Emrick's accompanying note highlighted first reading Nicholas Severstal's summation and the court's ruling.

The special masters had rendered a unanimous decision for federal compensation awards to the victims of CPI's cloned varicella immunization.

CPI's bastard scientists stole my precious son. Senseless illness snatched so many harmless children to death before they even had a chance to truly live.

Numb, Graywood swiveled the chair, back facing the monitor. Together, the past and present magnified the cataclysm ripping apart identity and blasted any desire to rebuild toward the crushing conversion he must pursue to live.

Once he'd hoped Bobby might find a normal life after Maren. He'd fretted her not claiming their son's existence because ADHD and Ritalin doubly marked the boy as something less.

A hundred years ago, there existed no ADHD in America—no arbitrary, blunt weapon to sort society's kids apart. Graywood bet none abided in the non-western world today.

Unfair to label a little kid with a disease if reading and classroom concentration are below average. Are poor people diseased because they're poor? Certainly not! Damn all oppressive standards!

Fair or not, Graywood could not reconcile how the definition for average had changed with time and culture, verily after every century.

Two years ago he'd fought to tolerate his loss of Bobby, but not now, not this way. Powerless, helpless, ashamed, and angry, he blamed himself. And self-hatred drilled purpose inward and into shards.

I can't live like this!

Recovery derailed by hopelessness. Without hope. No resurrection.

He drove from Elmendorf the final time.

Panic pumped the chest, squeezed the throat.

One more time to decide the century to be in, which culture to transplant to.

Graywood kicked open the front double door. The hallway mirror Maren had bought after the honeymoon only returned anguished eyes sunken within an ashen face.

Grasping the hockey stick, he smashed Bobby's room starting on the model F22 Raptor. Outside, he whacked limbs bare on the birch tree the boy and he had planted. Worn down, heart turgid and tarnished, he collapsed.

You killed your son.

I don't feel at home with the job of living.

You killed your son.

I can't ever grasp for hope at dawn.

You killed your son.

I … won't live.

Blistered fury, resolute jaw—*to* Seneca *and escape!*

Graywood had fallen into the fourth space, the anchorless abyss where no belief in God or science existed.

He handwrote letters to Rachel and Cub warning never to take a stimulant drug, legal or not.

For Bearhead he crafted a terse email to pop on five days hence:

Monroe,
I'm gone. Burn the pole. I caused my sweet child's death!
Judas

He craved vodka … just a shot. Two or three hasty ones would inflame a buzz, but the lubricating effects would come only after a half bottle.

Straight hell, Piper'd kick my ass to Juneau and back if he caught me flyin' plastered.

Phth!

Hell with him.

Yet Graywood kept the hidden cache closed. Liquor dulled pain, but he might do wrong by it. He needed wits. If blitzed, he'd back down and not go through with it.

He filed *Seneca*'s flight plan so not to tip off the real intent: Anchorage//Augustine Island—to the sheltered inlet on the west shore of Augustine's volcano abutting a hiking trail—Homer//Anchorage.

Good visibility, easy flying. He'd pilot *Seneca* to the sunset quickly enough to beat the low-pressure weather system forming off the Bering Sea.

Before exiting the air terminal, he mailed a postcard of a humpback whale breeching in majestic Glacier Bay. His internal autopilot dutifully switched on and scribbled:

Jen,
I'm leaving for good.
What's the me leftover without Bobby?
Remember what I told you in your office.
You know what to do.
Always,
Gary

He'd centered the world upon Bobby's grievous fate, a wretched outcome he'd fashioned. He'd severed all hunger for human connection.

There had been a time belief in God and the future had stemmed foremost from adoration for his child and medical science. But one had obliterated the other. The twin pillars that had defined his existence had smashed together like matter and anti-matter in the Hadron collider—leaving nothing. Life lost purpose. Cognition and spirit transmogrified to chaos. Living slated into the null.

Resolved.

Seneca taxied for takeoff. Destination: ram her down Augustine's throat.

Arching above Redoubt Bay swelled the Crescent River valley's emerald-hued optimism—a horizon the color of hope. And a mysterious instinct itched Graywood to play a pretend game of Bush Pilot Trivia with an imaginary Bobby.

He'd created the question and answer competition for entertainment whenever soaring toward Campsite. Each quizzed the other on historical facts and legends regarding famous Alaskan aviators.

At the same time, they might tackle a contest of Spot-and-Name the ships sailing Cook Inlet below. Wrestling with both passed the time and allowed Graywood to assess Bobby's ADHD-labeled capabilities to focus on two tasks at once. It didn't matter how excited the little guy got when he outscored his dad again and again. What mattered was strengthening the skills for concentration.

Graywood had made over a hundred trivia cards on history-making bush pilots. Before they left home, Bobby randomly picked twenty and dealt them into two equal piles. Each card had three printed factoids and assigned values: the easiest question received a point, the next hardest two, and three for the most difficult. A player carried his group of ten throughout the expedition. Bobby and Graywood took turns asking one question at a time. If a wrong response was given, its point value was deducted with the card sent to the stack's bottom. Whenever a quizzee had correctly answered all three questions, he got to keep the quizzer's card. The outright winner had to capture all the competitor's cards first. A round of play might consist of six back-and-forth turns. And to make it more interesting and test arithmetic, each game had a winner determined by total points scored at the end.

"Dad, I don't see any boats. I wanna play Pilot Trivia."

Graywood looped through his scanning routine on the control panel. "We've got stable conditions and good visibility ahead, Bobby. Don't you think *Seneca*'s just humming along?"

"She's fine. Can I ask first? Can I, can I? Please, please, please?"

"Okay. Pull out your card, partner."

"I'm ready, Dad. How many points?"

Graywood hesitated, teasing, "I better start off easy, so go with one."

"Yahoo! I like this one," Bobby enthused. "What was Merle Smith's nickname?"

"Oh, come on, that's a hard one," said Graywood in mocked pain. "Are you sure that's only a one-pointer?"

"Yep, it is."

"Well it should be three."

"Come on, Dad."

"At least two. "

"Dad!"

Graywood rubbed the back of his neck. "I think Mudflap."

"No, no, no … wrong answer." Gleefully, Bobby placed the card at the bottom of his pile. "It's Mudhole."

"Mudhole," repeated Graywood, in feigned disgust. "I ought to get partial credit for mud at least."

"You can't do that, Dad," defended Bobby.

"How about half a point?" pleaded Graywood.

"Nope, you lose a whole point," he judged. "It's the rules."

"Okay, so I'm already a point in the hole." Graywood checked *Seneca*'s gauges before quizzing from his card. "How many points you want to try?"

"Three, Dad"

With a touch of paternal pride for the cocky boy, Graywood said, "Where in 1928 did Carl Eielson fly that was the first ever to be done?"

"I know it, I know it." Excited, Bobby rubbed hands together to think harder. "Over the Arctic."

"You've almost got it," coached Graywood. "You still gotta tell me which country he flew to from Alaska, and I'll credit you the three points."

Rocking back and forth, Bobby glanced out the starboard window and then straight ahead. He veered pensive to his dad. "Can I get a hint, please?"

"Yeah, but just a little one." Graywood increased *Seneca*'s airspeed to 130 knots. "Choose from these four countries: Japan, Norway, Mexico, or Portugal."

"Oh, it's Norway," replied Bobby without dropping a beat.

"You're good. You knew it was Norway 'cause none of the other three have a border on the Arctic Ocean, right?"

"No, Dad, cuz Piper's told me 'bout flying to Norway."

"Do you even know which countries border the Arctic?"

"Yeah, Alaska."

Graywood left it at that. "Okay, you get three points."

"That makes me four points ahead."

"Stop braggin' and fire off your next question."

"How many points this time?"

"Better stick with one."

"Who founded Wien Air Alaska?"

"Phooey, I'll have to guess …"

Bobby won the round, eleven points to Graywood's eight.

Flying to adventure in a cloudless sky, the day held true for father and son.

There was something behind *Seneca.*

Compelled, Graywood's high-beam eyes pierced past the vacant copilot's seat … where Bobby would have sat.

Another aviator out there? A pilot's surrendered mortal wings, a ghost … or guardian angel? Their essences?

Not sure.

Approaches all clear 360?

Indeed, not a thing portside or starboard. No shadows of man or thing.

Graywood altered course to Tin Cup Lake.

Seneca skimmed the Sisters' treetops and set down beyond a furrow of drifted lake fog by Campsite's shore.

Atop the anchored starboard pontoon, Graywood stared into lucid waters, mirror-like. A different eternity opened. He disconnected the aircraft's GPS and Emergency Locator Transmitter.

To draw tighter to the lily-white underbelly of the cooling sky, Graywood scaled the ridge to the tallest Sister. He paused at a smooth hollow where defiant spring flowers, tipped in ice, had opened north … crystal petals of tiny forget-me-nots.

Swollen clouds rolled a shower only a tumble away. He backtracked to safety within *Seneca,* too late for a proper tent in bear country, and rounded the long day with a sleep.

CHAPTER TWENTY-FIVE

Event Horizon – June 2018

Breakfast.

He wanted none and shoved away in the ky-canoe … solitude in stout parka. Man and boat … forest relics of the past.

Toward the far side of the lake, sobbed each oar stroke. A mounding blister plagued the right palm more and more. Shoulders ached. Low in the craft as a lifeless Viking bobbling in a sea coffin, he ceased going on.

God, you know my pain. Will I ever find peace?

His mind formed the two words that had conceived every religion and philosophy, the plain reason that propelled the pilgrim on the journey to comprehension, the confused duple behind every birth and every death not in its time—WHY THIS?

What beckoned beyond the stony point, dressed thick in fresh alder? He stopped pulling and rested, paddle dripping.

A marbled murrelet surfaced before the bow. The underwater hunter's sharp launch into the air made Graywood's heart shudder. Graywood would have jumped out had he not been confined by the ky-canoe's hatch. Beak heavy with prey, its glistening wings elevated to a high nest somewhere in the old-growth forest. Transfixed, Graywood followed the bird's sortie toward its home built for breeding.

The murrelet circled back, opposite in character, to reveal how its winter white and black had fluxed to brown. It warned, "Kerr, kerr, kerr," and Graywood wished it an apology for intruding on its fishing grounds.

I bet you're a better diver than Maren ever was.

When the flying fisherman overcrossed the third time, it whistled, "Kee, kee, kee, kee," and swooped in a right angle to deceive the true course to its elusive nest.

Such secretive behaviors had dubbed the marbled murrelet the enigma of the Pacific. Graywood had never seen one in the air or rise up from the water. Were Bearhead here, he'd resurrect a story, which might have made sense.

Graywood aimed the bow at the shoreline's massive clutch of boulders—the ancient gravestones that marked a melted rock glacier. A headwind plagued progress. By instinct, he varied the stroke pace so as not to overheat.

"Eeh- eeh," amped from the woods.

Graywood focused to a tall spruce cluster.

"Eeh-eeh, eeh- eeh." A plaintive groan whined phantomlike.

Arms stopped. Ky-canoe slowed. The water's rhythms lapped it like driftwood.

Escaping the treetops, the murrelet set to sky. Awestruck, Graywood watched it curve and return to roost. By sound and flight, it had gone out of its way to broadcast its secluded home, inviting him in. The bewildering bird had forgiven the man's presence.

With ignited will, Graywood skimmed uplake. He remembered the time Bobby and Bearhead had witnessed a murrelet ascend out of the deep with a fish scissored in its beak.

A miniscule comfort soaked in … soothing balm not felt for so terribly long … hinting release … and peace.

He beached at the mouth of Bobby's stream and struck a fire in the old stone circle. Flames popped in clock-shop cacophony. Heaping wood on them, he watched the resin-laced smoke crest westward on the breeze … a small comfort, but short-lived.

Startled, the brown bear vented thirty yards from Graywood's side, not a warning growl or grunt, more a challenging snort. Ignorant to intention, two pairs of opposing eyes, ursine verses human, locked and engaged. Binary orbs searched far into the other. Motionless, Graywood now counted every breath a precious jewel.

Rising on hind limbs, the sow sniffed the liberated spice in the spruce-smoked air as she shielded two cubs, lined up behind. Too close to yell and wave arms without provoking a charge, Graywood held rigid, ready to drop to fetal position and appear threatless. For the moment, she deferred an attack, confident her family's security remained intact.

The yearling cubs squatted, mindful and strong. Graywood admired how well she'd brought them into their second verdant spring.

You're a good momma!

If slashed dead or not, he beamed pride for her.

She lumbered off uttering low-pitched drones, cubs in tow, to rock outcroppings on the hill rich with fattened moths. Graywood cherished the dewdrop his eye formed as she led her family away. Not blotting it, he breathed it in and yearned to inhale the moment forever.

Caked clouds tracked from the west and obliterated the sun. Graywood left the ky-canoe and hiked to Campsite's old alder tree with the embedded arrowhead.

Wind bursts pounded his frame as the sun dimmed, yet he remained a granite sentinel until spasms rippled his torso. Gulping oxygen freed from the chilled mists swirling over the lake, he wailed, "Oh God, let the earth take my tears. Let the ground take me!"

His right wrist hammered the exposed end of steel, then the left. He folded to the earth, both forearms streaked scarlet.

The merciful twilight covered all. Oncoming gentle rain lulled the air anew.

AAARK-aaww-AAARK pealed from a pair of courting northern fulmars. Awakened, Graywood couldn't fathom how long he'd been in borderland's crucible.

Blinking to clear the eyes, he wiped crusted blood on the beryl moss surrounding the tree's base and acknowledged life's ambiguity racing in circles.

In human time, doubt trumped stout convictions. But beyond dusk's boundaries, the life-and-death worlds simply showed two shades of creation. A mind anchored solely within the sciences comprehended a few grains in the greater universe. A heart meshed too tightly to biased morals surely fibrillated whenever stretched beyond its compassion for all things. Shackled by science and tethered to emotion, Graywood's head and soul blew him pell-mell into mirage … a grey zone of storms.

But uncanny fragments of forgiveness were present too. And clogged thoughts unblocked.

How to find forgiveness, give forgiveness, to oneself most of all? Growth would not happen if not watered by it.

Shall it come to him, or come from within? How even to measure it?

Funerals and dreams and tapestries of shattered glass … hovered together by all their laws, broken or not. Works of art perhaps … formless yet with form.

He pulled to his knees and bellowed air like an accordion. An overhead osprey whistled its watch had finished, and forest sovereignty passed back to the overlord.

Graywood realized he'd reached out for his child before his birth and had loved him completely without complete understanding. "Bobby, are you up there?" he uttered. "Are you on my side?"

Leg strength returned. He bandaged the wounds. Taking to tent, he slept the second night.

A racket from harlequin ducks splashing the water broke the morning. Oncoming azure washed the sky as the sun rose behind two crossed trees.

"My palms are ready to steal his nails," Graywood spoke.

Seneca swooped southwest atop the Aleutian Range. By the glorious dozens, whitened pinnacles reached skyward to hint their envy.

The wings shuddered unnaturally when an extraordinary updraft jolted the cabin. Never-before-known serenity whirled onto Graywood. Through lungs and skin and heart, he gathered it in. He nosed *Seneca* toward the Douglas River and the land of ice-filled ravines.

"He's a huge sleeping dragon who blows in the mist, and he lives beyond the greatest mountain in a secret cave …"

The miracle of life played out most heroically on the edges of a hanging glacier, fractured off an awesome peak. Cobalt-blue ice blended spectral essences. Always, death teetered nearby.

Notified Graywood had not returned to work, Piper and Bearhead organized the search party. Graywood's flight plan had indicated an intermediate destination on the western side of Augustine Island. Neither man remembered Graywood voicing inclinations ever to explore there—a strange dead end and the beginning of many. In time, Bearhead and Piper widened the effort to Graywood's favorite places: Campsite, each Seven Sister, the Valley of Ten Thousand Smokes, Tuxedni River, and others.

They discovered *Seneca-Sky Woman* upright and undamaged on Fourpeaked Glacier, fuel tank half full. Oil dripped from the engine and discolored the ice. Squalled snow had obscured the landing tracks. No sign of Graywood.

Residual indentations, more linear than random, hinted footprints parallel to the gaped crevasse two hundred yards southeast. Yet something dimpled the surface braid-like toward Shelikof Strait on Cook Inlet. Neither Bearhead nor Piper deduced a sure pattern.

Cub serviced *Sky Woman*'s piston rings and flew her to Anchorage. Maren sold it to Tailwind Talbot for parts. To forestall a similar fate to the Beaver, Piper only semi-retired his workhorse.

Piper and Cub mended the house on Snowline Drive and looked after it with Bearhead. When Cub repaired Bobby's unhinged bedroom door, Bearhead discovered Graywood's favorite book missing from the den—the Nobel Prize winning autobiography *Out of My Life and Thought* by Doctor Albert Schweitzer. Perhaps this story of humanity—a touchstone of history—had been loaned to a medical student who'd forgotten to return it. Or maybe Graywood had given away this guidepost to life's conduct before he vanished. Cub, Rachel, Piper, and Jennelle denied seeing it.

A year beyond Graywood's disappearance, Bearhead carved two ravens into the crown of the cedar mourning pole—a larger one watching over the smaller extend its wings. Cub and Piper loaded the twenty-foot totem onto a flatbed truck with building supplies hauled to Glennallen. Bearhead paid the teamster extra to deliver the monument to Chitina.

The Gunlocks, Bearhead, and little Brandy Belle flew in the Beaver to the village the afternoon prior to its arrival and prepared the standing site:

four yards angled off the front of Bearhead's lodge. With villagers pounding out raven drum cadences, they raised the honored remembrance.

Each evening, the new queen of the longhouse, Brandy Belle, stretched her elegance and then whiskered scent on the totem's base. Whenever she wished to curl and nap, she'd plop behind the portal's Dlam where Raven clutched the silver orb. Like Rum Tum, Brandy Belle had flown in the belly of a giant, metallic seagull and found a fresh home. As the Dlam cradled her head, perhaps she dreamt she and Raven had joined Bobby and Rum Tum and Aleutian girl to steal away the moon once more.

Jennelle forged a letter under Graywood's official Department of Justice seal and routed it to DEA: The contents specified details and sketches on Theo's drug network, uncovered when Graywood had verified Masi's Alaskan map. An anonymous victim stricken with Bobby's disease from an outlying village had revealed alleged evidence that Theo Nowell had killed Johnny Toofish.

Convicted of murder and banished to Kamchatka, Theo was elected Circle Three's prisoner mayor thirteen years after his Elmendorf flight to exile.

EPILOGUE: SEPTEMBER 2020

Parceling faded stamina, Bearhead trudged a curved, deliberate path inside the Klatt Road cemetery. Thinning clouds threatened no further rain, and enough time had elapsed to shrink the puddles.

Living through successive thaws and freeze-ups, his shoulders hunched higher from emphysema's glacial advance scouring the diminished air sacs in the lungs. He still had enough coveted membranes to supply oxygen to the legs for motion with slowed esteem.

He savored the ripe musk from fresh-turned dirt. There's beauty even in the saddest of places, but the eighty yards to the hummock holding Bobby tested endurance. This time he'd make it on his own and, with hope, the upcoming year as well. He hand carried two light stones—one for Bobby, one for Gary.

Authorities never recovered Graywood's body. They concluded it had wedged deep in the monster crevasse and, after a century or two, might reappear if enough ice had melted in retreat. Amused, Bearhead regarded such predictions' folly: Cashel Goodlette had pointed out portions in the Fourpeaked face had advanced 318 feet in the two years since Graywood's disappearance. It seemed a fool's errand to predict when frozen blocks might reverse.

Each month before the snows unleashed, Bearhead placed a pebble on his godson's grave. Gone by the following visit, the custodian or an intrigued bird likely had removed it. But today Bearhead, the old Raven, would leave two: one for missing Raven and one for missing Raven's son. Two meager stones to honor the branch ill pruned from his extended family.

Bearhead's dodder ceased.

A woman in a tan coat and cream silk headscarf hovered over Bobby's grave. She deposited white carnations on the headstone and snapped a digital of the beautified site. Arms to the sides, she kept on for some time as a pillar until gazing back pensive.

Bearhead discerned not what she wished to see—the lodgepole pines in file outside the cemetery, the distant opulence off the Chugach Mountains, or something farther? Expending immense effort not to disturb her, he suppressed an irregular cough and backpedaled four paces behind the pruned yellow cedar.

Kneeling, she bore an ivory envelope from under her wrap and positioned it on the memorial's marble base. Rising, she liberated a heavy sigh, loosened the scarf, and strolled away with calculated finesse. Enthralled, Bearhead observed her scrutinize the grand expanse beyond the hemlock grove.

He wended to her standing spot and set the two stones cairn-like beside the bouquet on Bobby's marker. Who was this woman? She didn't resemble one of Piper's wives, and Jennelle had returned to Atlanta more than a year ago.

Three white-fronted geese in *V*-formation swept the sky. Yellow-bright, channeled shafts opened the clouds and paralleled their far widening arcs.

A coughing paroxysm blunted Bearhead's chain of thought and forced sole concentration on inflating the chest. Once regular airflow returned, he muttered a curse for succumbing to cigarettes. Swallowing viscid phlegm, he inspected the envelope. Breaking the seal, a jasmine scent wafted, reminiscent of a birthday card Gary had displayed decades ago. Shocked, he read the single page of polished longhand, which tight-fisted his breathing worse than any emphysema bout:

I always kept your baby pictures and those sent when you were six.
I wish I could tell you my story.
My love,
Mother

Bearhead willed to inhale. The woman who'd been adrift sought a forgiveness lifeline at her son's tombstone. An edge of bravery had surfaced to vanquish her brittleness and showed her capable after all to express some selfless love. Bearhead prayed Maren cleaved to it forever. Now but a grain of sand in the world's giant clam, one day she might become a pearl of true beauty. Made in God's image and grace, she had the potential.

Bearhead resealed and centered the note.

He turned southward to the Chugach spine and prayed Gary had found mercy too. Had he discovered it on the ice floe? Had it reached up and cleaved him to its heart as well?

Buddha said it was fitting to die in a small place …

Graywood had rappelled from Spencer Glacier once with Piper. But atop vast Fourpeaked's ice floes, he was alone … alone with God. Did He lift him off? … Was He the midwife?

Buddha said it was fitting to die in a small place …

Opposite the hemlocks, Bearhead beheld the graveyard's eastern wall and spotted a western red cedar—the tree of hope.

"The end is where we start from," he whispered. "Let truth be your life, Gary, and you be your own lamp."

THE END

APPENDIX:

Pandora's Box Resides in Junk DNA

Nicholas Severstal, PhD, Assistant Director
National Institute of Allergy and Infectious Diseases

We find it misplaced that the accepted term for the majority of human DNA—DNA that appears to have no useful purpose—is called junk.

In the past, over 97 percent of the genome has been classified to have unknown functions, if ever any, and therefore conveniently labeled as junk.

We disagree and propose that most is essential for our orderly development from a fertilized ovum in the uterus prior to birth. Thus the majority, if not all, of our DNA is crucial to the development and perpetuation of our species.

We estimate it will take one to two decades to elucidate what every part in the human genome does; particularly throughout the critical stages of fetal development within the womb. Henceforth, we advocate no piece of the human genome is to be called junk: we believe every strand may prove critical for organ creation and maturation during the first and second trimesters of pregnancy.

To help understand the joint discovery by the National Institutes of Health and the Massachusetts Institute of Technology, we must briefly review the anatomical formation of a baby in the human womb—its embryogenesis—from fertilized egg into an embryo, from embryo into a fetus and then advancing to a newborn.

In pregnancy's first trimester, the processes for organ creation start from a few dividing, pluripotent stem cells that have developed out of the fertilized egg. By gestation's second week, a bilaminar, or folded, embryo is created. At day fifteen, the primitive streak of the embryo's outer layer, called the ectoderm, is formed, and closely thereafter, its neural tube derives what will become the baby's early brain and spinal cord.

Extensive physical changes continue at a rapid pace: The two-week-old embryo is remarkably unrecognizable by six weeks; the six-week-old is radically different from a twelve-week-old fetus; and so on. At six weeks, for example, the intestine is still located within the umbilical cord, the embryo has a stubby tail, and its toes are fan-shaped and webbed. One week later, the tail is absent, the toes are separated, and the head, trunk, and limbs have human characteristics.

By six months, at the conclusion of pregnancy's second trimester, the mother's womb supports a recognizable baby. The final three months of gestation fine-tunes and matures the baby's tissues and organs to markedly enhance its survival potential after birth.

All this embryological development is driven from extensive blueprints of genetic codes that are sequentially downloaded from the human genome's DNA. We propose that, throughout each developmental period in the uterus, a fresh genetic blueprint is clicked on by the previous set or sets of codes so as to perpetuate the processes that form the ultimate baby. Each interval may last as little as a few hours or as long as a week. When finished, that particular blueprint code is turned off, and the next in line is simultaneously activated to continue the progress.

The genetic bio-hardware, as well as the bio-software employed, also becomes extensive and complicated as more genetic memory is brought online—like switching over from a hand-held device to a desktop computer and then connecting to quantum supermachines. Development and maturation take congruent multiple layers of code because so much has to be completed in the limited nine months ordained from fertilized ovum to birth.

If from scratch we artificially attempted to duplicate in a test tube or petri dish the creation of a completed fetus from an egg, we estimate the required lines of downloaded computer code necessary to assemble it from raw materials would fill a supercomputer and more.

So where does this tremendous amount of downloaded code exist for the creation of a baby out of a fertilized egg cell? In essence, we hypothesize it comes from the so-called junk DNA within the genome: turning on and switching off in serial applications, our junk DNA directs the fertilized egg to become a fetus and mature into a newborn. Thus we believe junk DNA to be an extensive series of startup and maturation genetic programs—each has its critical turn in the ultimate development of a human being from only a few pluripotent stem cells.

In making a baby out of a fertilized egg, we cannot overemphasize the crucial progressions that switch on and off DNA sections in an ordered fashion. Narrowing our attention to the shutdown process in more detail, we will utilize the human branchial apparatus as a helpful example.

The branchial apparatus in the human embryo is confusing unless considered from an evolutionary viewpoint. In fish and larval amphibians, the branchial apparatus, also called branchial arches, form a system of gills for exchanging oxygen and carbon dioxide between the animal's blood and the surrounding water environment. In fish, the branchial arches ultimately form the supporting structures for gill development.

The branchial apparatus initially presents itself in the same way for human embryos, but because gills are not destined to remain in us, the branchial arches are either obliterated or transformed into other parts of the human face and neck. In an ordered manner, some tissues are modified, and some are instructed to atrophy away to produce the finalized form to the baby's face and neck. When these processes do not entirely work to human genetic specifications, babies are born with congenital malformations of the head and neck. Examples of these malformations are lateral cervical sinus, branchial fistula, or the more common cervical cyst lying free within the neck right below the jaw angle.

The timing of actions to obliterate the gill tissues formed in the human embryo is critical. If done too late or incompletely, one of the malformations mentioned above will occur.

In a similar manner, we propose all other redundant or unnecessary embryonic and fetal tissues—our stubby tails for instance—that represent primitive stages from our collective past with other life forms on our planet are turned off and absorbed.

How the turnoff process works:

We know infants born with cardioencephalomyopathy invariably die because their mitochondria are diseased. These unfortunate children possess a catastrophic genetic alteration in their cells that interrupts the normal metabolic functions within the mitochondria.

The mitochondria are the cellular powerhouses. They make the substance adenosine triphosphate, labeled ATP, the energy source each cell employs to maintain itself. ATP results from a chain reaction of chemical events involving sugars and oxygen.

Mitochondria also have their own genetic material—their inherent DNA—and they process and replicate independent from the rest of the cell. It is believed they evolved from simple bacteria that had come to reside within larger, more complicated cells two billion years ago. Since that time, they have remained permanent residents in all higher organisms, passed on from one generation to the next, and living in the ultimate symbiosis within every cell.

The most efficient way to shut down cells, such as the gill remnants in the human fetal neck for example, is to interfere with cellular metabolism by switching off their powerhouses—the mitochondria.

How the shutdown process is initiated:

Metabolism is hard-wired into our genes, and researchers have discovered the DNA in the cell's nucleus communicates with the DNA in the mitochondria through a feedback loop that employs agents called transcription factors.

We know there are genes that make transcription-factor agents. These agents are proteins, and they exist in all living creatures from single-celled bacteria to humans. They operate at the highest levels of the cell's internal control system. The agents bind to other DNA in the cell's nucleus and thus control the down-line activity or transcription processes for multiple other genes. Throughout embryonic and fetal development, these agents and the genes that produce them are very active.

Once an embryonic or fetal tissue not destined for retention has served its purpose, it is wasted away by turning off its mitochondria. A replacement tissue directs this process by manufacturing a message—a shutdown protein transcription factor—that is absorbed into the cell destined to be turned off. Once the message is received by that cell's nucleus, it makes its own chemical proteins to take its own mitochondria offline.

For example, in brain development, the protein transcription-factor agents probably assist to align the parts of the fetal brain correctly: They link groups of neurons as they should be and switch off those neural cells that are superfluous. All this copying, pasting, and erasing employ proteins that either direct the continuing development for the finalized neurons or, in the unneeded ones, deactivate their mitochondrial DNA. Disrupting the neural cell's energy source means there will be no ATP to help transmit electrical signals or maintain its cellular integrity. Such a neuron atrophies and dies.

We have discovered that these shutdown proteins block receptor signaling within the mitochondria by interfering with downstream ATP creation. The proteins are tiny molecular inhibitors at five hundred daltons in size. For comparison, the monoclonal antibodies our immune system produces to fight infection range as high as 150,000 daltons.

Returning to the human branchial apparatus as our model, we shall emphasize how these signaling proteins function in early neurological development within our mother's womb. In human embryos, there are redundant neurologic tissues that support the gills we are not destined to have. To make those tissues atrophy, signaling proteins are secreted by newer tissues that have come online. Initiating the shutdown mechanism will stop the progression of proto-gill development and inhibit maintenance for the neural axons within the branchial apparatus that support the primitive gill structures. Furthermore, it will trigger their eventual absorption into the future neck of the baby to be.

Every cell contains genetic material to turn itself off, like the shutdown function found in computer software. The shutdown genetic code is located in the vast areas we regrettably have called junk DNA, and its sites are variable among our two hundred different tissue types. Each cell type, from skin to muscle to gland to brain, possesses a distinct endpoint, different from the original, few, pluripotent stem cells in the fertilized egg;

thus, the shutdown genetic mechanism for each tissue is not located at the same chromosomal location. Consequently, we speculate there are two hundred or more shutdown genes scattered across our junk DNA.

This form of cellular regulation has been going on for two billion years, indeed, since mitochondria became junior partners to the larger complex cells. Each cell's nucleus dominates and may shut itself down by turning off its mitochondria.

Most important, in the cells that compose each finalized tissue, the shutdown program remains dormant.

Connection to Bobby's disease:

To produce their varicella vaccine, Cannes Pharmaceutical Internationale developed and harvested cloned human stem cells to incubate its viral substrate, in lieu of employing standard chicken embryos commonly used by other immunization manufacturers.

We wish to express we have no ethical issues about medical research that involves stem cells.

Regarding the brain, we concur with other scientists who have shown stem cells may trigger the brain's own self-repair mechanisms to decrease neural degeneration by pumping out molecules to boost nerve survival and related blood vessel development. The brain has the means to demonstrate plasticity and strives to function toward normal levels, even after one or more devastating assaults on its integrity: Stem cells may assist to diminish the harsh effects resulting from an acute or chronic neurologic disease or injury.

We prefer to think of stem cells as repair facilitators, in contrast to the hypothesis common at the time CPI manufactured its product: they believed stem cells were potentially transplantable replacements for injured or atrophied neurons. Coupled with supporting cells—astrocytes and other glial cells that produce nourishing chemicals for the neurons—we believe future significant advances may come with stem cell utilization in the management of debilitating brain afflictions, such as Parkinson's disease.

Yet stem cells can also be harmful. The malignancy neuroblastoma is an example of stem cells running wild within neural tissues. In this unfortunate disease, stem cells in an afflicted young child's sympathetic nervous system and adrenal cortex continue to multiply out of control.

Apparently one or more elements of cellular auto-regulation fail to switch them off.

We have hypothesized yet another type of unexpected outcome from stem cells for Bobby's disease—CPI's cloned stem cells. After several cloning iterations, the safeguards described above became degraded and failed to keep the shutdown program dormant after one was born. We contend once CPI's vaccine was injected, its varicella virus—nurtured on cloned human stem cells—unlocked a section of the shutdown program in the recipient's neural cells. When the neural cells were stimulated by methamphetamine or Ritalin, the shutdown program accelerated into high gear and produced the downstream signaling proteins that blocked the neuron's mitochondria. The neural cells' metabolic activity ground to a halt. Without an energy source, they died.

	CPI Vaccine	**No Vaccine**
Meth/Ritalin	+/ + Disease	- /+ No Disease
No Meth/Ritalin	+/- No Disease	-/- Healthy

In perhaps a manner similar to Shelley's Doctor Frankenstein, CPI brought one or more Franken-genes back to life. In the neural cells, CPI's human-cloned, varicella vaccine had tragically reactivated dormant Franken-genes located in the so-called junk sections of DNA. Unfortunately, the Franken-genes would not turn off—they never stopped—and their effects unknowingly were amplified whenever exposed to stimulants such as Ritalin or methamphetamine. Piecemeal, they switched off the victim's neurons and ultimately overwhelmed the brain's plasticity to shift cortical and sub-cortical functions from the damaged circuits to the still-viable ones. Why some parts of the brain were affected ahead of others is unknown at this time, but there is the possibility adolescent hormonal changes made some brain areas more inclined, and others more resistant, to these activated Franken-genes.

After spawning upstream, the neurological systems of sexually mature salmon are programmed to atrophy. Concurrently, we endeavor to locate the shutdown DNA snippets on salmon chromosomes to aid our exploration and comprehension regarding such loci within our own genome, so coded to shut down the human nervous system.

Bottom line, the disassembly instructions for neural cells were activated by the cloned CPI immunization. The reactivated Franken-genes retooled the affected cells into factories that churned out shutdown agents and Franken-proteins. Together they overwhelmed the brain's hardwiring to cause defaults in the neural operating systems. They acted much like a computer virus and lethally disabled the DNA sub-computer running the mitochondria.

Computers do what they're told to do. They obey the bad scripts of operating instructions as well as the good.